PREVENTING ANTISOCIAL BEHAVIOR

PREVENTING ANTISOCIAL BEHAVIOR

Interventions from Birth through Adolescence

Joan McCord
Richard E. Tremblay

Editors

THE GUILFORD PRESS
New York / London

© **1992 The Guilford Press**
A Division of Guilford Publications, Inc.
72 Spring Street, New York, NY 10012

Printed in the United States of America

This book is printed on acid-free paper.

Last digit is print number: 9 8 7 6 5 4 3 2 1

Library of Congress Cataloging-in-Publication Data

Preventing antisocial behavior : interventions from birth through adolescence / edited by Joan McCord, Richard E. Tremblay.
    p. cm.
   Includes bibliographical references and index.
   ISBN 0-89862-882-2
   1. Conduct disorders in children—Prevention—Con-gresses. 2. Conduct disorders in adolescence—Prevention—Congresses. 3. Juvenile delinquency—Prevention—Con-gresses.   I. McCord, Joan. II. Tremblay, Richard Ernest.
   [DNLM: 1. Antisocial Personality Disorder—in adoles-cence—congresses. 2. Antisocial Personality Disorder—in infancy & childhood—congresses. 3. Antisocial Personality Disorder—prevention & control—congresses. 4. Child Be-havior Disorders—prevention & control—congresses.
5. Social Behavior Disorders—in adolescence—congresses.
6. Social Behavior Disorders—in infancy & childhood—con-gresses. 7. Social Behavior Disorders—prevention & con-trol—congresses.   WS 350.8S6 P944]
RJ506.C65P74 1992
618.92'858—dc20
DNLM/DLC
for Library of Congress   92-1444
                                                CIP

Contributors

◆ ──────── ◆

Robert D. Abbott, PhD, Department of Educational Psychology, College of Education, University of Washington, Seattle

Jack Arbuthnot, PhD, Department of Psychology, Ohio University, Athens

Russell A. Barkley, PhD, University of Massachusetts Medical Center, Worcester

Kathryn E. Barnard, RN, PhD, Department of Parent and Child Nursing, University of Washington, Seattle

Hélène Beauchesne, MSc, Research Unit on Children's Psychosocial Maladjustment, University of Montreal, Quebec

Lucie Bertrand, MSc, Research Unit on Children's Psychosocial Maladjustment, University of Montreal, Quebec

Hélène Boileau, BSc, Research Unit on Children's Psychosocial Maladjustment, University of Montreal, Quebec

Cathryn L. Booth, PhD, Department of Parent and Child Nursing, University of Washington, Seattle

Richard F. Catalano, PhD, Social Development Research Group, School of Social Work, University of Washington, Seattle

Lucille David, MSc, Research Unit on Children's Psychosocial Maladjustment, University of Montreal, Quebec

L. Edward Day, doctoral candidate, Social Development Research Group, School of Social Work, University of Washington, Seattle

Thomas A. Dishion, PhD, Oregon Social Learning Center, Eugene

George J. DuPaul, PhD, University of Massachusetts Medical Center, Worcester

David P. Farrington, PhD, Institute of Criminology, Cambridge University, England

Ronald A. Feldman, PhD, School of Social Work, Columbia University, New York, New York

Denise C. Gottfredson, PhD, Institute of Criminal Justice and Criminology, University of Maryland, College Park

Gary D. Gottfredson, PhD, Center for Social Organization of Schools, Johns Hopkins University, Baltimore, Maryland

J. David Hawkins, PhD, Social Development Research Group, School of Social Work, University of Washington, Seattle

Kathryn A. Kavanagh, PhD, Oregon Social Learning Center, Eugene

Sheppard G. Kellam, MD, Prevention Research Center, Department of Mental Hygiene, School of Hygiene and Public Health, Johns Hopkins University, Baltimore, Maryland

Kenneth C. Land, PhD, Department of Sociology, Duke University, Durham, North Carolina

Marc LeBlanc, PhD, Research Unit on Children's Psychosocial Maladjustment, University of Montreal, Quebec

Phyllis Levenstein, EdD, Social Sciences Interdisciplinary Program, State University of New York at Stony Brook

Patricia L. McCall, PhD, Department of Sociology, Anthropology and Social Work, North Carolina State University, Raleigh

Joan McCord, PhD, Department of Criminal Justice, Temple University, Philadelphia, Pennsylvania

Colleen E. Morisset, PhD, Department of Parent and Child Nursing, University of Washington, Seattle

Diane M. Morrison, PhD, Social Development Research Group, School of Social Work, University of Washington, Seattle

Clifford R. O'Donnell, PhD, Department of Psychology and Center for Youth Research, University of Hawaii, Manoa

Julie O'Donnell, MSW, Social Development Research Group, School of Social Work, University of Washington, Seattle

Gerald R. Patterson, PhD, Oregon Social Learning Center, Eugene

George W. Rebok, PhD, Prevention Research Center, Department of

Mental Hygiene, School of Hygiene and Public Health, Johns Hopkins University, Baltimore, Maryland

Lee N. Robins, PhD, Department of Psychiatry, Washington University, St. Louis, Missouri

Lawrence J. Schweinhart, PhD, High/Scope Educational Research Foundation, Ypsilanti, Michigan

Susan J. Spieker, PhD, Department of Parent and Child Nursing, University of Washington, Seattle

Richard E. Tremblay, PhD, Research Unit on Children's Psychosocial Maladjustment, University of Montreal, Quebec

Frank Vitaro, PhD, Research Unit on Children's Psychosocial Maladjustment, University of Montreal, Quebec

David P. Weikart, PhD, High/Scope Educational Research Foundation, Ypsilanti, Michigan

Jay R. Williams, PhD, Department of Sociology, Duke University, Durham, North Carolina

Preface

◆ ──── ◆

The Reformatory Movement, begun in England around the middle of the 19th century, acknowledged the role of society in the production of crime and society's responsibility for its amelioration. One of the movement's leaders, Mary Carpenter (1864/1960) summarized this connection: "Dens of infamy are still tolerated in our cities, to give young children that schooling to vice, which no one gives them to lead them in the right way. . . . Society *is* responsible for all this, and therefore is bound to remedy as far as possible the evils arising from these various abuses" (p. 80).

Over the ensuing years, a variety of approaches have been used in an attempt to prevent children from following the path that leads to criminal behavior or to remedy that behavior before they become habitual criminals. These approaches have ranged from infant schools to residential treatment centers, from social training to psychological therapies. Evaluations have typically been little more than testimonials to current fashions, and fashions have been fickle.

The unique contribution of the 20th century, we believe, has been method. By introducing experimental approaches to the study of intervention strategies, enduring results can issue even from programs that have failed to achieve their therapeutic goals.

The scientific method, with its goal of replicability, permits outsiders to judge the usefulness of techniques that have seemed to warrant interference in the lives of others. The studies we selected for this work vary in the ways in which science has been applied. Some of the studies used blind treatment and control comparisons, others assigned subjects randomly to different conditions or to a treatment and a no-treatment group. Still others relied on complex designs so that both internal and external comparisons could be made. We hoped that by selecting variety in method, this book would provide readers with the opportunity to consider evaluation techniques while also enabling some readers to develop strategies for evaluating their own programs.

Our intention was not only to stimulate clearer consideration of evaluation strategies but also to show some of the imaginative interventions that have been designed to assist children at every age. The chapters include biological, social, emotional, and cognitive approaches. We have included interventions aimed at infants, at children, and at adolescents. The order of presentation follows, roughly, a developmental perspective in which the age of earliest intervention accounts for placement.

There may be critical ages at which particular approaches are likely to be successful, but in general, prevention seems to be more promising than treatment. Experience seems to show, however, that even effective prevention strategies will miss some of the people some of the time. That being the case, we are likely to need a variety of programs in order to help the variety of children in need of assistance. The chapters that follow describe programs that intervene in families, in schools, and in communities. Some target general populations at risk, while others focus on individuals.

Prevention of deviant behavior is a costly and often a heartbreaking enterprise. Those who embrace the task may be reluctant to spend either time or energy on what many regard as the "merely academic" task of evaluation. Some of the chapters in this book have been selected because they give poignant testimony to the importance of having clearly established, scientifically supportable evaluations. These are included, in part, to show that even exceptionally good intentions and high intelligence cannot guarantee the success of treatment. Once people recognize that psychosocial as well as chemical treatments can be harmful, they may be more willing to insist on careful evaluations.

The hard work of evaluating may be made easier if society were to recognize the simple truth that well-designed programs contribute the kind of information necessary to help improve the lives of others—whether or not the programs themselves are successful. When intervention programs are developed as a consequence of theory, their results can be used to refine that theory as well as to test it. When an experimental approach includes clear descriptions of process or outcome, the results are tests of assumptions about change that lie at the foundation of theories of human behavior. In either case, the contributions of prevention experiments extend beyond the borders of the client populations themselves.

This volume was planned following a symposium on longitudinal experimental studies organized by the editors for the Tenth Biennial

Meetings of the International Society for the Study of Behavioural Development, in Jyväskylä, Finland. We thank Professor Lea Pulkkinen, the host of that meeting, for providing the setting to initiate this enterprise. We also thank Chantal Bruneau and Debbie Banks who, respectively in Montreal and Philadelphia, provided the technical support. Finally, we thank all our contributors who were most helpful in meeting the deadlines we imposed.

Reference

Carpenter, M. (1969). *Our convicts*. Montclair, NJ: Patterson Smith. (Original work published 1864)

Joan McCord
Philadelphia

Richard E. Tremblay
Montreal

Contents

◆ ─────── ◆

PART I **INTRODUCTION**

CHAPTER 1 The Role of Prevention Experiments   3
in Discovering Causes of Children's
Antisocial Behavior
Lee N. Robins

PART II **PREVENTION EXPERIMENTS DURING**
INFANCY AND EARLY CHILDHOOD

CHAPTER 2 Infants at Risk: The Role of Preventive   21
Intervention in Deflecting a Maladaptive
Developmental Trajectory
Cathryn L. Booth, Susan J. Spieker,
Kathryn E. Barnard, and Colleen E. Morisset

CHAPTER 3 The Mother–Child Home Program: Research   43
Methodology and the Real World
Phyllis Levenstein

CHAPTER 4 High/Scope Preschool Program Outcomes   67
David P. Weikart and Lawrence J. Schweinhart

PART III **PREVENTION EXPERIMENTS DURING**
THE MIDDLE YEARS

CHAPTER 5 Social Interactions of Children with   89
Attention Deficit Hyperactivity Disorder:
Effects of Methylphenidate
George J. DuPaul and Russell A. Barkley

CHAPTER 6   Parent and Child Training to Prevent Early   117
             Onset of Delinquency: The Montréal
             Longitudinal–Experimental Study
             Richard E. Tremblay, Frank Vitaro, Lucie Bertrand,
             Marc LeBlanc, Hélène Beauchesne, Hélène Boileau,
             and Lucille David

CHAPTER 7   The Seattle Social Development Project: Effects   139
             of the First Four Years on Protective Factors and
             Problem Behaviors
             J. David Hawkins, Richard F. Catalano,
             Diane M. Morrison, Julie O'Donnell,
             Robert D. Abbott, and L. Edward Day

CHAPTER 8   Building Developmental and Etiological Theory   162
             through Epidemiologically Based Preventive
             Intervention Trials
             Sheppard G. Kellam and George W. Rebok

CHAPTER 9   The Cambridge-Somerville Study: 196
             A Pioneering Longitudinal–Experimental Study
             of Delinquency Prevention
             Joan McCord

PART IV   **PREVENTION EXPERIMENTS DURING**
             ADOLESCENCE

CHAPTER 10   The Interplay of Theory and Practice in   209
             Delinquency Prevention: From Behavior
             Modification to Activity Settings
             Clifford R. O'Donnell

CHAPTER 11   The St. Louis Experiment: Effective Treatment   233
             of Antisocial Youths in Prosocial Peer Groups
             Ronald A. Feldman

CHAPTER 12   An Experimental Test of the Coercion Model: 253
             Linking Theory, Measurement, and Intervention
             Thomas J. Dishion, Gerald R. Patterson,
             and Kathryn A. Kavanagh

CHAPTER 13   Sociomoral Reasoning in Behavior-Disordered   283
             Adolescents: Cognitive and Behavioral Change
             Jack Arbuthnot

CHAPTER 14 Theory-Guided Investigation: 311
            Three Field Experiments
            Denise C. Gottfredson and Gary D. Gottfredson

CHAPTER 15 Intensive Supervision of Status Offenders: 330
            Evidence on Continuity of Treatment Effects
            for Juveniles and a "Hawthorne Effect"
            for Counselors
            Kenneth C. Land, Patricia L. McCall,
            and Jay R. Williams

PART V   **CONCLUSION**

CHAPTER 16 The Need for Longitudinal–Experimental   353
            Research on Offending and Antisocial Behavior
            David P. Farrington

            Index   377

PART I

◆ — ◆

INTRODUCTION

If treatment success does not necessarily support a causal argument, what kinds of experiments do? The answer is the prevention experiment. Unlike treatment experiments, a prevention experiment cannot be irrelevant to causal hypotheses because prevention can occur only if exposure to risk factors has been reduced or if exposure to protective factors has been increased, making subjects less sensitive to the risk factor. That is not to say that an experiment that successfully prevents the development of behavior problems will always clearly support the *particular* causal hypothesis it was designed to test. Only when the experimenter can show that a specified risk factor has in fact been reduced or a specific protective factor has been provided to the experimental group but not to the control group, *and* that the two groups differ in no other ways, does the experimental group's lower rate of the outcome to be averted support the experimenter's causal theory.

These requirements for proving a particular causal hypothesis by experiment mean that the variable that is the hypothesized cause must be clearly specified and subject to accurate measurement, and the presence or absence of the outcome to be prevented must also be readily ascertainable. To obtain a definitive answer, the risk factor and the outcome must occur with high frequency in the control group, so that successful prevention of both will be observable. To increase the chances that the sample selected will be one in which the cause and outcome would both frequently occur without intervention, one must know what subpopulations are likely to have both. Thus, among the studies included in this book, the Cambridge-Somerville study considered poverty a risk factor for future delinquency among boys, and believed that social services would constitute a protective factor against many of the mechanisms through which poverty causes delinquency—even though poverty itself could not be prevented; the project with Montreal kindergarteners used poverty and low education of the parents to identify schools attended by children who would be at high risk both for aggression in kindergarten, the hypothesized risk factor for delinquency, and later on for delinquency itself. To know how long after the experiment is complete to assess final outcome, one has to know how long after exposure an effect is likely to be detectable. These requirements imply that the experiment should not be performed until substantial epidemiologic research and natural history observations of the occurrence of the disorder have preceded it. The earlier research is necessary to narrow the hypothesized causes to the one or very few that it is practical to manipulate in a prevention study, as well as to provide guidance as to the sample and protocol most likely to provide information. Indeed, the prevention experiment should usually be the last phase of a program of research.

PREPARING THE WAY FOR A
PREVENTION EXPERIMENT

The typical first step in that research program is either an ecological observation, such as noting that juvenile arrests are concentrated in the poorest areas of the city, or a clinical observation, such as a therapist's recognition that children's behavior problems are regularly associated with some other phenomenon, for example, school failure. When it occurs to the therapist that his or her patients' conduct problems might be a reaction to school failure, his or her next step should be to see whether this same association exists in other clinics. If it does occur in all or most children's clinics, next it is appropriate to ask whether it exists in the population as a whole, rather than being an artifact of referral practices. It could be only an artifact if children who had this pair of problems were much more frequently referred than children with conduct disorder but no school failure.

To learn whether the relationship is real rather than an artifact of selection for treatment, we need a survey of a general population of children. A sample can be obtained from an area sample (i.e., based on home addresses), from a survey of schools, or by follow-up of a birth cohort or school-entry cohort. The follow-up design is preferable to the first two because it will make us aware of children who do not live in households or who have dropped out of schools, and whose inclusion provides a more representative sample of the total population than do household or school samples. A general population sample provides information on how many youngsters fail, how many develop conduct disorder, what the demographic characteristics of both groups are, and the strength of the relationship between school failure and conduct problems in the population as a whole and also in those with the demographic characteristics associated with a high risk for failure. If we find that the association between school failure and conduct problems is strong in either the total sample or a subpopulation, we no longer have cause to doubt that the two are associated, but still have no evidence that school failure causes conduct problems. It might even be the reverse: conduct problems might lead to school failure.

We can rule out the possibility that the "cause" is in fact a consequence of the "outcome" by means of a longitudinal study. If such a study demonstrates that the school failure almost always comes first, we can stop worrying about whether failure might be a consequence of conduct problems. Longitudinal information can be obtained retrospectively, by asking mothers whether the behavior problems predated or followed school failure, or prospectively by selecting children without behavior problems early in their school careers, one group who has failed and a control group who has not, and following them for a year or two to see whether those who had failed more often develop behavior problems. The prospective design is preferable, because it will not put us at the mercy of the mothers' errors in recall. If conduct problems do follow school failure, the causal argument remains plausible but still unproven. Both the failure and the behavior problems could have been caused by some third prior variable—or some constellation of prior variables, such as low IQ, homes in which parents are constantly fighting, teachers who were ineffective and hostile, or parents who failed to teach both good study habits and obedience to rules. Such third variables can be the true explanation even when the "cause" almost always precedes the outcome. One event may precede the other simply because one is developmentally prior to the other. In this case, failing in first grade will precede delinquency simply because children are in first grade at age 6 or 7 and rarely become officially delinquent before age 10.

Although more rarely done, retrospection or prospective follow-up studies should also determine the order in which third variables statistically associated with both the cause and effect appear relative to the hypothesized cause and effect. By means of statistical controls for third variables that preceded both the failure and the conduct problems, we can rule out *these* particular alternative explanations if the relationship between the failure and antisocial outcome remains strong. But there will always be the possibility that we have failed to control on the factors that truly do explain both failure and antisocial behavior, and thus create the illusion that school failure is the cause.

It is an error to control on third variables that occur between the "cause" and the outcome, or that follow the outcome. In the latter case, the third variable may be a consequence of the antisocial behavior we are trying to predict. When the third variable occurs *between* the "cause" and the "outcome," it may be *another* result of the "cause," which, when controlled for, wipes out the effect of the cause, or it may be the mechanism through which the cause has its impact on behavior. It would be a serious mistake to discard our causal hypothesis because we had identified another of its effects or the mechanism through which it causes antisocial behavior. For example, school failure may lead to being moved to a special education class (a second effect) and to the child's low self-esteem. Low self-esteem may be the mechanism through which failure leads to antisocial behavior. Controlling on assignment to a "special ed" class and low self-esteem would probably make the relationship of failure to behavior nonsignificant, and might result in the false interpretation that school failure played no role in antisocial behavior. (Of course, it is useful to control on possible mechanisms such as low self-esteem in the search for ways to block the effect of the cause. If school failure caused antisocial behavior *only* if it led to low self-esteem, it might be more feasible to deal directly with the low self-esteem than to achieve academic success.)

The *plausibility* of a causal hypothesis can be established by showing that it precedes the outcome in the general population and can survive controls for preexisting correlates, and by replicating these findings in other samples in other places or other times, but the closest we can come to *proof* that a causal variable has been identified is through an experiment. As Susser (1991) pointed out, "Controlled . . . experiments yield the strongest assurances about association, time order, and direction. They allow the maximum mobilization and definition of change or activity in the determinant, since the exposure is wholly a creation of the design. . . . Then, given a priori hypotheses, an effect seen to follow an intervention can be inferred to be causal if it is not seen in a comparable group undisturbed by the same intervention" (p. 644).

Retrospective and prospective longitudinal studies can provide more help in designing experiments crucial to proving causes than just producing causal hypotheses to test. They can also give necessary information about the natural history of the relationship between the two events: Does a single failure have this effect, or must failure be pervasive? Are later failures less important than early ones, perhaps because the child failing later has already had some experience of success? The answers to these two questions tell us whether an experiment might succeed even if it does not prevent all school failures, but just reduces their number or postpones them. How long after the child becomes aware of his failure do the first behavior problems occur? Are they enduring or transient? Answers to these questions tell us when to do follow-up assessments and how narrow the window for follow-up assessment is within which an effect can be detected. Do subsequent successes change the pattern in the behavior variables? The answer to this question tells us whether it is reasonable to include children who have already failed for whom further failure might be prevented, rather than limiting the subjects to children who have not yet experienced a failure.

After carrying through the program of research outlined above, which has suggested causal hypotheses, ruled out as many competing explanations as possible, identified possible mechanisms through which the cause may operate, and described the natural history of the relationship between cause and outcome, it is time for the prevention experiment. The prevention experiment is the crucial test, but it would be foolhardy to enter on a prevention experiment without having traversed these earlier research stages. Without them, we would likely be testing causes that are not plausible, or we might well fail to prove the causal role by carrying out the study with an inappropriate sample or with one that is too small to demonstrate its power, by designing an experimental period too brief to provide a sufficient interruption of the causal variable, or by allowing too short a follow-up before final assessment to witness the effect of the causal variable on the control group.

Perhaps it is the lack of sufficient preparatory studies that accounts for the fact that as attractive as prevention experiments are in principle, it is difficult to find examples of ones that have succeeded in proving a causal theory of deviant behavior. The scarcity of prevention successes for behavior problems may also be attributable to a failure to have found some link in the chain of mechanisms between a root cause and the behavior that can be broken in the course of a relatively brief and affordable intervention. There are a number of successes in experimental *treatment* of childhood antisocial behavior, the use of behavior therapy (Krasner, 1969) or training parents how to modify disruptive behavior (Patterson, 1982), for example, but as noted above, it is not possible to infer from the fact that a particular intervention cured an undesirable behavior that the behavior was caused by the absence of that intervention.

EXAMPLES OF PREVENTION EXPERIMENTS THAT PROVED CAUSES

There are successful examples in preventive medicine, however, that the behavioral sciences can emulate. Snow (1855/1936) proved that bad water caused cholera, and Goldberger (Terris, 1964) proved that bad nutrition caused pellagra. There have been many experiments with vaccines showing that modified exposure to specific viruses protects against specific diseases. It is of particular interest that only in the case of vaccines was it necessary to specify the precise cause of the disorder. Snow had no idea which bacteria were responsible for cholera and Goldberger knew that a "good" diet was protective, but did not know the specific nutrient that was missing from the inadequate diets.

Goldberger's successful experiment is an inspiring model because it was indeed based on prior research that superbly ruled out alternative hypotheses and identified the populations at highest risk. He used all the types of data available for studying behavior problems: clinical observations, ecological correlations, general population surveys, and longitudinal studies. Clinical data showed that pellagra was common among long-stay patients of chronic hospitals and children in orphanages, but essentially absent among the hospital staff, making infectious contagion or exposure through insect infestations or poisoning by spoiled food unlikely causes. Records of orphanages also showed a strong age effect, with cases confined primarily to those aged 6 to 12 years. Goldberger faced the problem of inconsistent results across general population surveys, and brilliantly pointed out the errors in method that explained those that showed no correlation between pellagra and diet. One such survey had been conducted with one member of each household, who was asked about the frequency with which specific foods were served in that household. No attention was paid to individual dietary differences, no records of purchases were obtained, and seasonal variation in diet was ignored. A second survey had asked about diet in the year preceding the first attack, which often required recall from many years previous. Goldberger's own survey (Goldberger, Wheeler, & Sydenstriker, 1920) was longitudinal, with monthly clinical assessments of each family member to determine incident cases of the disorder. He obtained quantitative assessment of the household diet both by interview and purchase records during the 2 weeks when diet was most likely to be causal—a month or two before the typical late spring outbreak of pellagra—and converted the dietary elements into "adult-male equivalents" to take into account variation in the size of households and their age distributions. He was able to show that had he looked only at the *frequency* with which certain food groups were served, he would have failed to discriminate pellagrous from other households, just as the earlier studies did. However, he noted highly significant differences when the *quantity* of protein foods served was considered. In poor families (with poverty ascertained from wage records rather than self-report, and adjusted for family size) the persons mainly affected were women and school-aged children because milk was saved for the babies and meat for the working men.

Goldberger's experimental studies were of two kinds. One was designed to disprove the then-current theories of an infectious agent or effects of eating corn, and the second to prove the nutritional theory that his previous research had suggested. The first set of experiments involved eating the skin scrapings and excrement of affected patients to prove that pellagra was not infectious. That experiment was so distasteful and, if one believed the current views, so dangerous that Goldberger used only himself and his volunteer family members as experimental subjects. So heroic an experiment required a very strong conviction of the correctness of his hypothesis, but alone it only disproved the infection theory without supporting the nutritional deficit theory.

To prove the nutritional deficit theory, he needed a prevention experiment. His first attempt at prevention through improved diet showed a vast decline in the rate of the disorder in a population of residents in a mental hospital, but the success was not complete. Despite dietary supplements, a few cases occurred in persons who had had the disorder in previous years. He blamed this on the fact that the study was too poorly funded to provide enough meat for the patients. Rather than abandoning his solution as economically impractical, he continued to modify the experimental diet, honing it down to its essentials. By the end of his efforts, what was at first an extremely expensive solution—supplementation of the hospital diet with lots of meat, milk, and out-of-season fresh vegetables—became both simple and cheap, for he had only to add brewer's yeast to the diet.

THE REQUIREMENTS FOR A SUCCESSFUL PREVENTION EXPERIMENT

This remarkable success story, accomplished 70 years ago and hardly matched since, spells out all the necessary steps in first proving a cause and then putting it to use in formulating public policy. First, you have to have a good guess as to the cause's general nature through clinical observation. This guess is based on *who* is affected and *when* they become affected, and on noting how those affected differ from the rest in exposure to possible risk factors. The educated-guess phase is followed by population surveys with a longitudinal design, supplementing interview and observational data with record data. To follow surveys with an experiment requires causal variables that can be manipulated in well-matched control and experimental groups of adequate size, groups who do not currently have the disorder but who are known to be at risk for it, and who can be retained long enough to both experience the intervention *and* wait out the delay between undergoing the experiment and the expected development of the disorder. The experimental variable must be verified to have been experienced by the experimental group. It must also be shown that the control group did not inadvertently experience it as well, or at least not as uniformly and at as high a level as the experimental group. Finally, a valid assessment tool must be available that can reliably demonstrate the absence or presence of the disorder, to be used both initially to show that it is absent, and at the end, to show that it has occurred. For this purpose, the disorder must be one that is not so transient that cases occur and disappear between measurements. One successful experiment is seldom sufficient. The causal hypothesis must be validated by replication in other experiments, which can simultaneously attempt to specify the cause more narrowly so that it can gradually be reduced to its minimal dimensions. This increased specification adds to the scientific understanding of the causal process, while reducing costs of acting on the understanding when knowledge is translated into public policy.

IS CHILDHOOD DEVIANT BEHAVIOR RIPE FOR EXPERIMENTATION?

We have noted above that prevention experiments should build on a previous body of research. That research must provide one or more causal hypotheses strongly correlated with the outcome to be prevented, and, to be of practical importance, the cause should precede the outcome sufficiently often so that its successful prevention might significantly reduce the numbers who develop the outcome. The existing research should tell us in what population with respect to age, sex, and income group to carry out the experiment; how we are to measure the presence of the cause and the mechanisms through which it has its effects as well as the presence of the outcome; for how long the control group will need to be exposed to develop the outcome; and how long after exposure we should measure the outcome. Without this information, we are unlikely to be able to design a successful intervention.

There is probably no area of behavior or psychiatric disorder riper for an experimental design than conduct problems. We know the population at high risk: it is boys living in poor areas of inner cities in their first school years. We can measure the presence of conduct problems by a series of standardized questionnaires and interviews developed to be administered to the child, his parent, and his teacher during the early and middle school years. Conduct problems tend to be long-lasting, enduring often even into adulthood, and almost always beginning by the midteens, so evaluation of their occurrence can take place at any time from age 10 to 15 or 16.

We also have an abundance of hypothetical causal agents to consider as possible candidates for prevention. Children with conduct problems often have parents with adult antisocial behavior or substance abuse, whose parenting skills have serious deficits (Glueck & Glueck, 1950). Parents tend to be erratic and violent disciplinarians.

Many affected children are in one-parent homes, are only children, or in large sibships (Farrington, 1978; McCord, 1990; Offord, Alder, and Boyle, 1986). Their home life is chaotic, and may be characterized by a variety of persons living in the home who are not members of the typical nuclear family. Affected children often are brought up in poverty and live in neighborhoods where there is an abundance of antisocial role models (Clark & Wenninger, 1962; Hindelang, 1976). Early in life, many of these children have personal attributes that are reasonably good prognosticators of antisocial behavior, particularly attentional deficits, hyperactivity, a slightly low IQ, poor school success (Offord & Waters, 1983; White, Moffit, Earls, Robins, & Silva, 1990), a low tolerance for frustration and boredom, and mild neurological liabilities (Cadman, Boyle, Szatmari, & Offord, 1987; Offord, 1989; Rutter, 1977).

Despite this wealth of information, there are certain missing elements. We have not developed well-standardized ways of measuring conduct problems before age 6, and thus it is difficult to choose a group of young children in whom to carry out experiments who are at risk but clearly have not yet developed conduct problems. A solution to this difficulty is to carry out the intervention beginning at or near the time of birth (Robins & Earls, 1986). Protective factors are also not well identified (Rutter, 1979). There is some evidence that the presence of some competent adult is a help, and perhaps high IQ in the child. The better outcomes of children adopted away suggest that exposure to an orderly and predictable environment may be protective, although here the margin between absence of a risk factor and presence of a protective factor gets blurred.

Most of the correlates of conduct disorder that may be its causes are difficult to prevent, and few of the possible protective factors could be instigated without violating community standards. It is not easy, for example, to overcome poverty or to cure parents of their antisocial behavior; nor is it permissible to remove children from the parental home as a purely preventive measure; nor would it be easy to find good substitute families were it permissible. Still, a variety of strategies are possible. Parents can be trained in disciplinary techniques or treated for substance abuse. Children can be offered an orderly environment within daycare. Child caretakers can be trained to use principles of behavior modification to reward prosocial behavior and extinguish antisocial behaviors. Children with attentional problems and hyperactivity can be offered psychological and pharmacologic therapies. Enriched educational experiences in the preschool years might reduce risks of school failure. Foster grandparents or "Big Brothers" can attempt to provide a protective, competent adult figure. Examples of efforts to provide such interventions are presented in the chapters to follow.

In addition to our ignorance about what types of intervention would effectively change the risk factors, we also know little about the best timing for these activities. We do not know what the critical periods are for developing conduct problems, how long the intervention must last, how soon after exposure to a risk factor the conduct problems are likely to appear, nor what proportion of the affected population could be prevented by removing any particular risk factor.

WHY REAL CAUSES OF CONDUCT PROBLEMS REMAIN UNPROVEN

Not knowing how or when to intervene and when to measure the effect of an experiment creates a danger that we may end by discarding a sound causal theory because our experiment did not actually remove the risk factor or instigate the protective factor, or not for long enough, or not at the right stage of the child's development, or we measured outcomes too soon. Additional hazards that may lead to erroneous negative results include a poor match between experimental and control subjects initially or by time of follow-up due to dropouts from either group, and exposure of the control subjects to an alternative and equivalent intervention without our knowledge.

While the risk with survey and longitudinal studies looking for causes is typically a risk of overidentification of plausible causes through spurious relationships, bias on the part of the researcher, or bias on the part of the affected person who is trying to explain the outcome, the risk of error in prevention research, with its rules of blind assessment, random assignment, and use of sham treatments to avoid the Hawthorne effect (a general response to an interested and caring researcher) is almost always that of failing to prove a causal relationship that is in fact present. This is a special risk in studying causes of conduct disorder because antisocial behavior appears to have multiple causes, no one of which is a necessary cause. Experiments at best can try to prevent exposure to only a few of these. As a result, experiments in preventing conduct disorder are unlikely to show the near 100% success achieved by Goldberger when he enriched the diet. The smaller the proportion of sufficient causes an experiment can remove, the larger the study must be to demonstrate an effect. Large experimental studies are expensive to mount, and costs may dictate studies too small to be definitive. Failures can also occur because preventing the hypothesized causal factor was not entirely successful.

It is important to monitor the status of the risk factor to learn whether it has been prevented. And the final, and most chilling possibility, is that in preventing one cause, the experiment may have inadvertently created another that the child would not have been exposed to if we had not meddled.

A HELPFUL DESIGN

How then can we best undertake experiments to test a variety of causal hypotheses about deviant behavior without discarding them mistakenly? We can offer no guarantees, but there are some general principles that should help.

1. The intervention should be rewarding in the short run to both the subjects and the staff. Otherwise, the design may not in fact be carried out because of an excess of attrition of subjects and so much staff turnover that the program was only sporadically actually in operation. One method, when the experiment is not intrinsically appealing to the participants, is to pay both staff and subjects well for their participation. Human Studies Committees often object to paying subjects to participate in studies, claiming that payment constitutes coercion, that participation in research should be purely for the sake of science. (Luckily, they do not make the same stipulation requiring volunteer status for the staff!) This is a Catch-22 from the scientist's point of view. After he has gone to great lengths to get access to unbiased samples of the population at risk, he is then asked to exclude members who are not prepared to donate their time for the sake of science. Those at risk of conduct problems and their parents generally are particularly deficient in altruism and ill-informed about the scientific importance of low refusal rates. Indeed, a lack of altruism might not be a bad indicator of high-risk status!

2. The program should be generously designed in terms of the investment of time and manpower and the number of approaches used to prevent the targeted hypothesized cause. Because the experiment is intended to test a causal hypothesis, not to see whether a particular intervention program is acceptable and feasible in a particular community, there is no necessity for limiting the staff to the kinds of people who would be readily available for translating the results of this experiment into a large public program nor for limiting its costs to those the community is willing to underwrite for a large-scale project. The time for these practical considerations is later, after the causal factors are demonstrated and there is a decision to translate

their prevention into public policy. For a study to test causal hypotheses, the only economic concerns are to get the best possible information, given the number of dollars available to the researcher.

3. Although random assignment virtually guarantees equivalence of risk status among two very large groups, this is not the case for sample sizes typical of prevention experiments. By chance, random assignment to small control and experimental groups can result in groups that differ along important dimensions at entry into the intervention program. A variety of strategies can prevent this happening. A simple way is to rank all potential subjects by risk strata and then do random assignments within strata.

4. Multiple experiments assigned in pairs to different causal hypotheses can overcome some of the problems inherent in small experiments and the plethora of attractive causal hypotheses. Replicates provide two chances to demonstrate success, and, when procedures are closely matched, twice the sample size to test the hypothesis. Addressing multiple causal hypotheses allows seeing which appear most amenable to intervention.

5. Although a study is typically aimed at one or only a few of the plausible causes, the full range of viable causal hypotheses needs to be assessed in both experimental and control cases to be sure that some factors other than those being attacked do not account for differences or prevent the discovery of differences. Randomization helps to prevent this, but even randomization can fail. Studies typically claim that randomization has succeeded when there are no significant differences in demographic characteristics and in the particular risk factor to be influenced. But the constellation of risk factors for which no intervention is planned must be equal as well to give the targeted cause a fair trial.

6. The effectiveness of the intervention in preventing the hypothesized cause must be demonstrated throughout the experiment to ascertain not only whether the experiment ever successfully modified the risk factor, but for how long and how consistently. For example, parents may be taught better child management skills, but apply them too sporadically to make much difference.

7. Although it may not be possible to measure the outcome variable until the end of the study, it should be possible to measure a series of associated behaviors at regular intervals to see whether the intervention appears to be working. For example, while one cannot be certain whether one has prevented juvenile delinquency until the subjects are officially adults, that is, at age 16–18, an effective program is likely to have interim effects on behaviors known to precede delinquency. If, for example, interim comparisons with a control

group showed improved school performance, less attentional deficit and hyperactivity, less stealing, lying, fighting, and truancy, these data would be encouraging. If instead, these behaviors are higher in the experimental than the control sample, there should be a serious concern that the program is actually harmful rather than helpful, and discontinuation or major changes in the protocol must be considered.

8. When it is time to assess the final results, the investigator must again compare the experimental and control groups with respect to the characteristics assessed at the beginning of the study. Fewer of the control than experimental cases may still be available if there has been less contact with them over the years. That in itself is no great problem unless the differential loss affects the comparability of the two groups. Because loss is likely to be greatest among those initially at highest risk, greater attrition in the control group may mean that the controls available at the end of the experiment had a lower average level of risk initially than the remaining experimental cases. A lower initial risk profile for controls would reduce the chance of showing true positive results. Statistical adjustment or excluding experimental cases that are not well matched in the control group is needed to make the comparison sound.

9. Include "real-life" measures in the final assessment, taken from objective records such as school achievement tests, police records, and records of disciplinary action. This avoids positive bias resulting both from personal relationships the experimental families have developed with the study staff and from the researcher's attachment to his causal theory. It also avoids negative bias due to the study's having collected more complete information for experimental than control subjects because of the greater contact with them.

10. Effects in a positive direction that are less than those originally posited should be investigated, not written off because they are not statistically significant. A subgroup may have been helped, or all children in the experiment may have been helped a little, even if not as much as anticipated. A trend in the hypothesized direction should lead to better specification of the causal hypothesis or a more realistic prediction of the size of its contribution rather than discarding it.

WHAT TO DO NEXT WHEN AN EXPERIMENT SUCCEEDS

Let us assume that a study following all these prescriptions has been carried out, and that it has succeeded, that is, there are more conduct problems in the control than in the experimental group. The next step should be scrutinizing the results to see whether the causal variable can be more narrowly described, as Goldberger's findings of the effectiveness of a "good diet" was eventually pinpointed to require only the provision of niacin. Replications are then needed to validate the results of the initial successful study and to demonstrate that the more narrowly defined cause is also potent. If precise replication produces the same effects, experiments should be launched in samples with different risk profiles to see how broadly applicable the results are.

At this point we have specified the cause as precisely as we can, specified the populations to whom it applies, and proved beyond a reasonable doubt it is indeed a real cause because when it is prevented in the experimental sample, reliably fewer children develop deviant behavior than among controls. Now the extra dividends from the use of experiments in establishing cause can be enjoyed: the experiment can serve as a blueprint for a program that might reduce problem behavior in the general population, and study results can be explored for new causal hypotheses.

The search for new hypotheses begins with the experimental failures. Those children who became antisocial despite the intervention must either have had insufficient exposure to the effective intervention (perhaps they were ill or away during part of the experiment) or they had sufficient *other* risk factors to explain their outcome. Looking for characteristics that distinguish them from the successes may reveal what those sufficient risk factors are. But even though discovered in the course of an experiment, the status of the new hypotheses with regard to *proof* is no greater than of those discovered through nonexperimental studies. An experiment to test these new hypotheses is needed next, to elevate them to the status of highly probable causes.

REFERENCES

Cadman, D., Boyle, M., Szatmari, P., & Offord D. R. (1987). Chronic illness, disability and social well-being: Findings of the Ontario Child Health Study. *Pediatrics, 79*, 805–813.

Clark, J., & Wenninger, E. (1962). Socioeconomic class and area as correlates of illegal behavior among juveniles. *American Sociological Review, 27*, 826–834.

Farrington, D. P. (1978). The family backgrounds of aggressive youths. In L. Hersov, M. Berger, & D. Shaffer (Eds.), *Aggression and antisocial behavior in childhood and adolescence* (pp. 73–93). Oxford, England: Pergamon Press.

Glueck, S., & Glueck, E. (1950). *Unravelling juvenile delinquency*. Cambridge: Harvard University Press.

Goldberger, J., Wheeler, G. A., & Sydenstricker, E. (1920). A study of the relation of diet to pellagra incidence in seven textile-mill communities of South Carolina in 1916. *Public Health Report, 35*(12), 648.

Hindelang, M. J. (1976). With a little help from their friends: Group participation in reported delinquent behavior. *British Journal of Criminology, 16*, 109–125.

Krasner, L. (1969). Assessment of token economy programs in psychiatric hospitals. *International Psychiatric Clinics, 6*, 155–185.

McCord, J. (1990). Long-term perspectives on parental absence. In L. Robins & M. Rutter (Eds.), *Straight and devious pathways from childhood to adulthood* (p. 117). Cambridge: Cambridge University Press.

Offord, D. (1989). Conduct disorder: Risk factors and prevention. In D. Shaffer, I. Philips, N. B. Enzer, *The prevention of mental disorders, alcohol and other drug use* (pp. 273–307). Rockville, MD: U.S. Department of Health and Human Services. Washington, DC.: Alcohol, Drug Abuse, and Mental Health Administration.

Offord, D. R., Alder, R. J., & Boyle, M. H. (1986). Prevalence and sociodemographic correlates of conduct disorder. *American Journal of Social Psychiatry, 6*(4), 272–278.

Offord, D. R., & Waters, B. G. (1983). Socialization and its failure. In M. D. Levine, W. B. Carey, A. C. Crocker, & R. T. Gross (Eds.), *Developmental-behavioral pediatrics* (pp. 650–682). Philadelphia: W. B. Saunders.

Patterson, G. R. (1982). *Coercive family process*. Eugene, OR: Castalia.

Robins, L. N., & Earls, F. J. (1986). A program for preventing antisocial behavior for high-risk infants and preschoolers: A research prospectus. In R. Hough, V. Brown, P. Gongla, & S. Goldston (Eds.), *Psychiatric epidemiology and prevention: The possibilities* (pp. 73–83). Los Angeles: Neuropsychiatric Institute.

Rutter, M. (1977). Brain damage syndromes in childhood: Concepts and findings. *Journal of Child Psychology and Psychiatry, 18*, 1–21.

Rutter, M. (1979). Protective factors in children's responses to stress and disadvantage. In M. W. Kent & J. E. Rolf (Eds.), *Primary prevention of psychopathology: Social competence in children* (Vol. 3, pp. 49–74). Hanover, NH: University Press of New England.

Snow, J. (1855/1936). *On the mode of communication of cholera* (2nd ed.). London: Churchill, 1855. (Reprinted in *Snow on Cholera*. New York: Commonwealth Fund, 1936).

Susser, M. (1991). What is a cause and how do we know one? A grammar for pragmatic epidemiology. *American Journal of Epidemiology, 133*, 635–648.

Terris, M. (Ed.). (1964). *Goldberger on pellagra*. Baton Rouge: Louisiana State University Press.

White, J. L., Moffit, T. E., Earls, F., Robins, L., & Silva, P. A. (1990). How early can we tell? Predictors of childhood conduct disorder and adolescent delinquency. *Criminology, 28*, 507–533.

• — •

PART II

PREVENTION EXPERIMENTS DURING INFANCY AND EARLY CHILDHOOD

CHAPTER 2

◆ ——— ◆

Infants at Risk:
The Role of Preventive Intervention in Deflecting a Maladaptive Developmental Trajectory

CATHRYN L. BOOTH
SUSAN J. SPIEKER
KATHRYN E. BARNARD
COLLEEN E. MORISSET

As many of the chapters in this volume note, programs designed to prevent deviant behavior frequently have focused on the identification and treatment of children and adolescents who have already demonstrated problematic behavior. One advantage of this approach is that the provision of services is cost-effective in the sense that those children who are most likely to follow a path of continued deviance are targeted for treatment. In contrast to this approach, our work has focused on the early identification of family-relationship and environmental factors that place a child at risk for a variety of poor outcomes, including the development of deviant behavior. Inherent in this approach is a belief in the importance of early experiences in shaping the child's development. That is, the child's first years are viewed as formative ones during which preventive intervention services may alter the child's developmental pathway more easily than if services are provided later. Although such an approach targets a larger number of children, and is therefore more costly initially, it may be more beneficial in the long run.

In this chapter we will outline a risk model for one pathway leading to the development of deviant behavior, and we will describe our preventive intervention research program within the context of this model. We will provide data about the effectiveness of the intervention. Additionally, we will present evidence from the literature and from our own research to support the model.

THE DEVELOPMENT OF DEVIANT BEHAVIOR: A RISK MODEL

Setting Conditions

Our conceptual model begins with the assumption that children reared under *negative setting conditions* are at risk for a variety of poor outcomes. By "negative setting conditions," we mean ecological factors that may occur singly or together, including poverty, crowded living conditions, constant family crises, maternal depression, lack of social support, marital distress, and so forth. A considerable body of literature links these setting conditions with poor social-emotional and cognitive outcomes (e.g., Belsky, 1984; Crnic & Greenburg, 1990; Elder, Caspi, & Burton, 1987; Radke-Yarrow, Richters, & Wilson, 1988; Spieker & Booth, 1988).

In addition to negative setting conditions, the child's risk status may be exacerbated by a difficult temperament (e.g., Kagan, 1989; Thomas & Chess, 1977) or by medical risk factors such as prematurity (e.g., Bennett, 1987) that are more likely to occur in high-risk families. Interaction of these child factors with negative setting conditions places the child at even greater risk.

Negative setting conditions and endogenous child factors are considered distal indicators of risk in the sense that they do not directly describe the process by which risk is transmitted. That is, we need to explain the more proximal *process* relating these factors to child outcomes. It is assumed that this process involves the nature and quality of the relationship that develops between the mother and the child (Barnard, Hammond, Booth, Bee, Mitchell, & Spieker, 1989) (Note that we will be referring to "mothers" rather than "parents" hereafter. In so doing, we are not attempting to minimize the influence or importance of fathers. Typically, however, mothers are the primary caregivers, and, in the case of many of the families we have studied, the mother is the *only* caregiver.) We believe that the behaviors of both the mother and the infant are important in establishing this relationship. However, before describing these behaviors, we will discuss more general "adult" competencies that are affected by negative setting conditions and that, in turn, affect the mother's ability to develop a positive relationship with her child (see Mitchell, Magyary, Barnard, Sumner, & Booth, 1988). Our focus on these competencies grew out of our earlier preventive intervention research (Barnard, Booth, Mitchell, & Telzrow, 1988), in which we found that attempting to modify parental interactive skills was very difficult when multiple stressors impinged on the mother, especially when she had inadequate skills for coping with these stressors. That is, we found that a mother cannot "receive" information necessary to promoting a positive parent-child relationship when her own difficulties are her most immediate concern.

Adult Competence

Our clinical work with high-risk families has revealed the importance of the following competencies: (1) interacting with other adults in socially skilled ways, (2) managing emotional life, (3) managing stress and life change, and (4) gathering and using parenting information.

Social Skills

Social skills are important for the mother's management of her own life in her community—obtaining shelter, food, and other necessities, and dealing with various businesses, agencies, and institutions—and for her communication with others on the child's behalf—health care providers, other professional helpers, friends, and relatives. Poor social skills can interfere with the mother's ability to use these sources of information and support effectively.

In addition, a mother's skills in initiating, developing, and maintaining friendships and supportive relationships with others are essential to her social support. Many women from high-risk families lack basic communication and conversational skills. For example, we have observed that these women frequently break conversational "rules" involving orienting one's body to the partner, maintaining eye contact, responding appropriately to questions, taking turns, and using facial expressions and voice inflections to convey meaning. The lack of good social skills may undermine an important source of emotional support which, in turn, could exacerbate the deleterious effects of stress on parenting (Booth, Mitchell, Barnard, & Spieker, 1989).

Managing Emotional Life

Maternal depression and other disorders of emotional expression have been shown to negatively impact children's development (Houck,

Booth, & Barnard, 1991; Radke-Yarrow, Cummings, Kuczynski, & Chapman, 1985; Rutter & Garmezy, 1983; Spieker & Booth, 1988). The effects of temporary and less serious emotional problems are unclear, but they may contribute to levels of conflict and disorder in households. Emotional difficulties can be expressed in a range of poor parenting styles, including passivity, inconsistent responsivity, punitive control, and/or emotional unavailability. Thus, learning to cope with emotional issues and problems is important not only for the mother's own mental health, but also for her ability to provide appropriate parenting.

Managing Stress and Life Change

Many high-risk families undergo frequent life changes such as gaining or losing household members, changing jobs, marital separation, and the like. Additionally, these families experience minor daily stressors as well as major stressors stemming from chronic difficult life circumstances, such as living with an alcoholic family member or being harassed by creditors. The demands associated with such stressors can interfere with good parenting, especially when social support is lacking (Crnic & Booth, 1991; Crnic & Greenberg, 1990; Sarason, Johnson, & Siegel, 1978).

Gathering and Using Parenting Information

Learning basic facts about child care and development may be difficult for mothers who cannot read or who are poorly skilled. Even a task as simple as mixing formula may be problematic without the appropriate knowledge or skill. More complex concepts such as learning to facilitate the child's development via appropriate play behaviors may be impossible to grasp without direct guidance. Although books and classes about child development are widely available, poorly educated women in disorganized families are much less likely to know about or to take advantage of these resources.

To summarize, the mother's lack of adult competencies may interfere with her ability to develop a positive relationship with her infant. That is, a mother who is uninformed, unable to cope effectively with stress and life change, overwhelmed with emotional problems, and/or unskilled in obtaining support, is less able to devote sufficient energy to parenting. Consequently, the child's risk of poor outcomes may increase.

Mother–Child Relationship Components

In the previous section we explored mothers' adult competencies that may place the child at risk. Now let us move to an even more proximal level and outline our view of the maternal interactive skills that are important in more directly affecting child outcomes.

Although our primary focus is on the mother in this chapter, we have found it useful in our work to conceptualize the mother and infant as mutually dependent interactors in a dyadic system. Optimally, mother and infant engage in a process of *mutual adaptation*, resulting in the development of a positive relationship that fosters the child's growth and development (Barnard, Booth, Mitchell, & Telzrow, 1988; Booth, Lyons, & Barnard, 1984). Mutual adaptation depends upon the capabilities and behaviors of the mother and the infant. Characteristics of the mother that are important are her (1) sensitivity to her child's behavioral cues, (2) responsivity to her child's distress, (3) ability to foster social-emotional growth, and (4) ability to foster cognitive growth.

The mother's sensitivity to cues depends upon her ability to accurately read the signals given by the infant. This sensitivity is in part a learned skill and can be improved by giving mothers specific information about the behavior and the behavioral cues of young infants. Yet the ability to interpret infant states and communications does not guarantee sensitive caregiving. Concerns about work or finances, emotional problems, or marriage stresses may interfere with a mother's ability to care for her infant in sensitive ways.

A second dimension in mother–child interaction involves the mother's response to distress. A mother's effectiveness in alleviating distress depends on several factors. First, the mother must recognize that distress is occurring; second, she must know the appropriate action to alleviate the distress; and third, she must be able to put this knowledge to work. Again, a mother under a great deal of stress may simply not have the time or energy to deal satisfactorily with the infant's distress. The consequences of consistent contingent responding may be especially important in the development of a secure or insecure attachment relationship of child to mother (Ainsworth, Blehar, Waters, & Wall, 1978; Bell & Ainsworth, 1972). We will return to this idea later.

The mother's social-emotional growth fostering occurs in the context of caregiving interactions as well as play. By sensitively facilitating the infant's early interactions, the mother helps the child to understand social contingencies and rules of interaction. As the child develops, the mother's role in this context changes to one of fostering emotional regulation and labeling emotions, and encouraging appropriate expressions of autonomy and independence. To be skillful in fostering social-emotional growth, the mother must be aware of her child's level of development and be able to adjust her behavior accordingly. Once again, this may depend upon how much motivation, energy, and information the mother has.

The mother's ability to foster cognitive growth depends upon her ability to gauge her child's developmental level accurately, and to provide stimulation that is just above the child's level of understanding (without overstimulating the child). To do this, the mother must have a good grasp of the child's abilities and understanding, and she must be able to guide the baby's exploration and play without being intrusive (Houck, Booth, & Barnard, 1991).

Mutual adaptation also depends on the infant's contribution, specifically, the infant's clarity of behavioral cues and responsiveness to the mother. Infants give behavioral signals when they are sleepy, fussy, hungry, or satiated. If an infant gives ambiguous or confusing cues, these cues can interfere with the mother's ability to read the infant and adapt her behavior accordingly (Thoman, 1975).

Infants also differ in the extent to which they are responsive to the mother's attempts, for example, to soothe them or help them achieve an alert state. If the infant is unresponsive and/or gives unclear cues, parenting may become especially difficult. For a mother who is already stressed, it may be nearly impossible to devote the extra attention and energy needed to assist the infant in developing organized behavioral patterns and becoming appropriately responsive (Vaughn, Egeland, Sroufe, & Waters, 1979; Waters, Vaughn, & Egeland, 1980).

A large body of literature documents the importance of the early mother–child relationship for the child's development. In general, high-quality interactions between mother and infant during the first year of life have been linked positively to the child's subsequent cognitive and linguistic competence, and to a more secure attachment relationship with mother (see Barnard, Hammond, Booth, Bee, Mitchell, & Spieker, 1989, for a review). It is the child's security of attachment to mother, as affected by the quality of their early relationship, that we are most concerned about in this chapter.

Security of Attachment

According to attachment theory, the quality of the early mother–child relationship determines the child's attachment security in relation to mother. Thus, children who are responded to sensitively and contingently during the first year of life are most likely to develop a secure attachment relationship with mother. In contrast, children who are responded to insensitively (either through overstimulation, psychological unavailability, or inconsistent responsiveness) are more likely to develop an insecure attachment relationship. These results, originally reported by Ainsworth et al. (1978), have been replicated numerous times (e.g., Bates, Maslin, & Frankel, 1985; Belsky, Rovine, & Taylor, 1984; Grossmann, Grossmann, Spangler, Suess, & Unzer, 1985).

Secure children are able to use their mother as a base from which to explore and as a source of comfort when distressed. Physical contact with the mother fully comforts secure children who, once soothed, are able to turn their attention fully to the environment in order to explore and learn. This exploration-attachment balance does not function in the same way for insecure infants, who show various maladaptive patterns when stressed or frightened. Some insecure infants may inhibit their expression of distress and not approach the mother for comfort and reassurance. Others heighten their display of attachment behaviors like crying and clinging, and yet are not really soothed by contact with the mother.

Sequelae of Attachment Quality

What is the significance of attachment quality for the child's subsequent development? A growing body of theoretical and empirical work has begun to accumulate, indicating that the child's security of attachment may have far-reaching implications for the child's relationships with peers and others.

The connection between the quality of the mother–child relationship and the development of social competence has been conceptualized in terms of the child developing, through the primary attachment relationship, an "internal working model" of the self in relation to others (Bretherton, 1985; Bowlby, 1982; Main, Kaplan, & Cassidy, 1985). That is, through continuing transactions with the attachment figure, the child develops complex mental representations, or internal working models, of the attachment figure, and of the relationship between self and other. These internal working models, in turn, provide rules that help direct the child's behavior not only with the attachment figure, but also with others.

There is some evidence that insecure attachment is associated with and predictive of children's socially maladaptive behaviors with peers. For example, it has been found that insecure attachment to mother in infancy is predictive of hostile and aggressive behavior directed to peers during preschool years (Egeland & Sroufe, 1981; Sroufe, 1983; Troy & Sroufe, 1987). Other researchers have found that insecure attachment to mother is related to the development of passive withdrawn behaviors in early childhood (LaFreniére & Sroufe, 1985; Renken, Egeland, Marvinney, Mangelsdorf, & Sroufe, 1989). In contrast, secure attachment is associated with later assessments of ego-resiliency (as rated by adults) and of interpersonal problem-solving ability (as assessed by hypothetical-reflective interviews) (Sroufe, 1983).

Although not all insecurely attached children develop maladaptive behaviors with peers, insecure attachment appears to be an additional risk factor for maladaptive peer behaviors. It has been suggested that children who feel insecure in their social relationships interact with their peer group "by shrinking from it or doing battle with it" (Bowlby, 1973, p. 208). Those children who shrink from their peer group are deprived of a rich learning environment in which they develop the skills to interact appropriately and positively with their peers. Those children who do battle with it are learning maladaptive behaviors that typically lead to rejection and isolation (see Rubin & Coplan, in press).

Continuing along the risk trajectory, we find that peer rejection has been shown to predict academic difficulties, truancy, and high school dropout (e.g., Barclay, 1966; Ullman, 1957). Aggression toward peers predicts adolescent crime and delinquency (e.g., Farrington, 1991; Kupersmidt & Coie, 1990; Parker & Asher, 1987), and is an antecedent of externalizing problems in adulthood (see Pepler & Rubin, 1991). Social withdrawal has been indicated as an antecedent to internalizing problems (Hymel, Rubin, Rowden, & LeMare, 1990; Rubin & Mills, 1988, 1991).

Summary

Reviewing our model as a whole, we view setting conditions and infant characteristics as distal factors that affect the more proximal relationship between mother and infant. The relationship that develops between them depends on mutual adaptation, a process that involves behaviors of both the mother (e.g., sensitivity, response to distress) and the infant (e.g., responsiveness to mother). Under negative setting conditions, mutual adaptation can be impeded by the mother's lack of competence in interacting with her infant, as well as the mother's lack of competence in coping with her stressful life circumstances, getting the support she needs, and managing other aspects of her life. One outcome of these interfering factors may be insensitive or inconsistently responsive parenting, which can lead to an insecure infant–mother attachment relationship. Insecure attachment places the child at risk for the development of maladaptive behaviors with peers, such as aggression or social withdrawal. Peer-directed aggression, in particular, has been shown to predict delinquency and deviant behavior in adolescence.

It is important to understand that the model we have presented is a *risk* model, and describes only one of many potential pathways to deviance. At any point in time, factors within the child, within the family, and outside the family may change so that the child's risk status improves or deteriorates. In providing preventive intervention services for these families, we hoped to modify the risk trajectory from early in development.

PREVENTIVE INTERVENTION

In our first preventive intervention research project, Newborn Nursing Models (Barnard, Booth, Mitchell, & Telzrow, 1988), our goal was to provide high-risk families with nursing services during the first 3 months after birth. These 3 months of intervention, averaging 11 hours of nurse home visiting, were not effective with the families who had multiple social problems. Moreover, we found that certain mothers were hesitant to get involved in the intervention process. Further analysis revealed that women who did not respond to the nurse intervention had few friends, little support, and many problems in their lives. This discovery prompted us to reconceptualize our intervention model to include treatment designed to improve the mother's adult competence as well as to foster a positive mother–child relationship. That is, the new treatment included a focus on helping the mother develop adult social skills, to maintain social relationships, to manage her emotional life, and to cope with stress. We then tested this new intervention by evaluating it in comparison with a program of typical services provided by public health nurses. We refer to this project as Clinical Nursing Models (CNM; Barnard et al., 1988; Booth et al., 1989; Mitchell et al., 1988).

Subjects

The subjects in the CNM project were 147 high-social-risk women who sought prenatal services from health department clinics. A public health nurse interviewed potential participants to determine their life circumstances. Women who were 22 weeks pregnant or less and had

one or more of the following characteristics were invited to participate (percentage of sample in parentheses): (1) alcohol or drug addiction (8%), (2) psychiatric diagnosis (4%), (3) previous child maltreatment (3%), (4) both low educational level and low social support
(48%), (5) young and low social support (16%), (6) low income and
low social support (67%), and (7) low educational level, young, and
low income (24%).

The women's mean age was 21.2 (± 4.0) years and they had
completed an average of 11.0 (± 1.5) years of school. Ninety percent
of the women were Caucasian. Only 25% of the women were married
and living with their spouses. Thirteen percent were working outside
the home. The average yearly family income was in the range of
$5,000 to $7,500.

The study infants were primarily fullterm, with a mean gesta-
tional age of 39.7 (± 1.6) weeks. Most were delivered vaginally (78%);
49% were male, and 50% were firstborns.

Procedure

The research design involved the following: (1) pretreatment (ante-
partum) assessments of the mother; (2) provision of preventive intervention services (two types) from midpregnancy to the child's first
birthday; (3) assessments of the child during treatment; (4) immediate
posttreatment assessment of the mother, the child, and the mother–
child relationship around the child's first birthday; and (5) delayed
posttreatment assessments around the child's second birthday.

Assessments of the mother included measures of stress, social
support, depression, social skills, and intelligence. The quality of the
mother–child relationship was assessed by various observation measures both in the lab and at home. Of particular interest to this report
was that the security of the child's attachment relationship to mother
was assessed in the lab immediately posttreatment (at 13 months), as
well as 7 months later (at 20 months). Finally, child assessments
reflecting various aspects of social, cognitive, and linguistic development were performed.

Treatment—Mental Health Model

The CNM project compared two different approaches to providing
nursing services. The two programs shared several important features.
First, both programs shared the ultimate goal of preventing poor
social-emotional and cognitive outcomes in the children. Second, both
provided services by a single consistent nurse-caregiver in the home.

Third, the two programs were both organized by written protocols delineating specific goals and objectives.

The primary differences between the two models were in their philosophy and specific content. The *Mental Health* (MH) model, which we hypothesized would be the most beneficial, focused on the mother's adult competencies (as outlined in our model) and mother–child relationship skills. The MH nurses' primary objective was to develop a therapeutic relationship with the client, and through this relationship to provide support and to demonstrate ways of dealing with interpersonal situations and problems. Treatment was individualized in the sense that it was based on assessment of the mother's strengths and weaknesses. Assessment of the mother's adult competencies (e.g., her social skills, her coping strategies) and later, her parenting skills, assisted the nurses in identifying areas of primary concern. The nurses utilized Brammer's (1973) Helping Relationship model. That is, they viewed their role as working within the framework of what the mother wanted help with, rather than dictating a course of treatment without her input. In other words, the mother was viewed as an active participant rather than as a passive learner or resource user.

An important aspect of the intervention was that it began prior to the birth of the child. We reasoned that our best opportunity for improving child outcomes was to develop a relationship with the mother and begin working on her adult needs and issues (as well as helping her prepare for the baby) before her attention was focused on coping with a newborn. Therefore, the intervention began in the second trimester of pregnancy and continued until the child's first birthday. We ended the intervention at one year primarily for pragmatic reasons of funding. Ideally, the intervention would continue until the child's capabilities of locomotion and language were well established.

The nurses providing the MH intervention had masters' preparation in parent-child nursing. The nurses developed the intervention objectives and provided ongoing consultation to each other about the implementation of the intervention. A caseload of 25 active families was considered a full-time responsibility. The nurses were free to set their own context (home, clinic, or elsewhere), schedule, and focus, within the framework of intervention objectives.

During pregnancy the major goals of the MH intervention were to: (1) increase the support of the mother's network; (2) foster decision making about delivery options; (3) deal successfully with situational anxieties and needs; (4) increase the mother's self-image and confidence in parenting; and (5) enhance mother-infant attachment. For each objective, behavioral outcome criteria were outlined. For example, in relation to the goal of enhancing mother-infant attachment, the nurse assessed maternal-fetal attachment by having the mother complete an inventory and discussing her feelings and preparation for the baby. The nurse helped the mother identify and feel fetal body parts. She encouraged the mother to practice communicating with the fetus through massage and talking. She encouraged discussion about parenting values, beliefs, and expectations.

During the intrapartum period there were three major treatment objectives: (1) ensuring the mother's affiliative support; (2) enhancing mother–infant acquaintance; and (3) promoting an environment that enhances self-regulatory behaviors of the mother and infant. Again, each objective involved specific behavioral criteria that were monitored by the nurse assigned to the mother. The majority of mothers, for example, achieved part of the first objective by having a support person with them during labor and delivery. In some cases, this person was the nurse. During the immediate postbirth period, through 3 months of age, the objectives included maintaining a focus on the mother's support system, and were expanded to include mothering and the baby's adjustment. There was considerable focus on enhancing the quality of mother-infant interaction. The specific behavioral criteria for this objective included developing the mother's awareness of infant cues; encouraging the mother to vocalize to the infant, respond contingently, and provide appropriate stimulation; and teaching the mother to have appropriate expectations about the infant's capacity to see, hear, show awareness, and learn from the environment.

During the remainder of the first year the parenting objectives were to (1) maximize the mother's affective involvement with the infant; (2) assist the mother in providing temporal organization and varied stimulation for the infant; (3) increase the mother's understanding of reciprocal interaction; (4) ensure the mother's realistic developmental expectations for her child; (5) increase a sense of trust in mother and child; (6) promote a safe environment; and (7) avoid restrictive caregiving.

Throughout the first year, the objectives relating to the mother's adult competencies were to (1) increase maternal social competence and affiliative relationships with others; (2) facilitate participation in community resources offering child care support; (3) facilitate use of personal and community resources according to need; and (4) facilitate adaptive and coping behaviors that minimize disruption of parenting.

Treatment—Information/Resource Model

The comparison group for this study had nursing follow-up that was typical of public health nursing in the United States during the early

1980s. The model was labeled "Information/Resource" (IR) to signify that a major objective of public health nurses in serving clients during pregnancy and early parenting is to provide the client with information and to make the client aware of community resources. The nurses providing care for this group were employed by the Seattle-King County Public Health Department. For this project we developed goals and client behavioral criteria in keeping with current practice. The major objective of this model was to provide information—facts, procedures, and practices—to the mother in a straightforward way. Examples of IR's specific objectives were to have the mother demonstrate (1) knowledge of infant illness, basic home-health-care techniques, and when to seek medical care; (2) knowledge of birth-control methods; (3) knowledge and use of appropriate type and amount of infant stimulation through toys, activities, and socializing; and (4) attachment behaviors to infant and pleasure in infant-related care activities and play.

Along with direct teaching, the nurse also provided referrals to other agencies, so that she served as a resource coordinator as well as caregiver. The IR model focused on health promotion and disease prevention and represented the closest approximation to existing community nursing services for clients during pregnancy and early child-rearing years. There was no nontreatment (control) group in the CNM study, due to ethical concerns about withholding services to a high-risk population.

Assessing Attachment Security

Infant–mother attachment was assessed at ages 13 and 20 months in the laboratory using the Strange Situation paradigm (Ainsworth et al., 1978). The Strange Situation, involving the usual series of mother-infant separations and reunions, occurred at the end of the lab visit following other videotaped assessments of mother–child interaction and child competence. At 13 months, the "stranger reunion" segment was omitted because we noted that the additional stress to the infant was not necessary to code the episode.

All videotapes of the Strange Situation were coded by observers in accordance with conventions outlined by Ainsworth et al. (1978) and Main and Solomon (1990). Attachment classifications were assigned as follows: Children were classified as securely attached (B) if, upon reunion with the mother, they greeted her and initiated interaction (if not distressed) or approached her and sought contact (if distressed). Children who avoided their mothers upon reunion were classified as insecure-avoidant (A). Children who showed angry resistant behavior in combination with proximity-seeking were classified as insecure-resistant (C). Children with disordered temporal sequences of behavior, dazed affect, stereotypes, and moderate-to-high levels of avoidance and resistance in the same reunion episode were classified as insecure-disorganized-disoriented (D). For purposes of this report, we have grouped the three insecure classifications together.

Different sets of blind observers coded the 13- and 20-month tapes. Agreement among the coder pairs was 78–79%. Disagreements were resolved by consensus among the coders. Additionally, agreement with Mary Main on 18 of the tapes was 89%.

Results

Group Differences—Treatment Process

Mothers in the Mental Health group had more contact with their nurses than did the mothers in the Information/Resource group (25 vs. 12 hours). The MH mothers also achieved more of the goals of the program (72% vs. 62%), and reported greater satisfaction with the services received. Empirical analysis of each nurse-client contact indicated that the "nursing acts" in the MH group involved more support, therapeutic acts, and goal setting, while nursing acts in the IR group involved more monitoring and providing information.

Group Differences—Treatment Outcomes

Although the MH treatment was successful in terms of client retention, client satisfaction, and goal completion, the real test of program effectiveness was whether the program had affected the mother–child relationship and child outcomes in a positive way, and to a greater extent than did the IR program. Initial statistical comparisons of the two groups revealed very few differences between them on these outcome measures (see Barnard, Magyary, Sumner, Booth, Mitchell, & Spieker, 1988).

Of particular interest for the present report are the attachment results, which also did not differ by treatment group. In the MH group, 43% of the children were rated as securely attached to mother at 13 months, compared with 47% of the children in the IR group. At 20 months, 56% of the MH group were securely attached, compared with 52% of the IR group. The stability of secure attachment (from 13 to 20 months) was 32% in the MH group and 31% in the IR group. None of these differences was statistically significant.

Our next step in analyzing the data was to evaluate group differences in relation to the presenting characteristics of the mothers (see Barnard et al., 1988; Booth et al., 1989). As previously indicated, the attrition rates in the two groups were markedly different: 80% of the MH mothers remained in the program, compared with 53% of the IR mothers. We found that mothers who began the treatment with the most problems—those who were depressed, who had low social support, and/or lower intellectual capacity—were more likely to drop out of the IR program, but to continue with the MH program. Thus, posttreatment differences between the groups were diminished by these initial characteristics.

Given these findings, we hypothesized that treatment type would interact with initial characteristics of mothers. Specifically, we expected that for the mothers with the most problems, treatment outcomes would be better in the MH group than in the IR group. To test this hypothesis, we split the mothers into groups based on their initial characteristics, for example, IQ below 90 (the sample mean) versus IQ equal to or above 90; depressed versus not depressed, and so forth (see Barnard et al., 1988). In general, the results supported our expectations: less competent mothers had better outcomes in the MH group and more competent mothers had better outcomes in the IR group. With respect to the attachment data, the results were as follows: For the MH model, the rate of secure attachment at 13 months was 48% in the low-IQ group and 38% in the higher-IQ group. For the IR model, the rates of secure attachment were 33% and 60%, respectively. A significant difference also was found for stability of secure attachment between 13 and 20 months. For the MH model, 39% of the children were securely attached at both ages in the low-IQ group, versus 25% in the higher-IQ group; for the IR model, the rates of secure attachment at both ages were 17% and 45%, respectively. These results indicated that secure attachment and stability of secure attachment were most likely in the low-IQ MH group and the higher-IQ IR group.

The proportion of insecure infants in this sample as a whole is somewhat higher than has been reported in several other studies of high-social-risk mothers and infants (reviewed in Spieker & Booth, 1988) and the stability from 13 to 20 months is lower (e.g., Vaughn et al., 1979). It is possible that our use of the "D" classification category, not used in previous studies of similar samples, resulted in our detecting higher rates of insecurity (because many of these children would have been misclassified as secure or "unclassifiable"). The lower stability of attachment may be due, in part, to the continued readjustments made in these families in the year after termination of the intervention. We are currently investigating this possibility in other analyses.

Discussion

Taken together, the findings illustrate one of the major lessons of the CNM project: the evaluation of preventive intervention effects is not a matter of simple group comparisons. Mothers with differing initial characteristics may be responsive to different treatments, and may vary in the extent to which they are able to make life changes quickly enough to benefit the child. In evaluating our results, we realized that the most appropriate question was "*For whom* was the MH intervention effective?," rather than "*Was* the intervention effective?" In general, the MH intervention was most effective for mothers and children in the most problematic families—those at highest risk for poor outcomes. Due to the lack of a control group, we cannot evaluate what these children would have been like without any treatment. However, we do know that the MH treatment generally was more effective than standard PHN services (in the IR group) for the most problematic families.

Despite the apparent success of the MH treatment, a relatively low percentage of children were classified as securely attached, compared with what we would expect in a low-risk stable sample. Looking at the CNM sample as a whole, approximately half of these children would be considered still at risk for subsequent attachment-related difficulties.

To investigate the consequences of insecure attachment for these high-risk children, a follow-up study of peer-directed social competence was conducted at age 4 years.

ATTACHMENT SECURITY AND SUBSEQUENT PEER-DIRECTED BEHAVIOR

At age 4 years, a small number of CNM subjects (32) (as well as other children who had been studied longitudinally) were brought back into the laboratory to evaluate their peer-directed social behavior (see Booth, Rose-Krasnor, & Rubin, 1991). As indicated by our model and by previous research, we hypothesized that those children who had been insecurely attached to mother at age 20 months would show more maladaptive behavior in relation to an unfamiliar same-aged peer at age 4 years, when compared with children who had been coded secure in infancy.

Subjects at Follow-Up

Subject characteristics were as follows: Mean maternal age was 27 ($\pm$ 4.0) years; mean years of education was 11.2 ($\pm$ 1.5) years. The mothers were predominantly Caucasian (90%); 40% were married. Half of the children (50%) were firstborn; 55% were boys.

Each child was paired with an unfamiliar, same-age ($\pm$ 3 mos), same-gender peer, on the basis of attachment classification at 20 months. From the pool of longitudinal participants, we formed 20 pairs of children. Each pair comprised a "focal" child and a "control" child. The control children were securely attached; half of the focal children were insecurely attached and half were secure (thus forming secure-secure and insecure-secure focal/control pairs, based on 20-month Strange Situation classifications). Only the behaviors of the focal children were coded from the videotapes. (Some of the control children participated twice.)

Procedure

Children and their mothers were observed and videotaped in a laboratory playroom during a variety of tasks: (1) warm-up free play (focal child and mother), (2) free play (both children and both mothers), (3) block-building task (both children and focal child's mother), (4) free play (both children and focal child's mother), (5) novel toy (children only), and (6) cookie sharing (children only).

The Novel Toy segment is the primary focus in this context. The segment occurred when the focal and control children were alone in the playroom. After interacting with the same set of attractive free-play toys throughout the laboratory session, the experimenter introduced *one* novel toy for the children to share—a "He-Man" action figure for the boy dyads and a "She-Ra" action figure for the girl dyads. The experimenter entered the room with the novel toy in her purse. She requested that the children sit on the floor with her, one on each side. Then she told them that she had a very special toy for them, removed the figure from her purse, and placed it on the floor between, and equidistant from, the two children. The experimenter then left immediately, leaving the children alone in the playroom. The Novel Toy segment was designed to create a social challenge for the children: competing for possession of a desired object and the resolution of object conflict. If one or both children became too aggressive, the segment was terminated (this happened once).

The focal child's behaviors in the Novel Toy segment were coded by observers who were blind regarding 20-month attachment status and other subject characteristics. The coding scheme utilized a social problem-solving taxonomy in which the focus was on the child's goals, the means by which he or she attempted to accomplish these goals, the degree to which these strategies were successful, and the affect associated with goal-directed attempts. All socially directive behaviors were coded as problem-solving attempts, using an event recording procedure. Kappa values expressing the degree of inter-observer reliablity ranged from .82 to .91.

Results

The results indicated that the secure and insecure focals did not differ in their types of goals. However, as predicted, insecurely attached children used more aggressive strategies and engaged in more negative affective interchanges in attempting to accomplish their goals. Interestingly, insecure children were as successful as secure children in getting their goals met, although the former group tended to have fewer total goals. Overall, it would appear that insecurely attached children tended to be successful by using aggressive strategies. Although these strategies may be beneficial to the child in the short term, the use of aggression to solve social dilemmas is costly in terms of resulting peer rejection (e.g., Rubin & Daniels-Beirness, 1983).

CONCLUSIONS

The results of the follow-up study provided support for part of our model: children at risk due to insecure attachment tended to behave in maladaptive ways with peers that are predictive of subsequent deviance. As we continue to study these children at age 7, we hope to shed more light on the extent to which early childhood risk factors, including setting factors and maternal competencies, continue to predict a pathway to deviance.

Regarding our method of preventive intervention, we conclude that it was partially successful in modifying the risk trajectory for some children. Our results suggest that in the future, increased study of the process of matching treatments to clients may prove more beneficial than designing new treatments that are uniform for everyone.

ACKNOWLEDGMENT

Research reported in this chapter was supported by grant no. MH36894 from the National Institute of Mental Health, grant no. NR01635 from the National Center for Nursing Research, and grant no. HD27806 from the National Institute of Child Health and Human Development. The first three authors are affiliates of the Child Development and Mental Retardation Center at the University of Washington.

REFERENCES

Ainsworth, M. D. S., Blehar, M. C., Waters, E., & Wall, S. (1978). *Patterns of attachment*. Hillsdale, NJ: Erlbaum.

Barclay, J. R. (1966). Sociometric choices and teacher ratings as predictors of school dropout. *Journal of Consulting and Clinical Psychology, 53*, 500–505.

Barnard, K. E., Booth, C. L., Mitchell, S. K., & Telzrow, R. (1988). Newborn nursing models: A test of early intervention to high-risk infants and families. In E. Hibbs (Ed.), *Children and families: Studies in prevention and intervention* (pp. 63–81). Madison, CT: International Universities Press.

Barnard, K. E., Hammond, M. A., Booth, C. L., Bee, H. L., Mitchell, S. K., & Spieker, S. J. (1989). Measurement and meaning of parent-child interaction. In F. J. Morrison, C. E. Lord, & D. P. Keating (Eds.), *Applied developmental psychology* (Vol. 3, pp. 39–80). New York: Academic Press.

Barnard, K. E., Magyary, D., Sumner, G., Booth, C. L., Mitchell, S. K., & Spieker, S. J. (1988). Prevention of parenting alterations for women with low social support. *Psychiatry, 51*, 248–253.

Bates, J. E., Maslin, C. A., & Frankel, K. A. (1985). Attachment security, mother-infant interaction and temperament as predictors of behavior problem ratings at age three years. In I. Bretherton & E. Waters (Eds.), *Growing points of attachment theory and research* (Monograph of the Society for Research in Child Development, Vol. 50 [1–2], Serial No. 209, pp. 167–193). Chicago: University of Chicago Press.

Bell, S. M. & Ainsworth, M. D. S. (1972). Infant crying and maternal responsiveness. *Child Development, 43*, 1171–1190.

Belsky, J. (1984). The determinants of parenting: A process model. *Child Development, 53*, 83–96.

Belsky, J., Rovine, M., & Taylor, D. (1984). The Pennsylvania Infant and Family Development Project II: Origins of individual differences in infant–mother attachment: Maternal and infant contributions. *Child Development, 55*, 706–717.

Bennett, F. C. (1987). The effectiveness of early intervention for infants at increased biologic risk. In M. J. Guralnick & F. C. Bennett (Eds.), *The effectiveness of early intervention for at-risk and handicapped children* (pp. 79–112). Boston: Harcourt Brace Jovanovich.

Booth, C. L., Lyons, N. L., & Barnard, K. E. (1984). Synchrony in mother-infant interaction: A comparison of measurement methods. *Child Study Journal, 14*, 95-114.

Booth, C. L., Mitchell, S., Barnard, K., & Spieker, S. J. (1989). Development of maternal social skills in multiproblem families: Effects on the mother–child relationship. *Developmental Psychology, 25*, 403-412.

Booth, C. L., Rose-Krasnor, L., & Rubin, K. H. (1991). Relating preschoolers' social competence and their mothers' parenting behaviors to early attachment security and high risk status. *Journal of Social and Personal Relationships, 8*, 363-382.

Bowlby, J. (1982). *Attachment and loss: Vol. 1. Attachment* (2nd ed.). New York: Basic Books.

Bowlby, J. (1973). *Attachment and loss: Vol. 2. Separation, anxiety, and anger*. New York: Basic Books.

Brammer, L. M. (1973). The helping relationship process and skills. Englewood Cliffs, NJ: Prentice Hall.

Bretherton, I. (1985). Attachment theory: Retrospect and prospect. *Monographs of the Society for Research in Child Development, 50* (Nos. 1-1, Serial No. 209).

Crnic, K., & Booth, C. L. (1991). Mothers' and fathers' perceptions of daily hassles of parenting across early childhood. *Journal of Marriage and the Family, 53*, 1042-1050.

Crnic, K., & Greenberg, M. T. (1990). Minor parenting stresses with young children. *Child Development, 61*, 1628-1637.

Egeland, B., & Sroufe, L. A. (1981). Development sequelae of maltreatment in infants. In R. Rizley & D. Cicchetti (Eds.), *Developmental perspectives in child maltreatment* (pp. 77-92). San Francisco: Jossey-Bass.

Elder, G. H., Caspi, A., & Burton, L. M. (1987). Adolescent transitions in developmental perspective: Historical and sociological insights. In M. Gunnar (Ed.), *Minnesota symposia on child psychology* (Vol. 21, pp. 151-179). Hillsdale, NJ: Erlbaum.

Farrington, D. P. (1991). Childhood aggression and adult violence: Early precursors and later life outcomes. In D. J. Pepler & K. H. Rubin (Eds.), *The development and treatment of childhood aggression* (pp. 5-30). Hillsdale, NJ: Erlbaum.

Grossmann, K., Grossmann, K. E., Spangler, G., Suess, G., & Unzer, J. (1985). Maternal sensitivity and newborns' orientation responses as related to quality of attachment in northern Germany. In I. Bretherton & E. Waters (Eds.), *Growing points of attachment theory and research* (Monograph of the Society for Research in Child Development, Vol. 50 [1-2], Serial No. 209, pp. 233-256). Chicago: University of Chicago Press.

Houck, G. M., Booth, C. L., & Barnard, K. E. (1991). Maternal depression and locus of control orientation as predictors of dyadic play behavior. *Infant Mental Health Journal, 12*, 347-360.

Hymel, S., Rubin, K. H., Rowden, L., & LeMare, L. (1990). Children's peer relationships: Longitudinal predictions of internalizing and externalizing problems from middle to late childhood. *Child Development, 61,* 2004–2021.

Kagan, J. (1989). *Unstable ideas: Temperament, cognition and self.* Cambridge: Harvard University Press.

Kupersmidt, J. B., & Coie, J. D. (1990). Preadolescent peer status, aggression, and school adjustment as predictors of externalizing problems in adolescence. *Child Development, 61,* 1350–1362.

LaFreniére, P., & Sroufe, L. A. (1985). Profiles of peer competence in the preschool: Interrelations between measures, influence of social ecology, and relation to attachment history. *Developmental Psychology, 21,* 56–69.

Main, M., Kaplan, N., & Cassidy, J. (1985). Security in infancy, childhood, and adulthood: A move to the level of representation. In I. Bretherton & E. Waters (Eds.), *Growing points of attachment theory and research* (Monographs of the Society for Research in Child Development, Vol. 50 [1–2], Serial No. 209, pp. 66–104). Chicago: University of Chicago Press.

Main, M., & Solomon, J. (1990). Procedures for identifying insecure-disorganized/disoriented infants. In M. Greenberg, D. Cicchetti, & E. M. Cummings (Eds.), *Attachment in the preschool years: Theory, research and intervention* (pp. 121–160). Chicago: University of Chicago Press.

Mitchell, S. K., Magyary, D. L., Barnard, K. E., Sumner, G. A., & Booth, C. L. (1988). A comparison of home-based prevention programs for families of newborns. In L. A. Bond & B. M. Wagner (Eds.), *Families in transition: Primary prevention programs that work* (pp. 73–98). Beverly Hills, CA: Sage.

Parker, J. G., & Asher, S. R. (1987). Peer relations and later personal adjustment: Are low-accepted children at risk? *Psychological Bulletin, 102,* 357–389.

Pepler, D. J., & Rubin, K. H. (Eds.). (1991). *The development and treatment of childhood aggression.* Hillsdale, NJ: Erlbaum.

Radke-Yarrow, M., Cummings, E. M., Kuczynski, L., & Chapman, M. (1985). Patterns of attachment in two- and three-year-olds in normal families and families with parental depression. *Child Development, 56,* 884–893.

Radke-Yarrow, M., Richters, J., & Wilson, W. E. (1988). Child development in a network of relationships. In R. A. Hinde & J. Stevenson-Hinde (Eds.), *Relationships within families: Mutual influences* (pp. 48–67). Oxford: Clarendon Press.

Renken, B., Egeland, B., Marvinney, D., Sroufe, L. A., & Mangelsdorf, S. (1989). Early childhood antecedents of aggression and passive-withdrawal in early elementary school. *Journal of Personality, 57,* 257–281.

Rubin, K. H., & Coplan, R. (in press). Peer relationships in childhood. In M. Bornstein & M. Lamb (Eds.), *Developmental Psychology: An advanced textbook.* Hillsdale, NJ: Erlbaum.

Rubin, K. H., & Daniels-Beirness, T. (1983). Concurrent and predictive correlates of sociometric status in kindergarten and grade 1 children. *Merrill-Palmer Quarterly*, *29*, 337–351.

Rubin, K. H., & Mills, R. S. L. (1988). The many faces of social isolation in childhood. *Journal of Consulting and Clinical Psychology*, *6*, 916–924.

Rubin, K. H., & Mills, R. S. L. (1991). Conceptualizing developmental pathways to internalizing disorders in childhood. *Canadian Journal of Behavioral Science*, *23*, 300–317.

Rutter, M., & Garmezy, N. (1983). Developmental psychopathology. In P. H. Mussen & E. M. Hetherington (Eds.), *Handbook of child psychology: Vol. 4. Socialization, personality, and social development* (pp. 775–911). New York: Wiley.

Sarason, I., Johnson, H., & Siegel, M. (1978). Assessing the impact of life changes: Development of the life experience survey. *Journal of Consulting and Clinical Psychology*, *46*, 932–946.

Spieker, S. J., & Booth, C. L. (1988). Maternal antecedents of attachment quality. In J. Belsky & T. Nezworski (Eds.), *Clinical implications of attachment* (pp. 95–135). Hillsdale, NJ: Erlbaum.

Sroufe, L. A. (1983). Infant-caregiver attachment and patterns of adaptation in preschool: The roots of maladaptation. In M. Perlmutter (Ed.), *Minnesota Symposia on Child Psychology* (Vol. 16, pp. 41–83). Hillsdale, NJ: Erlbaum.

Thoman, E. B. (1975). How a rejecting baby affects mother-infant synchrony. In *Parent-Infant Interaction, Ciba Foundation Symposium* (Vol. 33, n.s., pp. 177–200). Amsterdam: ASP/Elsevier

Thomas, A., & Chess, S. (1977). *Temperament and development*. New York: Brunner/Mazel.

Troy, M., & Sroufe, L. A. (1987). Victimization among preschoolers: Role of attachment relationship history. *Journal of the American Academy of Child and Adolescent Psychiatry*, *26*, 166–172.

Ullman, C. A. (1957). Teachers, peers, and tests as predictors of adjustment. *Journal of Educational Psychology*, *48*, 257–267.

Vaughn, B., Egeland, B., Sroufe, L. A., & Waters, E. (1979). Individual differences in infant–mother attachment at twelve and eighteen months: Stability and change in families under stress. *Child Development*, *50*, 971–975.

Waters, E., Vaughn, B. E., & Egeland, B. R. (1980). Individual differences in infant–mother attachment relationships at age one: Antecedents in neonatal behavior in an urban, economically disadvantaged sample. *Child Development*, *51*, 208–216.

CHAPTER 3

◆ ——— ◆

The Mother-Child Home Program:
Research Methodology and the Real World

PHYLLIS LEVENSTEIN

Social scientists had become aware before the middle of this century of a major linkage between low levels of education and people's active involvement in socially and personally dysfunctional activities: crimes of various sorts, drug addiction, juvenile delinquency, teenage motherhood ("children having children"), to name a few. However, it was not until the gradual advent of the technological society in this country, starting in the 1940s, that the related link in the United States to another kind of problem also became painfully prominent: the growing unemployability of persons who could not meet the minimum literacy demands of working in that society (Myrdal, 1962). A high school diploma usually became a necessary passport to even entry-level jobs. Those who could not meet this standard because they dropped out of high school before graduation were likely to be doomed to permanent states of jobless poverty or of welfare dependence. They became what Myrdal called the "underclass." They also became vulnerable to the temptations of using illicit means of alleviating their impoverished lives. It was for social as well as humane reasons that in the mid-60s President Lyndon B. Johnson launched a "War on Poverty." Money became available, both federal and from private foundations, for research on the causes of the educational disadvantage that seemed to be associated with poverty and was apparent in children's earliest school grades.

This research led to recognition of economically disadvantaged children's need for preschool enrichment and gave rise to a number of well-researched preschool interventions (Lazar & Darlington, 1982). Most preschool programs to prevent educational disadvantage added cognitive emphases to relatively traditional nursery school procedures and were "center-based," that is, they were conducted within a classroom. The experimental method was the wise choice for measuring the short-term impact of intervention programs specially constructed and researched in the 1960s for low-income preschool children considered to be at risk for educational disadvantage. Few of these experimental preventive interventions obtained support long enough to follow up their subjects through high school. At least one that did, David Weikart's Perry Preschool Project in Ypsilanti, Michigan, found positive results for its graduates and a substantial savings in dollars from their decreased need for special school or social services, aside from the program's personal benefits to graduates (Berrueta-Clement, Schweinhart, Barnett, Epstein, & Weikart, 1984).

THE MOTHER-CHILD HOME PROGRAM

Goals

Although the Mother–Child Home Program (MCHP) was part of the preschool intervention movement at the time it was created in 1965 by the Verbal Interaction Project (VIP), the program was unusual for being a *pre*-preschool educational/mental health intervention that was entirely home-based, rather than center-based. The family, rather than a center-based setting, was chosen for its locus because recent empirical research had traced the educational problems of schoolchildren to short supplies of conceptual-verbal exchange between young children and members of their economically disadvantaged families. It seemed sensible to try to prevent children's school disadvantage by centering intervention in their families. The MCHP focused particularly on families with the most depressed, least educated and least motivated parents, usually single-parent (often bilingual) mothers, and their very young children. It shared with the many home-based educational programs that arose in its wake only its comparatively inexpensive home-based locus of operation and also one of its two major goals: the ultimate prevention of educational disadvantage in children. The other major goal was the transformation of low-income mothers from being "Hesitaters"—defined as passive and feeling hopelessly out of control of their lives and those of their children—to becoming "Strivers"—defined as possessing the self-respect and ability to influence their children toward good intellectual development and resulting school success. As the means for attaining these goals, the program's immediate objective was to stimulate conceptually rich verbal interaction between the child and his or her mother, the person likely to be the child's closest and most enduring parent in impoverished families.

The Verbal Interaction Project, Inc. (under the aegis of State University of New York at Stony Brook and—in its early years—the Family Service Association of Nassau County, New York) spent 16 years, with 10 yearly cohorts of mother–child dyads, to develop its model of the MCHP and to investigate through experimental research this intervention's effectiveness in achieving its short-term and long-range goals.

Theoretical Background

The MCHP was built on a multidiscipline theoretical and empirical foundation, which demonstrated the importance to children's intellectual development of early positive verbal and social-emotional interactions in the family. Many systematic empirical investigations antecedent to the program (e.g., Bernstein, 1961, 1965; Deutsch, 1965; Hess & Shipman, 1965; John & Goldstein, 1964) had shown the profound influence of verbal (and thus conceptual) interaction within the family on the early cognitive development of children and on their school-age academic skills. Later research, published some time after the MCHP began, upheld these findings (e.g., Gottfried, 1984; Schacter, 1979).

Such empirical studies supported the earlier conjectures of Bruner, Olver, and Greenfield (1966) that the symbolic mode of representing the world of reality in language is the highest and most necessary linguistic-conceptual skill for dealing with the complexities of industrial society. Bruner's thinking reached back to the philosophical arguments of Cassirer (1944), who argued that symbolic language is unique to man, that he alone among the animals is "animal symbolicum"; to Sapir's (1921) declaration that language is the perfect symbol system for the human ability to generalize from concrete experiences; and especially to Vygotsky's (1962) empirical evidence for the efficiency of language as a verbal symbol system.

From the convergence of philosophy and research, it became obvious to the creators of the MCHP that the family, as the basic unit of social organization, is as responsible for children's early verbal and cognitive development as for teaching the social-emotional behavior acceptable in their society. Both current conventional wisdom and accumulated scientific knowledge agree that mother is the very young child's first and best teacher. Mothers' behaviors toward their children in their early years have profound effects on the children's cognitive as well as their social-emotional growth. For one thing, the mother is probably in those years the object of the child's closest emotional attachment; her love and approval are powerful external motivators. Further, in low-income families the mother is often the only enduring parent. Therefore it is with her that her child is most likely to play what Roger Brown (1965) called the "Original Word Game," the exchange of language between parent and child in which the child learns to acquire words, first as labels for the concrete objects of his world and then gradually as words that summarize similarities among the labels—verbal symbols of concepts. He or she learns that a little wooden chair meant for him or her to sit upon, a blue upholstered chair big enough for his or her mother, a chair that grownups draw to the table—all are like each other in one essential way: their "chairness." He or she has identified the "chairness" among them and learned, from his or her basic human symbolic ability, to use the word "chair" as the verbal symbol for this chairness. His or her mother has reinforced the concept by her example. In Bruner's (1964) vivid analogy, he or she has learned to change the pennies, nickels, and dimes of labels into bigger denominations of symbolic language: a verbalized concept, "chair," that goes beyond the label "chair."

In low-income homes the small change of labels is more likely to be available than the larger denominations of verbalized concepts. For one thing, because of the environmental privation, there are fewer labels available for generalization, or "category availablity," as it was called by Roger Brown (1958). For another, low-income mothers are often too harrassed by the time-consuming tasks of poverty—the long waits at clinics, the making do with insufficient heat, hot water, clothing, or food, and so forth—to pay much attention to anything but their children's basic physcal needs. Still another reason for the scarcity of concept-building language exchanged between child and mother in poverty-handicapped families is that non-college-educated mothers (i.e., most low-income mothers) have what might be called Victorian ideas about child rearing: children should be seen and not heard. Therefore dialogue between mother and child tends to be short and "telegraphic" (Bernstein, 1961). Moreover, there are few objects, the "props" as Cazden (1970) called them, to encourage conversation between child and mother. As the VIP's early interviews with representative mothers found, books were scarce in their homes, and what unbroken toys there were (often originally selected from TV commercials) offered little intellectual challenge.

McCord and McCord's (1959) follow-up data from the Cambridge-Somerville Youth Study showed with poignant clarity the benign or disastrous effects of family, and particularly maternal, influences, on children's turn toward criminal or noncriminal lives. Neither their research nor the VIP's indicated that the attachment between mother and child was any less in low-income families than in other families. Nor was there any reason to believe that low-income mothers and their children lacked what seem to be the universal internal (as distinguished from external) motivational drives described by Harvard psychologist Robert W. White (1959, 1963). On the basis of research evidence from dozens of studies, White demonstrated that competence resulting in a feeling of efficacy (heightened self-esteem) is developed through an individual's drive and ability to master the environment, which he called "effectance." Low-income mothers, often Hesitaters who feel helpless and depressed because of being unable (it seems to them) to control their own fates, are badly in need of internal sources of self-esteem, of feeling the power to effect positive changes in themselves and their children. On the other hand, children at the beginning stages of intellectual development need, for optimum development, to feel the excitement of mastering their environments through their own efforts—in short, to have repeated experiences of efficacy that build self-confidence to master ever more challenging tasks, including eventually the challenges of academic tasks.

Affect-laden motivation and mother–child attachment are probably so entwined, it was felt at the inception of the MCHP, that both must be as much a part of the MCHP as the all-important verbal interaction that leads to the child's conceptual and therefore cognitive development. It was clear from previous theory and research, supported later by more recent empirical data (e.g., Clarke-Stewart, Vanderstoep, & Killim, 1979), that an intervention to prevent children's later school failure must include stimulation of conceptual conversation between mother and child and utilize their motivational drives interacting "hand-in-glove," to quote Bronfenbrenner (1974).

What should be the age of the child for a preventive intervention? At the time the MCHP began as a pilot project in 1965, the age of 4 years was considered the "natural" time for intervention. Cassirer (1944), however, had noted that the emergence of the infant-toddler into "reflective intelligence" was signaled and reinforced by rapid language development, which Hebb (1949) and Bayley (1965) agreed as occurring at about the age of 2 years. This coincides with the intensified attachment to the child's mother (Ainsworth, 1973), with his or her curiosity and insistence on learning labels for objects in the environment. Thus the age of 2 years was chosen for the start of the MCHP and about age 4 for its termination, as the VIP's early research indicated that while most of the gains occurred by the end of the first MCHP year, a second Program year was needed to stabilize them.

Intervention Method

The MCHP incorporated not only this theoretical foundation but also took advantage of some basic human motivational features in the program's approach to mothers and their children. The program's procedures drew on the previous person-intensive experience of its staff (in clinical psychology, social work, teaching, and parenthood) for informed guesses about features that were likely to motivate "Hesitater" mothers to join and stay with the program for its full 2 years. Interviews with mothers had already revealed their universal goal: to better their children's lives through education. The MCHP added other motivational elements: respect for mothers' and children's dignity, independence, and right to privacy; permanent assignment of high-quality program materials; stress on the voluntary nature of mothers' participation; the program's delivery to their own homes; and finally, the program's emphasis on mothers' roles as the main members of a team to help their children.

The program's method was explicitly nondidactic. The intervention (detailed in the program's manual and in Levenstein, 1988) started when the child reached age 2, with twice-weekly half-hour Home Play Sessions continuing with child and mother together for 2 successive school years. "Toy Demonstrators" (trained home visitors, either paid paraprofessionals or unpaid volunteers) brought books or toys (Verbal Interaction Stimulus Materials or "VISM") as permanently assigned curriculum materials: high-quality, commercially available books and toys that were intrinsically attractive to both child and mother. Twelve books and 11 toys were the "props" in each of the two MCHP years for verbal interaction between mother and child and were important incentives for mothers to join the program. However, their main purpose was to be the focus for a developmentally suitable cognitive curriculum outlined on simply written "Guide Sheets" given to the Toy Demonstrators and shared with mothers. Each Guide Sheet contained the program's entire cognitive curriculum of core concepts, illustrated by the current toy or book, and grouped under five major reminders to the Toy Demonstrator.

Cognitive Curriculum Centered Around Toys

For toys, the first reminder was *Name, and encourage the child to name* (concepts listed vertically at the left side of the Guide Sheet): labels, colors, shapes, sizes, textures, spatial relationships, number, categories and "causing things to happen" (consequences).

The second reminder was *Describe your actions, encourage the child to describe his actions* (concepts listed vertically at left side): general actions, matching, fitting, creating sounds.

The third reminder was *Remind him to think about what he does* (concepts listed vertically at left side): to give his attention, to make a choice, to have self-control, to remember other related experiences, to pretend, to do things in the right order.

The fourth reminder was *Remember, throughout the home session, to:* encourage him to talk (ask him questions, listen to his answers, answer his answers); encourage his curiosity, his imagination, his independence; encourage him to want to learn, praise him when he does well, try to ignore his mistakes, help him when he really needs help.

The final reminder was *Have a good time with [toy], the child, and the mother.*

Cognitive Curriculum Centered Around Books

The curriculum Guide Sheet for each book was structured in a manner relevant to introducing a book and reading to the child in a Home Session. It started with concrete instructions for what to model for the mother:

Invite the child to look and listen
Try to sit with the child between you and the mother
Show and read the title page of the book
Show and describe how to turn the pages and treat the book
Read in a clear, easy voice
Stop at most illustrations to:
  Invite him to point out labels name and ask him to name colors, shapes and sizes, number, texture, relationships, and categories, causing things to happen.
  Invite the child to tell about related personal experiences
  Ask questions about the illustrations to help the child reason things out
Encourage the child to join in on familiar words
Enjoy the book yourself

The final instruction was:

Invite the mother to take over the reading .

Roles of Toy Demonstrators and Mothers

In play with child and mother together, the Toy Demonstrators modeled for parents, without verbal teaching, the cognitive curriculum of verbal interaction with the children, focused around the VISM, as well as an affective "curriculum" to foster mothers' parenting skills and children's social-emotional development. They involved the mothers actively from the beginning and withdrew into the background as soon as possible in each Home Session. The Toy Demonstrators' training emphasized the importance of self-effacement in assisting the mother in her primary role as her child's first teacher. They were taught to be friendly but not friends or counselors for the mothers. However, they informed their program Coordinators, as part of their mandatory written reports of every Home Session, of mothers' seeming to reach for help with problems. The Coordinators (already known to all mothers from the initial enrollment procedures) promptly responded with a visit to a mother and with whatever aid was needed from herself or from community agencies.

The Toy Demonstrators were trained for their role in an introductory 8-session Training Workshop and in continuing weekly group supervision throughout the program year.

By the end of the 2-year program, each participant family had accumulated a library of 24 books and 22 educational toys. At that time all mothers were invited to become paid Toy Demonstrators, a role that required little education and no prior work experience but had standards spelled out for such work behavior as reliability, constructive use of supervision, preservation of the privacy and autonomy of participant families, and comprehension of job goals. The program's creators felt that the Toy Demonstrator's role could be an ideal step toward entry-level jobs as a first rung in the private sector ladder.

Experimental Research of the Mother-Child Home Program

Research Method and Subjects

The experimental method has for many years been considered to be superior to all others as the research method of choice for the study of educational or social programs. In this method people, or units of people (Campbell & Stanley, 1963, p. 22), all similar to the target population intended to receive the program, become members of a "subject pool" that is then randomly divided by subject, or units of subjects, into treatment groups: "experimental" subjects to receive the intervention, or "control" subjects to receive no intervention, or to receive a placebo intervention. The members of all the randomized groups are believed to be equal in every way, since they have fallen into one group or the other purely by chance. If only the intervention group is found to benefit in the experiment, it seems reasonable to conclude that the intervention is indeed effective within the groups tested. If it thus meets the test of "internal" validity and then also of "external" validity, because the subjects truly represent the target population, the intervention should be generalizable, that is, successful with that population.

Unit-Randomized Experimental Research of the Mother-Child Home Program

For cohorts entering the research from 1967 to 1972, the VIP used the unit-randomized experimental research method to evaluate the effects of the MCHP (a method used later by Slaughter, 1983, in research of this program). As short-term evaluation measures, it used standardized intelligence tests found to be most reliably predictive of the children's later school performance. For the long-range effects of the intervention in the real world, it followed the children into school, surveyed their teachers about their school accomplishments ("blind" ratings), and tested the children's reading and arithmetic achievement, while continuing tests of their intellectual status.

In 1967 three widely separated low-income housing projects were randomized (by coin toss) for 54 families with 2 year olds living in the housing projects to receive either the MCHP, or a placebo, or only evaluations, by their location in one of the three housing projects (randomization by unit). The three housing projects had the same requirements for tenants' eligibility, primarily the low level of the family income. This unit-randomized experimental method assured that the low-income mothers of 2 year olds in each housing project, almost all of them of below-12th-grade education as well as similar on many other background variables (e.g., mothers' age, grandparents' education, number receiving welfare support), would be offered one of the three specific programs, according to the one randomly assigned to her own housing project: only yearly evaluations for their children; yearly evaluations plus a placebo program of giving the mothers "respite time" by not being present for nonverbally stimulating home visits and gifts (intended to control for the Hawthorne effect: improvement resulting from families being singled out for special attention); or yearly evaluations plus the MCHP.

The short-term intellectual and social-emotional effects on children and the positive parenting behavior of their mothers were measured year after year in each of five new yearly cohorts following the 1967 unit-randomized pattern from 1968 to 1972, for a total of 129 mother–child dyads either in the 2-year program ($n = 78$) or in control groups ($n = 78$), the latter including a 1972 control group of 27 six-year-old disadvantaged children recruited at the same age and school grade as children who had been in the 1968 cohort. An average 85% of the 1967 to 1972 mothers accepted the treatment assigned to their housing project through the unit-randomized design, whether it was for evaluations only, for the placebo treatment plus evaluations, or for the MCHP plus evaluations.

Subject-Randomized Experimental Research of the Mother–Child Home Program

Beginning with the cohort entering in 1973, and continuing with the 1974, 1975, and 1976 cohorts, the research method was changed to a subject-randomized rather than a unit-randomized experimental research design. Mothers were invited individually to enter what was, in effect, a lottery in which the prize would be to receive the MCHP: "Will you agree to take a chance on being randomly selected to receive either the Mother–Child Home Program along with yearly evaluations of your child, or to receive only yearly evaluations for your child?" The mothers were thus invited to be subjects in an experiment rather than offered a specific treatment. It is not surprising that for the 4 years of recruiting mothers for this subject-randomized design, the overall average acceptance rate was 52%, with the acceptance rate declining in each yearly cohort, until by the 1976 cohort (the last in this subject-randomized research design) the acceptance rate was down to 27%. It was clear that there was much self-selection among the total of 166 mothers who accepted the invitation (55 in the 1976 cohort). This was in marked contrast to the average 85% (indicating limited self-selection) of the 1967 to 1972 mothers who accepted the treatment assigned to their designated housing project through the unit-randomized design, whether it was for evaluations only, for the placebo treatment plus evaluations, or for the MCHP plus evaluations.

MOTHER-CHILD HOME PROGRAM
RESEARCH RESULTS

Positive Outcomes in Unit-Randomized Experimental Cohorts

The VIP used, as short-term evaluation measures of the effects of the MCHP, tests for 2 and 4 year olds that were considered to be most reliably predictive of the children's later school performance. The yearly evaluations consisted of developmentally suitable standardized tests yielding IQ and achievement scores. Starting in 1973, a VIP-created video-based instrument called "Maternal Interactive Behavior" was added immediately postprogram and in follow-up to measure the amount of mothers' verbal and other interaction with their children. For the long-range effects of the intervention in the real world, the program's ultimate cognitive goal for children, the researchers followed the children into school, surveyed their teachers about their school behavior, and tested the children on their reading and arithmetic achievement.

1. The short-term and long-range outcome IQ scores for all six cohorts of the 1967 to 1972 unit-randomized program graduates were consistently superior to the untreated or placebo-treated control groups, and to their own pretest IQ scores. Their average gain after 2 years of the MCHP was 17 IQ points, placing the scores at or slightly above United States norms for the standardized tests that were used (Cattell, Stanford-Binet, and Wechsler Intelligence Scales for Children) (see Levenstein, 1988, Table 5.1).

2. These postprogram scores endured into fifth and eighth grades. They, and their scores on academic achievement tests, predicted school success that would endure long enough for a majority of MCHP graduates to graduate from high school (see Levenstein, 1988, Table 5.2; Madden, Levenstein, & Levenstein, 1976; Royce, Darlington, & Murray, 1983).

3. Fifty-two younger siblings of program children entered the MCHP at age 2 with IQ scores significantly higher, by 8 points (or half an IQ score's standard deviation), than the pretest scores of their older brothers and sisters, suggesting that mothers fostered their younger childen's intellectual development through parenting skills learned in the program (Phillips, 1973).

4. The mean posttest IQ of 10 MCHP graduates at the age of 4 years was compared to that of their untreated siblings at the same age. The mean IQ of the MCHP-treated children reached national norms, significantly above that of their older siblings, who had not had the program (Levenstein, 1988).

5. Three related kinds of outcome data were highly pertinent to the goals of the program. First, significantly improved maternal child-rearing behaviors, including verbal interaction, were demonstrated by the 1972 program mothers' observed behavior, measured at children's age 2 and again near the end of the program at the children's age 4, on a VIP-created instrument called "Parents And Children Together" or PACT. Second, significant concurrent correlations were found between maternal verbal interaction within the same PACT scores and the children's observed social-emotional behavior as seen on another VIP-created instrument called "Child's Behavior Traits" or "CBT," measured within the program. And third, children's CBT ratings correlated significantly with their postprogram IQ scores, arrived at independently by psychologists, as well as with their mothers' verbal interaction ratings in PACT. This was a triadic pattern of relationships that seemed to indicate the close association among mothers' positive verbal interaction, their children's social-emotional status, and the children's cognitive status (Levenstein, 1979).

6. Of even greater support for the hypotheses and goals of the MCHP was the correlation between the early maternal verbal interaction seen on "Parents and Child Together" (PACT) and the children's later positive classroom attitudes when they reached elementary school. Mothers' verbal interaction at children's age 4 predicted the program children's social-emotional attitudes and behavior in the school classroom, as rated on "Child's Behavior Traits" (CBT) by their first grade teachers. The latter were unaware of the children's program participation. The CBT, developed by the VIP, had been tested for reliability and validity (Levenstein & Staff, 1976). Table 3.1 (from Levenstein, 1979) shows the relationships between the mothers' early verbal interaction with their children and the children's academically functional school behavior traits in first grade. Further, a later study demonstrated that mothers' significantly improved verbal interaction scores demonstrated postprogram on videotape endured for at least 2 years, into kindergarten (Levenstein & O'Hara, 1983; Levenstein & O'Hara, in press).

These long-range positive effects on children's school performance of the model program's promotion of enduring maternal verbal interaction is one of the MCHP's most important accomplishments.

Positive Outcomes from Research in Replications of the Model Mother-Child Home Program

The MCHP passed in 1978 the exacting standards of the federal Joint Dissemination Review Panel, and thus became a member of the

TABLE 3.1. Correlations of Maternal Verbal Interaction at Child's Age 4 with Child's Social-Emotional Competencies in First Grade, at Age 6 (Pearson's r, $n = 39$)

Child's social-emotional competencies	Mother	
	Responds verbally	Tries to converse
Requests help appropriately	.38	.38*
Protects own rights	.33*	
Is self-confident	.47***	.49***
Seems cheerful, content	.33*	.39*
Is spontaneous, not explosive	.42**	.47***
Completes tasks		.35*
Enjoys mastering new tasks	.48***	.54***
Is well organized	.39*	.41**
Expresses ideas in language	.48***	.48***
Discerns fact from fantasy	.61***	.61***
Is creative, inventive	.40*	.52***

*$p \leq .05$
**$p \leq .01$
***$p \leq .005$

National Diffusion Network of successful educational interventions. The program's description has appeared, since the 1979 edition, in the yearly *Educational Programs That Work* (1991). In the program's present 26 replications, all trained by the Verbal Interaction Project's Center for Mother–Child Home Program to be exact duplicates of the original model, the philosophy and method of the MCHP continue to be the same as in the early model program, except for very minor local variations. When mothers and children from the target population were admitted to replications of the program, significant positive program effects were found, although not through the use of randomized experimental designs.

1. The first four replications of the MCHP used before-after research designs to show IQ gains for their program graduates that paralleled those in the model program (Levenstein, 1972).
2. Of 80% of the first children to participate in the program in a White Plains, New York, low-cost housing project who could be found, *all*, unlike their parents, had graduated from high school, and many had entered college (Greene & Hallinger, 1989).
3. A Canadian replication, conducted by a child/family service social agency serving Canadian Native Americans, used a pre-post time series evaluation method and VIP's "PACT" to measure a mother's interaction with her child (McLaren,1988). The results with these

mothers, whose educational mean was eighth grade, showed a statistically significant difference from pretest to posttest, at the .01 probability level, in their positive interaction with their children, besides a commitment to the MCHP as shown in the mothers' 100% enrollment in the MCHP for its second year. McLaren commented: "At a relatively low cost, relationships between mothers and children were improved in families where other interventions had not been successful. . . . As the mothers interacted with their children, they became more aware of the children's needs, more responsive and more understanding. They realized that they could influence their children's learning and felt a sense of accomplishment on their own behalf and on behalf of their children. Perhaps most importantly, they now enjoyed their children. All of these developments reduced the risk of abuse and neglect."

McLaren's data were informally duplicated through anecdotes from the Coordinators of almost all other replications of the MCHP, whether conducted in other child/family social service agencies or in school systems.

4. Of 32 five year olds who had completed a MCHP replication in the schools of Union, South Carolina, less than half were found, on the basis of their DIAL-R posttest scores, to require the schools' remedial services although all had shown their at-risk eligibility for such services at pretest (Springs, 1990).

5. The most impressive and far-reaching research of a replication's school effects on children, surpassing that of the VIP itself, were the follow-up studies through high school of a MCHP replication in Pittsfield, Massachusetts. Not only did this research measure the program's academic effects on its child participants through high school, but it was an out-of-house evaluation not of the original model program but of a certified replication of that program. Thus it testified both to the exportability of the MCHP and to its effects on children's school performance. Moreover, it was conducted by an evaluation team unknown to the VIP and headed by the evaluation director of the Rhode Island State Education Department, Dr. Pasquale J. DeVito.

Most of the graduates of the Parent-Child Home Program (as it was called in Pittsfield, Massachusetts) showed significant short-term gains after the program, erasing their original eligibility for Chapter 1 services based on the fact that their low-income status predicted school problems. They retained their gains (DeVito & Karon, 1984). Their academic work was normal throughout school, and they graduated from high school at the same rate as the nondeprived students of Pittsfield, Massachusetts (DeVito & Karon, 1990). Table 3.2 (from

TABLE 3.2. Total Scores, California Achievement Test, for PCHP Group and Chapter 1-Eligible Comparison Group, in Combined Grades 6-8 (Pittsfield Schools replication of the Mother-Child Home Program)

Group	Mean	t-value	Probability
PCHP ($n = 25$)	52.24		
		4.13	0.001
Comparison ($n = 24$)	36.08		

DeVito & Karon, 1984) shows the typical academic performance of the first MCHP participants to reach sixth through eighth grade in the Pittsfield school system as compared to that of students who had been eligible for the program under Chapter 1 standards but had not been included in the program.

DeVito and Karon (1984) noted that the California Achievement Test Scores of the students who had been in the program reached or were higher than the national norms for these tests. The evaluators commented at the end of their earlier evaluation:

> In summary, the Parent-Child Home Program appears to be successful in sustaining the effects achieved during participation in the program and in preparing students to use the increased cognitive development for future school endeavors. The project selects those students for participation who appear to be most "at-risk" at two years of age and for whom the prognosis of adequate performance throughout their school years is doubtful. Overall, it appears that program intervention for these students as two and three year olds had lasting effects since as a group throughout school they met or exceeded national achievement scores and generally outperformed the groups to which they were compared. (DeVito & Karon, 1984).

They recommended in their last evaluation, which examined the program children's performance through high school, "The results of this study should be disseminated widely to state, local, and other sources since longitudinal investigations of this scope are relatively uncommon for Chapter 1 ECIA programs" (DeVito & Karon, 1990).

Problematic Outcomes in Subject-Randomized Research of the Mother-Child Home Program

1. The program results for the four subject-randomized cohorts entering the VIP's experimental research of the model program from 1973 to 1976 were different from the positive results found for the

unit-randomized subjects. Measurement of the program's short-term IQ effects on the children in subject-randomized experimental designs (1973, 1974, 1975, and 1976 cohorts) showed a significant short-term positive effect only for the 1976 group (Madden, O'Hara, & Levenstein, 1984). The average IQ results for both control and program children, even in the 1976 cohort, were at or above the national norms for the IQ tests! Further, in their follow-up IQs, the control and program children showed no score differences—all were above national norms. On the other hand, subject-randomized program mothers were very significantly superior to control mothers in a video-taped measure ("Maternal Interactive Behavior" or "MIB") of the mothers' positive interactive behavior with their children (Levenstein, O'Hara, & Madden, 1983). Further, 2 years after the original MCHP, program mothers showed retention of this superiority through their children's entrance into first grade. It seemed that even self-selected subject-randomized program mothers learned to improve their interactive behavior with their children in the MCHP.

2. A subject-randomized experiment to investigate the MCHP in a valid Bermuda replication yielded nonsignificant short-term effects for the program group (Scarr & McCartney, 1988). In an earlier presentation of their study (Scarr & McCartney, 1987) the authors had described their sample as "not on average socioeconomically disadvantaged" (p. 20) and had commented: "Children in Bermuda were not found, as a group, to be at educational risk." Both observations were supported by data in the 1988 journal article: both program and control children started with almost identical IQs close to 100 (99.8 and 99.3), and most of the parents had education above high school. Almost all of the mothers accepted the initial invitation to a research "lottery" and stayed in the study until the end of the program. The program children's postprogram short-term IQ of 106.6 was numerically higher than that of the control group's 103.1, but the difference was not statistically significant.

3. In 1972 an experiment intended to be subject-randomized was established, to evaluate the effects of 10 school replications of the MCHP in a New England state. At the outset each replication's Coordinator formed two supposedly randomized groups of disadvantaged, Chapter 1–eligible (low-income) children at age 2 years, with their mothers; one group received the MCHP, and the other did not. At the end of the program's 2 years, the IQs of both groups were found to meet national norms, with little difference between the group scores, indicating that the MCHP had had no effect on the treated group and bringing its benefits into question (personal communication from the state's Chapter 1 director).

Probable Reasons for Outcome Problems in Subject-Randomized Experimental Research

1. In the VIP's subject-randomized research, it will be remembered, the mothers were invited to enter a kind of lottery in which the prize would be to receive the MCHP. "Will you agree to take a chance on being randomly selected to receive either the Mother–Child Home Program along with yearly evaluations of your child, or to receive only yearly evaluations for your child?" This disclosure of the research plan to the mothers (federally required by 1973) may well have seemed strange to the mothers, resulting in a much lower rate of acceptance of their being subjects in an experimental research project than of their receiving a specific treatment. There was no guarantee that they and their children would receive the MCHP; and a "yearly evaluation" may have sounded like a consolation prize of dubious value. The 1976 subject-randomized mothers had shown the highest degree of self-selection in agreeing to be research subjects (27% acceptance of the random pool's "lottery"), so this cohort was selected for a close scrutiny of many factors that might explain the puzzling discrepancy from unit-randomized short-term and follow-up results. The majority of the 1976 mothers who had agreed to be in the experiment's "lottery" were discovered to be high school graduates, in numbers significantly superior to the mothers who had accepted specific treatments in the unit-randomized design and whose education was usually well below high school graduation. The majority of mothers in the 1976 cohort were also "Strivers," as shown by their unusually quick assumption of leadership in home sessions, if they were program mothers. In both program and control groups, their children's near-100 initial and normal postprogram IQs were also superior to those of the unit-randomized children (Levenstein, 1988). (The IQs of economically disadantaged 2 year olds were typically betweeen 80 and 90, predicting educational disadvantage when they reached elementary school.)

It appeared that neither the subject-randomized program nor control children actually needed the intervention to fend off school disadvantage, an impression supported by both the program and control children's normal school progress into second grade. Self-selection for the experiments at the outset should have predicted this; self-selected subjects, and presumably their children, tend to have above-average IQs (Rosenthal & Rosnow, 1975; Thorndike,1977).

2. Most of the parents invited into the subject-randomized experiment research of the MCHP in Bermuda (Scarr & McCartney, 1988) had education above high school and sometimes college, al-

though the education ceiling for the target population was twelfth grade (most mothers in the unit-randomized research and in program replications reached grade levels far below that ceiling). The Bermuda children started the experiment with an average IQ of almost 100, and their results perhaps spurred Scarr and McCartney to comment in a 1987 report: "the program is not effective in a group of children with 2-year-old scores that averaged 100." As noted above, there were no significant statistical differences in the postprogram IQs of the program and control groups of children. Both groups started with approximately normal IQs and ended 2 years later with somewhat higher IQs. Neither group had been, on average, at risk for educational disadvantage and thus did not belong to the MCHP's target population. Clearly, as in the model program's subject-randomized experiment, neither treatment nor control children needed the MCHP to prevent educational disadvantage (Levenstein, 1989). (It should be noted that later personal communications with the senior author revealed the fact that the minority of child subjects whose parents had below–high school education started with much lower IQs than the subjects' general initial IQ of 100. As might be expected, the children of these below–high school educated mothers made gains in the program.)

3. In the 1972 subject-randomized experiment with Chapter 1-eligible (low-income) families in 10 school replications of the MCHP in the New England state, the program Coordinators' misunderstanding of the design's requirements was found to be a prominent feature in the experiment and brought its results into question. As has already been noted, the results indicated no significant difference between the outcome scores of control and program children's outcome scores, which met national norms for both groups. At the beginning of the experiment each replication's Coordinator had formed two supposedly randomized groups of disadvantaged children at age 2 years; one group received the MCHP and the other did not. At the end of the intervention's 2 years, the IQs of both groups were found to meet national norms, with little difference between the groups' scores, indicating that the program had had no effect on the treated group. However, soon after the "no effect" was reported, it was discovered (personal communication from the state's Regional Coordinator) that an understandable human factor had entered the research picture: the Coordinators of the experimental replications had misunderstood the randomization requirements and had assigned the most seriously disadvantaged and nonverbal children and their lowest-educated single-parent mothers to the MCHP groups, leaving the more verbal children (group mean pretest IQ score: 98.1) and their better educated mothers

(actual high school graduation) for membership in the control groups. The control children apparently did not need the MCHP to achieve school readiness. On the other hand, the program group had been assigned to the MCHP because they showed serious at-risk indicators. It was likely that without the program their group mean pretest below-normal IQ score (89.2) would not have changed and would have accurately predicted their school disadvantage. Instead, their participation in the MCHP enabled them to catch up with children who did not need the program.

DISCUSSION

The primary aim of the MCHP was not to produce normal IQs for its graduates. Its goals were to foster real world school achievement for children who were unlikely to achieve it without the program's intervention, and to promote the maternal behavior to support such functioning through enhancing mothers' verbal interaction behavior and probably their sense of competence leading to increased self-esteem. The MCHP success in the real world was demonstrated through its effectiveness in meeting real-world expectations both in the model program (with a unit-randomized research design), and in the program's replications:

1. Almost all mothers recruited either for the model program or its replications accepted participation in the MCHP and usually continued to the end.
2. When test measures were used with children and mothers truly representative of the disadvantaged target population, the test scores predicted normal academic functioning for most graduates of the MCHP.
3. Where measured, the program demonstrated that it fostered verbal and other positive interaction of mothers with their preschoolers, which lasted into school years and was related to the children's later school competencies as a supportive "mother–child network." In addition, the model program and most of the replications have contributed anecdotal evidence of the program's beneficial effects on the mental health and achievement-supportive behavior of participating mothers (Levenstein, 1988).
4. When program graduates' actual school results were measured through all school grades, including high school, most graduates of the MCHP clearly demonstrated their escape from the educational disadvantage predicted by their preprogram test scores at the age of 2

years and graduated from high school at the same rate as their nondisadvantaged school mates.

The apparently unfavorable outcomes in three subject-randomized experiments had probably resulted less from experimental methodology than from a more homely and often unpredictable influence coming to bear on various subcategories of that method. This rogue research element is the tendency of human beings in the real world to roil, unintentionally, the research waters. Reaching beyond the Heisenberg Uncertainty Principle, succinctly summed up by McKerrow and McKerrow (1990), "observers, by their very presence, always change what is observed," this can perhaps be called "the Human Factor." Field research away from the laboratory, and thus in the real world, necessary for most social/educational interventions, is particularly vulnerable to problems arising from the Human Factor, and this was found to be true in the experimental research of the MCHP.

The human factor problems that obscured some of the results from the MCHP can be generalized, for possible consideration by other researchers:

1. In parent-involving subject-randomized experiments to study an intervention with very young children, the knowledge by parents who are of low education and motivation that they and their children will be entering a kind of lottery (the chance of receiving the intervention or not) is likely to cause enough question and hesitation to lead to refusal to participate in the experiment. Rosenthal and Rosnow (1975) have shown that self-selection, which may occur in any research involving the voluntary cooperation of human beings, can produce sample bias. In their review of hundreds of experiments, they demonstrated that volunteer subjects may be different from the group for which the treatment is intended. They are likely to be superior to the general population in their motivation, education, and even intelligence. Such sample bias arising from self-selection can result in the sample's lack of representativeness and is thus a threat to the generalizability of the study's effects. It had apparently affected even the 1972 norming of the Stanford-Binet Test of Children's Intelligence (Thorndike, 1977).

2. Methodologically naive administrators impair the randomization required by the experiment when they assign the neediest subjects to treatment groups so that those most at risk can get the predicted benefit of the treatment. The inevitable consequence is that the best functioning subjects, who may hardly need the intervention, end up in the control group, and only those most in need of the intervention

receive it. This may represent justice in the real world but it is devastating to investigators' research conclusions: at the end of the intervention, the treated subjects may achieve greatly improved scores on outcome measures, but they will probably be no different from those of the more advantaged control group. The result of administrators' misunderstanding of the experimental research design is that the experimental treatment can be thought to have failed because no significant differences between the two group outcome scores can be demonstrated.

3. If an experimental investigation of a social/educational intervention is not conducted with subjects representative of the target population, it is not possible to generalize the research outcomes to that population.

The research problems of the MCHP have been described in this chapter as examples of some hazards that the best planned experimental field research may encounter in actual practice. Investigators who study social programs by using the experimental method—the research design rightly favored as an ideal by most research methodologists—should be aware (and accordingly vigilant) that this method's results may at times be threatened by unanticipated human factors in evaluation of a social intervention in, and for, the real world.

REFERENCES

Ainsworth, M. D. (1973). The development of infant–mother attachment. In B. M. Caldwell & H. N. Ricciuti (Eds.), *Review of child development research: Vol. 3. Child development and social policy* (pp. 1–94). Chicago: University of Chicago Press.

Bayley, N. (1965). Comparisons of mental and motor test scores for ages 1–15 months by sex, birth order, race, geographic location and education of parents. *Child Development, 75,* 48–88.

Bernstein, B. A. (1961). Social class and linguistic development: A theory of social learning. In A. H. Halsey, J. Floud, & C. A. Anderson (Eds.), *Education, economy and society* (pp. 67–92). Glencoe, IL: Free Press.

Bernstein, B. A. (1965). Socio-linguistic approach to social learning. In J. Gould (Ed.), *Penguin survey of the social sciences* (pp. 27–54). Baltimore: Penguin.

Berrueta-Clement, J. R. B., Schweinhart, L. J., Barnett, W. S., Epstein, A. S., & Weikart, D. P. (1984). Changed lives: The effects of the Perry Preschool Program on youth through age 19. *Monographs of the High/Scope Educational Research Foundation, 8.* Ypsilanti, MI: High/Scope Press.

Bronfenbrenner, U. (1974). *Is early education effective: A report on longitudinal evaluations of preschool programs.* (Vol. 2., U.S. DHEW, OHD 74-25). Washington, DC: U.S. Government Printing Office.

Brown, R. (1958). *Words and things.* Glencoe, IL: Free Press.

Bruner, J. S. (1964). The course of cognitive growth. *American Psychologist, 19,* 1–15.

Bruner, J. S., Olver, R., & Greenfield, P. (1966). *Studies in coginitive growth.* New York: Wiley and Sons.

Campbell, D. T., & Stanley, J. C. (1963). *Experimental and quasi-experimental designs for research.* Chicago: Rand McNally.

Cassirer, E. (1944). *An essay on man.* New Haven: Yale University Press.

Cazden, C. B. (1970). The situation: A neglected source of social class differences in language use. *Journal of Social Issues, 26,* 35–60.

Clarke-Stewart, K. A., Vanderstoep, L., & Killim, G. (1979). Analysis and replication of mother–child relations at two years of age. *Child Development, 50,* 777–793.

Deutsch, M. (1965). The role of social class in language development and cognition. *American Journal of Orthopsychiatry, 35,* 78–88.

DeVito, P. J., & Karon, J. P. (1984). *Parent-Child Home Program. Chapter 1, ECIA. Pittsfield Public Schools. Longitudinal evaluation. Final report.* Photocopy. Pittsfield, MA, Public Schools.

DeVito, P. J., & Karon, J. P. (1990). *Parent-Child Home Program longitudinal evaluation.* Pittsfield, MA: Chapter One Program. Pittsfield, MA, Public Schools.

Educational programs that work. (1991). (17th ed.). Longmont, CO: Sopris West.

Gottfried, A. W. (Ed.). (1984). *Home environment and early cognitive development.* Orlando, FL: Academic Press.

Greene, B. S., & Hallinger, C. (1989). *Follow-up study of initial group of children of Mother–Child Home Program.* White Plains, NY: Westchester Jewish Community Services. (Photocopy)

Hebb, D. O. (1949). *The organization of behavior.* New York: Wiley and Sons.

Hess, R. D., & Shipman, V. C. (1965). Early experience and the socialization of cognitive modes in children. *Child Development, 36,* 869–886.

John, V. P., & Goldstein, L. S. (1964). The social context of language acquisition. *Merrill-Palmer Quarterly, 10,* 265–275.

Lazar, I., & Darlington, R. (1982). Lasting effects of early education: A report from the Consortium for Longitudinal Studies. *Monographs of the Society for Research in Child Development, 47* (2–3, Serial No. 195).

Levenstein, P. (1972). But does it work in homes away from home? *Theory into Practice, 11,* 157–162.

Levenstein, P. (1979). The parent-child network. In A. Simmons-Martin & D. R. Calvert (Eds.), *Parent-child intervention* (pp. 245–267). New York: Grune and Stratton.

Levenstein, P. (1988). *Messages from home: The Mother–Child Home Program and educational disadvantage.* Columbus, OH: State University of Ohio Press.

Levenstein, P. (1989). Which homes? A response to Scarr & McCartney. (1988). *Child Development, 60*, 514–516.

Levenstein, P., & O'Hara, J. M. (1983). *Tracing the parent-child network* (Final Report, Grant No. NIE G 8000042). U.S. Department of Education. National Institute of Education, Photocopy Center for MCHP, Wantaugh, NY.

Levenstein, P., & O'Hara, J. M. (in press). The necessary lightness of mother-child play. In K. B. MacDonald (Ed.), *Parents and children playing.* Albany, NY: SUNY Press.

Levenstein, P., O'Hara, J., & Madden, J. (1983). The Mother–Child Home Program of the Verbal Interaction Project. In Consortium for Longitudinal Studies, *As the twig is bent . . . lasting effects of preschool programs* (pp. 237–263). Hillsdale, NJ: Erlbaum.

Levenstein, P., & Staff of Verbal Interaction Project. (1976). Child's behavior traits. In O. G. Johnson (Ed.), *Tests and measurements in child development: Handbook 2* (Vol. 1, pp. 415–416). San Francisco: Jossey-Bass.

Madden, J., Levenstein, P., & Levenstein, S. (1976). Longitudinal IQ outcomes of the Mother–Child Home Program. *Child Development, 47*, 1015–1025.

Madden, J., O'Hara, J. M., & Levenstein, P. (1984). Home again. *Child Development, 55*, 636–647.

McCord, W., & McCord, J. (1959). *Origins of crime.* New York: Columbia University Press. (Reprinted as No. 49 in Reprint Series in Criminology, Law Enforcement, and Social Problems. Montclair, N.J.: Patterson Smith, 1972.)

McKerrow, K. K., & McKerrow, J. E. (1990) . Naturalistic misunderstanding of the Heisenberg Uncertainty Principle. *Educational Researcher, 20*(1), 17–20.

McLaren, L. (1988). Fostering mother–child relationships. *Child Welfare, 67*, 353–365.

Myrdal, G. (1962). *Challenge to affluence.* New York: Pantheon Books.

Phillips, J. R. (1973). *Family cognitive profile study. Final report to the Foundation for Child Development.* Freeport, NY: Verbal Interaction Project. (Mimeo).

Rosenthal, R., & Rosnow, R. L. (1975). *The volunteer subject.* New York: Wiley-Interscience.

Royce, J. M., Darlington, R. B., & Murray, H. W. (1983). Pooled analyses: Findings across studies. In Consortium for Longitudinal Studies, *As the twig is bent . . . lasting effects of preschool programs* (pp. 411–459). Hillsdale, NJ: Erlbaum.

Sapir, E. (1921). Culture, language and personality. Berkeley and Los Angeles: University of California Press.

Scarr, S., & McCartney, K. (1987). *Far from home: An experimental evaluation of the Mother–Child Home Program in Bermuda.* Paper presented at the Biennial Meeting of the Society for Research in Child Development, Baltimore.

Scarr, S., & McCartney, K. (1988). Far from home: An experimental evaluation of the Mother–Child Home Program in Bermuda. *Child Development, 59*, 531–543.

Schacter, F. F. (1979). *Everyday mother talk to toddlers*. New York: Academic Press.

Slaughter, D. T. (1983). Early intervention and its effects on maternal and child development. *Monographs of the Society for Research in Child Development, 48* (No. 4, Serial No. 202).

Springs, C. (1990). *Chapter I, Mother–Child Home Program Children: Evaluation results*. Union, SC: Union County School Board Fact Sheet.

Thorndike, R. L. (1977). Causation of Binet decrements. *Journal of Educational Masurements, 74*(4), 197–202.

Vygotsky, L. S. (1962). *Thought and language*. Cambridge: MIT Press.

White, R. W. (1959). Motivation reconsidered: The concept of competence. *Psychological Review, 66*, 297–333.

White, R. W. (1963). Ego and reality in psychoanalytic theory. *Psychological Issues, 3*, Monograph 11. New York: International Universities Press

CHAPTER 4

◆ ———— ◆

High/Scope Preschool Program Outcomes

DAVID P. WEIKART
LAWRENCE J. SCHWEINHART

The field of early childhood education has received increasing attention because the power of intervention during the preoperational period has been (and continues to be) demonstrated by a series of longitudinal studies. While most of these studies are presented in the final summary volume of the Consortium of Longitudinal Studies (1983), those specific to Head Start are given in a separate synthesis study by McKey et al. (1985). Though these studies report a range of outcomes, the essential finding is that high-quality early childhood education programs for 3- and 4-year-old disadvantaged children can significantly alter their later performance in both school and life through improved educational attainment and performance; increased employment with better wages and longer periods of job holding; and reduced social problems of crime and delinquency, teen pregnancy, and welfare utilization. While results differ markedly from program to program, the findings indicate that the issue is not the capacity of children to benefit from such intervention services, but the ability of adults to deliver the assistance. This chapter will look at the several studies of the High/Scope Foundation conducted over the past 30 years to examine the issues. The details of the projects will be presented and then their implications will be discussed.

THE HIGH/SCOPE PERRY PRESCHOOL STUDY

The High/Scope Perry Preschool study identified young children living in poverty, randomly assigned them to preschool and no-preschool groups, operated a high-quality child development program for the preschool group at ages 3 and 4, and thereafter collected data on both groups of children throughout their childhood, adolescence, and young adulthood. The preschool group surpassed the no-preschool group in intellectual performance from ages 4 to 7. Probably because of this intellectual boost and attendant changes in language, motivation, and sense of self-control, the preschool group achieved greater school success than the no-preschool group: higher school achievement and literacy, better placement in school, stronger commitment to schooling, and more years of school completed. Probably because of this greater school success, the preschool group surpassed the no-preschool group by age 19 in socioeconomic success and social responsibility measured in terms of higher rates of employment and self-support, a lower welfare rate, fewer acts of serious misconduct, and a lower arrest rate. Table 4.1 summarizes Perry Preschool study findings. Berrueta-Clement, Schweinhart, Barnett, Epstein, and Weikart (1984) verified the paths from preschool education through school success to socioeconomic success and social responsibility. Analysis of financial costs and benefits revealed that the program provided a substantial return on public investment.

Design

The longitudinal sample consists of 123 persons identified by surveying all households in the attendance area of the Perry Elementary School in Ypsilanti, Michigan. This sample was accumulated over a 4-year period, beginning with 28 four year olds and 17 three year olds in 1962, followed by 26 three years olds in 1963, 27 in 1964, and 25 in 1965. These children were invited to join the study sample because their families lived in poverty, as assessed by parents' years of schooling and employment status, and because the children scored low on intelligence tests given at age 3 (age 4 for the oldest wave of children). Their mothers had completed a median of 9.7 years of schooling and their fathers 8.8 years. In 58% of the families, at least one parent was employed, usually in unskilled labor. Half the families received welfare assistance; 47% had no father living with them. All members of the study sample were black, as was virtually everyone living in the attendance area of the Perry Elementary School.

The internal validity of the study rests on the rare accomplish-

TABLE 4.1. High/Scope Perry Preschool Study Outcomes through Age 19

Outcome	Age at measurement	Preschool group	No-preschool group
Stanford-Binet mean IQs	4	96	83
	5	95	84
	6	91	86
	7	92	87
School performance			
Achievement (% of items)	14	36%	28%
Literacy (% of items)	19	62%	55%
School placement			
Ever mentally impaired (records)	19	15%	35%
Years in special ed. (records)	19	16%	28%
Commitment to schooling			
High value placed on schooling	15	75%	62%
Enjoys talk about school (parent)	15	65%	33%
Does homework	15	68%	40%
"Smarter than classmates"	15	85%	59%
Schooling completed			
High school graduation	19	67%	49%
Postsecondary education	19	38%	21%
Adolescent socioeconomic success			
Employment	19	50%	32%
Self-support	19	45%	25%
Welfare	19	18%	32%
General Assistance (records)	19	19%	41%
Adolescent social responsibility			
Mean acts of serious misconduct	15	2.3	3.2
Mean number of arrests (records)	19	1.3	2.3
Ever arrested (records)	19	31%	51%
Adolescent problems[a]	19	1.3	1.8
0 problems	19	38%	14%
1 problem	19	21%	28%
2 problems	19	19%	29%
3 problems	19	23%	22%
4 problems	19	0%	7%

Note. Self-report unless otherwise indicated. For all entries, the preschool group performed better than the no-preschool group, with a nondirectional probability less than .05.
[a]Score 1 each for ever classified as handicapped, ever arrested, dropped out of high school, and on welfare.

ment of random assignment to groups: neither parents nor teachers had a choice about whether their children did or did not attend the preschool program. All families that were asked elected to accept the invitation to participate in the assigned study group. Each year from 1962 to 1965 project staff randomly assigned members of the class of children who joined the study sample either to the preschool group who received the Perry Preschool Program or to the no-preschool group who received no preschool program. Pairs of children with similar initial intelligence-test scores were randomly assigned to either of two groups; these assignments were reversed until the two groups had the same girl/boy ratio and the same average socioeconomic status. One group was randomly assigned to attend the preschool program and the other was designated the no-preschool group. As new classes were added to the study sample in 1963, 1964, and 1965, 23 younger siblings were assigned to the same group as their older siblings, to eliminate the possibility of the preschool program indirectly affecting a child in the no-preschool group. The preschool group had 58 members and the no-preschool group had 65.

Confidence that postprogram group comparisons reflect preschool program effects is justified also by the near absence of statistically significant group differences on background characteristics. There were no statistically significant differences (with a probability of less than .05) between the preschool group and the no-preschool group at project entry on mean Stanford-Binet Intelligence Test score, mean socioeconomic status, parental unemployment rates, percentage of fathers absent, mean school years completed by mothers and fathers, girl/boy ratio, mean family size, or mean birth order of the participating child. The only statistically significant difference between groups was in maternal employment rate at program entry (9% in the preschool group, 31% in the no-preschool group); but this difference did not recur when maternal employment was measured again 11 years later. Statistical tests have detected no bias attributable to maternal employment or any other background characteristics.

The Perry Preschool Program staff developed the High/Scope Curriculum—a developmentally appropriate curriculum approach that promotes intellectual, social, and physical development by providing an open framework in which children initiate their own learning activities with teacher support (Weikart, Rogers, Adcock, & McClelland, 1971; Hohmann, Banet, & Weikart, 1979). Children plan, carry out, and review their own activities. Teachers extend support to children during their plan-do-review cycle, and they employ key developmental experiences as a basis for observing and understanding child growth. Each year, four teachers taught a class of 20 to 25 three and four year olds—a ratio of one teacher for every five to six children. Although these group sizes exceeded the 16 to 20 children later found optimal by the National Day Care study (Ruopp, Travers, Glantz, & Coelen, 1979), the staff-child ratios were below that study's recommended 8 to 10 children per adult.

The program only employed teachers certified in both special education and elementary education with an endorsement in early childhood education. In those days of teacher shortage, the first qualified persons who applied were hired. They received supportive supervision, studied early childhood development, participated in special training sessions with invited speakers, and together with the director and research staff developed the High/Scope Curriculum. The school district paid them according to its teacher salary schedule. One teacher remained throughout the 5 years of the project; three remained over 2 years; and six remained over 1 year. Two of the teaching positions were consistently occupied by black females and two by white females. The project director was a white male and the school principal was a black male.

The teachers worked in partnership with parents; a teacher visited each mother and child in their home once a week for about 90 minutes to discuss the child's developmental progress, and to model adult-child activities like those in the school program. The class sessions for children ran 2.5 hours, weekday mornings. The program year ran 30 weeks from mid-October to late May, once at age 4 for the 13 oldest children (1962–63), twice at ages 3 and 4 for the remaining 45 preschool-group children. Since part-time programs of at least 30 weeks have been found effective, it is reasonable to assume that full-time programs lasting at least that long would be at least as effective (Berrueta-Clement et al., 1984; Westinghouse Learning Corporation, 1969).

Sources of data include parent interviews when children were 3 and 15; annual intelligence and language tests from ages 3 to 10 and at age 14; annual achievement tests from ages 7 to 11 and at ages 14 and 19; annual teacher ratings from ages 6 to 9; participant interviews at ages 15 and 19; school record information collected at ages 11, 15, and 19; and police and social services records information collected at age 19. Age-28 interviews and records data have been collected and are now being analyzed. The median percentage of missing cases across all data sources is under 5%, exceeding 25% on only four measures. Only two cases were missing for the crucial age-19 interview.

Findings

We report only those findings whose probability of chance occurrence is less than .05 based on the conservative two-tailed test. This procedure renders fewer significant results, eliminating findings of academic motivation and achievement in the elementary school years, age-15 college aspirations, teen pregnancies, and age-19 job satisfaction. Some readers may wish to consider these findings statistically significant as well.

Improved School Success

On average, the preschool group outperformed the no-preschool group on the Stanford-Benet Intelligence Scale at ages 4, 5, 6, and 7. The average intelligence-test scores of the two groups differed by 12 points at ages 4 and 5, by 6 points at age 6, and by 5 points at age 7. The two groups had the same mean intelligence-test scores prior to the preschool program and again at ages 8, 9, 10, and 14.

The average score of the preschool group on the California Achievement Test was substantially higher than the average score of the no-preschool group at age 14, overall and in reading, arithmetic, and language. Achievement test scores at age 7, 8, 9, and 10 favored the preschool group, but were not quite statistically significant. At age 19, the preschool group outscored the no-preschool group in basic literacy on the Adult Performance Level Survey, overall and on subscales representing occupational and health knowledge and reading.

The preschool group's high school grade point average of 2.1 exceeded the no-preschool group's average of 1.7. At age 15, the preschool group attached greater importance to high school than did the no-preschool group; almost two-thirds of the preschool-group parents, but only one-third of no-preschool group parents, reported that their children enjoyed talking about school; two-thirds of the preschool group reported doing homework, as compared to only two-fifths of the no-preschool group; and 85% of the preschool group, but only 59% of the no-preschool group, considered themselves smarter than their classmates.

Despite the fact that subjects' intelligence test scores at age 3 theoretically placed them on the borderline of mental impairment at that time, a minority were subsequently classified as mentally impaired and the percentage was significantly lower in the preschool group, 15%, as compared to 35% of the no-preschool group. Preschool-group members averaged 2 years in special education for all types of handicaps as compared to 3.6 years for no-preschool-group members. Some children may have received compensatory education services supplementing their regular education classes instead: preschool-group members averaged 1.0 school year receiving compensatory education classes as compared to 0.4 school year averaged by members of the no-preschool group. Compensatory education is a less costly and less stigmatizing form of assistance developed for children who need extra help but not special education. Combining the two types of special services, preschool-group members averaged 3.0 school years in special and compensatory education, while no-preschool group members averaged 4.0 school years ($p > .10$).

Sixty-seven percent of the preschool group, but only 49% of the no-preschool group, graduated from high school. The preschool group's graduation rate equaled that of all black 19 and 20 year olds in the U.S. in 1980 (U.S. Bureau of the Census, 1980). At age 19, 38% of the preschool group, but only 21% of the no-preschool group, were receiving postsecondary education, either academic or vocational.

Greater Success as Adolescents in the Community

Half the preschool group, but only one-third of the no-preschool group, were employed when interviewed at age 19. Between leaving school and being interviewed at 19, the preschool group had averaged 4.9 months without work, while the no-preschool group averaged 10.3 months. Forty-five percent of the preschool group but only 25% of the no-preschool group said they supported themselves by their own and/or their spouses' earnings.

When interviewed at age 19, 18% of the preschool group, but 32% of the no-preschool group, reported they were currently receiving welfare assistance. According to the records of the Michigan Department of Social Services, 19% of the preschool group, as compared to 41% of the no-preschool group, had *ever* received their own General Assistance (a state welfare program for those not qualifying for Aid to Families with Dependent Children [AFDC]); most of these people also received Food Stamps. Groups did not differ in their overall use of Food Stamps, AFDC, or Medicaid.

At age 15, the preschool group reported fewer acts of misconduct than did the no-preschool group, including fewer acts of *serious* misconduct—a mean number of 2.3 offenses per person as compared to 3.2. At age 19, although similar differences in self-reported misconduct were not statistically significant, the preschool group reported fewer involvements in serious fights, gang fights, inflictions of injuries needing medical attention, and run-ins with the police than did the no-preschool group (Schweinhart, 1987).

Police arrest records confirm this pattern. Only 31% of the preschool group, but 51% of the no-preschool group, were *ever* arrested, as juveniles or as adults. The 2.3 arrests per person in the no-preschool group were nearly twice as many as the 1.2 arrests per person in the preschool group. The preschool group had fewer adult arrests, for both major and minor charges. The rate per person of property and violence charges was 0.8 for the preschool group, as compared to 1.2 for the no-preschool group (Schweinhart, 1987, p. 142).

To assess how many participants were helped in various ways by the preschool programs, "adolescent problems" combined four yes/no variables: ever identified as handicapped, ever arrested, dropped out of high school, and on welfare. The preschool group averaged 1.3 problems as compared to 1.8 for the no-preschool group. Thirty-eight percent of the preschool group, but only 14% of the no-preschool group, had no problems. Consequently, the preschool group had higher percentages than the no-preschool group at three of the four remaining levels. In other words, the preschool program appears to have helped an extra 24% of participants avoid all these problems by helping them avoid one, two, or four problems.

Return on Investment

Although programs that contribute to young people's success and social responsibility should be of the highest national priority, it is nevertheless desirable that they demonstrate their worth in economic terms. In fact, taxpayers received substantial returns on their investment in the Perry Preschool Program: $3.00 for every dollar invested in the 60-week program at age 3 and 4 and $5.95 for every dollar invested in the 30-week program at age 4. The dollar figures reported in this section are the per-child costs and benefits exressed in 1988 constant dollars discounted at 3% annually. The ledgers of the Ypsilanti Public Schools provided a thorough accounting of program costs for personnel, overhead, supplies, child selection, and building space. Due largely to the high teacher-child ratios, the costs were high, about $6,500 per child-year, though not dissimilar from other special education programs. Reducing the ratios of teachers to children from 1:6 to 1:10 would have reduced the cost per child-year to $3,900 and probably would not have reduced program quality or effectiveness.

The program recounted herein generated $39,278 per child in financial benefits to taxpayers. Taxpayers saved $7,005 per child because of reduced special education costs, $4,252 because of reduced crime costs to victims and the criminal justice system, and $22,490 because of reduced welfare payments. The program cost taxpayers $964 per child because more of the preschool group than the no-preschool group received postsecondary education, but this higher educational attainment meant that the preschool group would have higher lifetime earnings and therefore pay $6,495 in additional lifetime taxes.

Children who received the 30-week program generated essentially the same benefits as did children who received the 60-week program. Thus, the 30-week program was a better investment. But even if the investment return had been only dollar for dollar, the investment would have been made worthwhile by the obvious nonfinancial benefits of preventing school failure, crime, and need for welfare assistance.

The High/Scope Perry Preschool study focused on the question "Does early childhood education make a difference in the lives of children?," but it did not look at specific contrasting curriculum methodology. In order to study the impact of different major curriculum approaches to early education, a second major study was established.

HIGH/SCOPE PRESCHOOL CURRICULUM STUDY

The High/Scope Preschool Curriculum study (Schweinhart, Weikart, & Larner, 1986; Weikart, Epstein, Schweinhart, & Bond, 1978), operating in the public schools of Ypsilanti, Michigan, served children 3 and 4 years old between 1967 and 1970 who lived in families of low socioeconomic status and who, according to test scores, were at risk of failing in school. Children were assigned to one of the three curriculum models described below by a random-assignment procedure that was also designed to assure the initial comparability of the groups. The curriculum models were all operated under similar administrative conditions to high standards of quality.

A wide range of academic performance, school participation, and social behavior were examined for the curriculum study sample by self-reports at age 15, official records, and individual tests. The central finding of these data is that one curriculum approach group, the direct instruction group, engaged in twice as many delinquent acts as did the other two curriculum groups, including five times as many acts of property violence and twice as many acts of drug abuse and such status offenses as running away from home. Other areas of social behavior corroborate this pattern of relatively poor social performance by the direct instruction group—poor family relations, less participation in sports, fewer school job appointments, lower expectations for educational attainment, and less reaching out to others for help with personal problems. For most of these variables, the sharpest contrast was with the High/Scope group, whose social behavior was relatively positive. The curriculum groups performed similarly to each other in the spheres of employment and money, academic performance, measured self-esteem, and perceived locus of control.

Design

The preschool curriculum models used in the project represented three major theoretically distinct approaches to preschool programs. These approaches differ with respect to the degree of initiative expected of the child and the teacher: whether the child's primary role in the program is to initiate or respond and whether the teacher's primary role is to initiate or respond (Kohlberg & Mayer, 1972; Weikart, 1972).

The programmed-learning approach, in which the teacher initiates activities and the child responds to them, was represented by the direct instruction preschool program developed by Bereiter and Engelmann (1966). In this approach, classroom activities are prescribed by behavioral sequences of stimuli, responses, and positive reinforcements. Objectives are clearly defined academic skills. The underlying psychological theory is behaviorist.

The open-framework approach, in which teacher and child both plan and initiate activities and actively work together, was represented by the High/Scope Curriculum (Hohmann et al., 1979). In this approach, children in the classroom develop activities through a plan-do-review approach. They are supported by teachers who use developmentally appropriate key experiences to understand and interact with the children to promote intellectual and social development. The underlying psychological theory is cognitive-developmental, as developed in the work of Jean Piaget.

The child-centered approach, in which the child initiates and the teacher responds, was represented by a nursery school program that incorporated the elements of what has historically constituted good nursery school practice. In this approach, classroom activities are the teacher's responses to the child's expressed needs and interests, and the teacher encourages children to actively engage in free play. Since the 1930s, the underlying psychological theory has been psychoanalytic.

All three programs in the study were part of the same research project, with the same director (Weikart), funding source, personnel policies, and position in the school system. All three programs in the study had two components: classroom sessions and educational home visits. Classroom sessions lasting 2.5 hours were held 5 days a week, Monday through Friday. A teacher visited each mother and child at home in 90-minute sessions every 2 weeks, at a time when the class was not meeting. During the home visits the teacher encouraged the mother to engage her child in learning activities that fit the curriculum approach used in that type of classroom.

Classes, operating between 1967 and 1970, had 15 or 16 three and four year olds and two teachers, making the typical ratio of teachers to children about 1 to 8. In addition, each class had a teacher assistant/ bus driver and a high school special-education student who helped take care of the children, especially on bus rides to and from school and on field trips. The teachers were all highly motivated to demonstrate that their curriculum model could be successful. (See Weikart [1972] for an account of the experiences of individual teachers in the study.)

Each of the three teaching teams engaged in daily evaluation and planning sessions, reviewing activities and the progress of individual children, but the teams did not engage in joint planning or meetings. A staff supervisor provided guidance to all three teams and used the daily evaluation and planning sessions to help them maintain curriculum-model goals and meet the needs of individual children. While the director or supervisor had the opportunity to exhibit subtle biases for or against a particular curriculum model, elaborate managerial procedures militated against such bias. Each program was frequently reviewed for faithfulness of curriculum implementation by nonteaching staff and outside consultants who observed the classroom and met with the teachers and supervisor.

The teaching team implementing the direct instruction model received training from University of Illinois consultants trained and employed by the Bereiter-Engelmann curriculum development team. The team implementing the High/Scope model engaged in the development of that model and continued to work with High/Scope curriculum consultants on further refinement. The team implementing the nursery school model developed it themselves, drawing upon their early childhood education training, experience with children, and teacher intuition, a resource highly valued in this approach.

Sixty-eight children met the study's criteria for inclusion based on their residency, age, low socioeconomic status, and high risk of school failure according to test scores. They were born in Ypsilanti between 1964 and 1966, attended preschool program at ages 3 and 4 between 1967 and 1969, and responded to interviews at age 10 between 1974 and 1976 and again at age 15 between 1979 and 1981. Most of the participants were interviewed again at age 22. However, the findings from this phase of the study are not yet available.

Each September from 1967 to 1969, the 3 year olds in these families took the Stanford-Binet Intelligence Scale (Terman & Merrill, 1970). Children with IQs between 60 and 90, with no evidence of physical disability, became eligible for enrollment in the preschool programs of the study. The mean IQ of the sample at program entry was 78.3.

Each year, the children in a new wave were randomly assigned to three groups, with reassignments until the three groups were comparable in race, gender, and mean IQ at program entry. The three groups were then randomly assigned to the three preschool curriculum models. In a departure from random assignment affecting 9 of the 68 children, siblings were assigned to the same curriculum models to prevent confusion of the effects of two curriculum models within families. The procedure for assignment to curriculum models ensured that each member of the sample had an equal chance of being assigned to any of the curriculum models, while keeping the groups as similar as possible on key background characteristics.

Each school year, the preschool programs brought together a wave of 4 year olds and a wave of 3 year olds. Because of this feature, two additional waves of children participated in the preschool programs with the study participants—one wave of children prior to the study sample, one after—but were not part of the study.

At program entry, of the 68 children in the program sample, 65% were black and 54% were female. Their families lived in poverty; one out of three received welfare assistance; 75% of families had fathers in residence; almost all of these fathers and 38% of the mothers were employed as unskilled labor; fathers averaged 9 years of schooling, mothers 10; the average household had 6.7 persons, or one person per room.

Curriculum groups were similar on the key characteristics of gender, family socioeconomic status, and child IQ at program entry. The only statistically significant group difference in background characteristics was that the nursery school group mothers had 10.9 years of schooling, the direct instruction group mothers had 9.6 years, and the High/Scope group had 9.1 years; this difference could bias outcome comparisons against the High/Scope group. However, analyses of variance in outcomes controlling for sex, race, mother's education and employment, and single-parent family status showed that none of these background variables had an effect on the results reported here.

Findings

The goal of the High/Scope Curriculum study was to compare the effects of theoretically distinct preschool curriculum models, so throughout this report the key analyses test for differences in outcome measures among the three preschool curriculum groups. Percentages or frequencies of categorical variables are presented for each group, with differences evaluated by chi-square analysis. Means of continuous variables are presented, with group differences tested by analysis of variance.

Effects on Intellectual and School Performance

When the mean IQs of the three preschool curriculum groups are compared, the differences between them are quite small. During the first year of the preschool program, mean IQs rose between 23 and 29 points, moving the groups of children out of the at-risk category. During the second preschool year, mean IQs of the High/Scope and nursery school groups dropped 9 to 10 points, whereas that of the direct instruction group dropped only 3 points and thereby achieved the only statistically significant intellectual assessment advantage among groups at any testing. Curriculum groups did not differ in mean IQs after kindergarten and stabilized in the range of 90 to 100.

The achievement scores gathered on all the children were the California Achievement Tests (Tiegs & Clark, 1963) at the end of first, second, and fourth grades. While each of the groups gained between 50 and 60 points between testings (using the same test form), the groups were not significantly different from one another at either time. This is to be expected, since the early IQ differences that separated the groups diminished by kindergarten and disappeared by the second grade. The modest early advantage that the direct instruction group had over the other two groups was not translated into superior achievement in elementary school.

Rounding out our understanding of the achievement abilities of the youths in the study is the Adult Performance Level Survey given at age 15, which measures a person's competence in solving real-world problems and coping with the cognitive demands of adult life. The APL total and subscale scores of the three preschool groups show that the direct instruction group scored the lowest on 9 of the 11 APL scales, to a statistically significant extent for occupational knowledge and approaching a statistically significant extent for writing. Table 4.2 summarizes all High/Scope Curriculum study findings at age 15.

Effects on Social Behavior

The average member of the direct instruction group engaged in 13 self-reported delinquent acts; the average Nursery School group member engaged in seven; and the average High/Scope group member engaged in five. On 17 items of the 18-item scale, the direct instruc-

TABLE 4.2. Curriculum Study Outcomes at Age 15

Outcome	Direct instruction	High/Scope	Nursery school
Delinquent acts	12.8	5.4	6.9
Property damage offenses	1.7	0.3	0.4
In-family offenses	3.0	1.6	1.2
Occupational knowledge	2.4	3.7	3.7
Family feels you're doing poorly	33%	0%	6%
Never participate in sports	56%	6%	28%
Appointed to school office	0%	12%	33%

Note. Adapted from "Consequences of Three Preschool Curriculum Models through age 15," by L. J. Schweinhart, D. P. Weikart, and M. B. Larner, 1986. *Early Childhood Research Quarterly, 1*, pp. 33, 35, 37–38. All the group differences presented here are statistically significant with a probability of less than .05. Copyright 1986 High School Educational Needs Foundation.

tion group reported the highest frequency, or one of the highest frequencies, of the three groups.

The 18-item delinquency scale is divided into five subscales: personal violence, property violence, stealing, drug abuse, and status offenses. The direct instruction group engaged in twice as many acts of personal violence as the other two groups, but this difference was not statistically significant because of the large variation among individuals within groups, particularly the direct instruction group. The direct instruction group had the highest frequencies of the three groups on each of the five items in that subscale.

The direct instruction group engaged in five times as many acts of property violence as did the other two groups, reporting 1.7 acts per person as compared to only 0.3 acts per person in the other two groups. The direct instruction group had the highest frequencies of the three groups on each of the three items in that subscale; the difference in the arson category approached statistical significance. Groups did not differ statistically in frequencies reported for the stealing subscale.

The direct instruction group reported engaging in twice as many acts of drug abuse as did the other two groups, in use of both marijuana and other illegal drugs. The direct instruction group reported engaging in twice as many "status offences": fights with parents, trespassing, and running away from home.

Although curriculum groups at age 15 did not themselves report different arrest rates, 0.5 times per person overall, group differences in arrest rate may appear in future years. Gold (1970) also reported that group differences in self-reported delinquency did not yet show up in arrest-rate differences for 15 year olds.

Effects on Other Social Variables

The one statistically significant group difference in the family domain was that 1 out of 3 members of the direct instruction group said their families felt they were doing poorly, a response made by only 1 out of 36 members of the other two curriculum groups. Similarly, though not to a statistically significant extent, 1 out of 5 members of the direct instruction group reported getting along poorly with their families, a response made by no one in the High/Scope group. One out of three members of the High/Scope group reported contributing to household expenses, while fewer than 1 out of 6 members of the direct instruction group did so. Given the substantially higher rates of delinquent behavior reported by the direct instruction group, their greater frequency of poor family relations should come as no surprise.

Nearly all of the High/Scope group participated in sports, whereas fewer than half of the direct instruction group did so. Compared to members of the direct instruction group, twice as many members of the High/Scope group had recently read a book.

No one in the direct instruction group had ever been appointed to an office or special job at school. The strongest contrast here was with the nursery school group, which reported 1 out of 3 members with some school appointment. Only half of the direct instruction group expected to pursue postsecondary education, while two-thirds of the nursery school group and three-quarters of the High/Scope group expected to do so.

Clearly, final decisions about curriculum model effects cannot be determined by one carefully done study of an unusual longitudinal nature. The loud protests of those who have developed the direct instruction approach used in the High/Scope Curriculum study indicate the extent to which opinion differs on various theories of child development and this study. (See Gersten and White, 1986, for an aggressive example.) However, several other long-term studies have suggested similar outcomes (Karnes, Schwedel, & Williams, 1983; Miller & Bizzel, 1983).

SUMMARY OF FINDINGS

In the Perry Preschool study, the preschool group surpassed the no-preschool group in intellectual performance from ages 4 to 7. Probably because of this intellectual boost, the preschool group achieved greater school success than the no-preschool group: higher school achievement and literacy, better placement in school, stronger commitment to schooling, and more years of school completed. Probably because of this greater school success, the preschool group surpassed the no-preschool group in teenage socioeconomic success and social responsibility: higher rates of employment and self-support, a lower welfare rate, fewer acts of serious misconduct, and a lower arrest rate. Analysis of financial costs and benefits revealed that the program provided a substantial return on public investment.

In the Preschool Curriculum Comparison study, the mean IQ of the children who had attended these three high-quality preschool programs rose a dramatic 27 points during the first year of the program, from 78 to 105, and at age 10 was 94. The three preschool curriculum groups differed little in their patterns of IQ and school achievement over time. According to self-reports at age 15, the group that had attended the direct instruction preschool program engaged in twice as many delinquent acts as did the other two curriculum groups, including five times as many acts of property violence. The direct instruction group also reported relatively poor relations with their families, less participation in sports, fewer school job appointments, and less reaching out to others for help with personal problems. Although these findings, based on one study with a small sample, are by no means definitive, they do suggest possible consequences of preschool curriculum models that ought to be considered.

CONCLUSIONS

Most importantly, these long-term studies demonstrate that disadvantaged children, on average, can be helped to achieve greater success in school and community. While making it clear that high-quality early childhood education is far from a cure for poverty, they also repudiate the pessimists who view the War on Poverty as a colossal policy blunder with no redeeming successes (e.g., Murray, 1984). Given the power of such approaches, they should be added to the means at hand to aid in the development of a more productive and just society.

Specifically, these studies point to several policy issues that need to be considered as the nation resolves to create solutions to the social problems that challenge our ability to provide a decent social and personal environment for all our citizens.

First, the outcomes of high-quality early childhood education need to be employed in the broader social context of our nation. For example, there is application of these findings to "least cost alternatives" in expenditures of public money (Cavanagh, 1986). In thinking about energy policies, a number of economists have developed what is called a "least cost alternative" approach to investment. For example, it will cost x billion to build a new electric generating plant with current gas, coal, or nuclear technology. However, by using "green" (conservation-sensitive) lightbulbs, high-efficiency appliances, insulation upgrades, and so forth, the cost for "generating" such power is actually $(x - y)$ billion dollars. Therefore, the least cost alternative is not the purchase of new construction but the purchase of conservation and energy-efficient devices. The argument is not made based on the ethics of conservation or the image of nuclear power, and so forth, but on the relative costs of investment. This same kind of thinking can be applied to the Perry study outcomes.

While not all participating children gained equally from the experience of high-quality education, significant numbers did reap personal and social benefits. Given the power of such an approach to work, should education be added to the means at hand to aid in the development of a more productive and just society? For example, we know that about 50% of black males experience being arrested by the age of 20. Currently, of every 100,000 black males in our population, 3,109 are now incarcerated. (The general U.S. rate is 426 per 100,000; the USSR rate is 268; the South African rate is 333; data are from the Justice Department's Sentencing Project.) The cost of a year in prison varies by state but a typical expenditure is $25,000 per year. Extending high-quality early education programs to all disadvantaged black males should reduce these rates significantly, using the Perry outcome data, leading to a reduction in police and prison expenditures. While nothing is so straightforward in any social policy area, it certainly calls for a serious planning and implementation effort by states wishing to improve the quality of life for its citizens, and permitting state expenditures toward more constructive efforts.

A second important outcome of these findings is that only high-quality programs work. There is no evidence that average or mediocre programs assist in reaching the desired goals. Further, such programs must be so constructed that children develop a sense of control over themselves and their environment. This objective can be reached only when a program permits children to state intentions, to self-generate action, and to engage in verbal reflection. Such child-initiated learning occurring in developmentally appropriate settings leads to the types of high-quality programs that permit the outcomes found in the High/Scope projects. The public should demand that early childhood programs have the characteristics needed for lasting effectiveness. Anything less is a waste of valuable human resources.

Parents and the public should be willing to pay much more to ensure that all early childhood programs meet the high standards of quality that lead to effectiveness. Early childhood teachers in the U.S. now earn on average only $9,363 annually (Whitebook, Howes, & Phillips, 1989) and 41% of daycare staff leave their jobs each year. This situation is simply not acceptable in a nation that values its young children and cares about its future.

Third, these studies point out the limited utility of intelligence tests as predictors of success. Although the Perry Preschool group's mean IQ returned to the low level at which it started a few years after the program, significant percentages of this group surpassed the no-preschool group in their eventual school and socioeconomic success and social responsibility. Similarly, although the mean IQs of the three curriculum groups differed little, favoring the direct instruction group at only one measurement, these groups differed substantially on self-reported delinquency at age 15, with the direct instruction group reporting the largest number of delinquent offenses. Intelligence tests did not relate to outcomes found in these projects.

Early childhood education for disadvantaged children has developed extensively over the last 30 years. Now that we have models that work, the obligation is to apply the knowledge and experience to benefit children as well as their families and society at large. When the early research on such programs first began, it was thought that the children could not benefit because they did not have the "ability" or the "culture" to learn. Now, with the probject data at hand, the issue is to arrange for the adults to deliver. The children can benefit; the problem is with the adult society. We need to act, and now.

REFERENCES

Bereiter, C., & Engelmann, S. (1966). *Teaching the disadvantaged child in the preschool.* Englewood Cliffs, NJ: Prentice Hall.

Berrueta-Clement, J. R., Schweinhart, L. J., Barnett, W. S., Epstein, A. S., & Weikart, D. P. (1984). Changed lives: The effects of the Perry Preschool program on youths through age 19. *Monographs of the High/Scope Educational Research Foundation, 8.* Ypsilanti, MI: High/Scope Press.

Cavanagh, R. C. (1986). Least-cost planning imperatives for electric utilities and their regulators. *Harvard Environmental Law Review, 299,* 315.

Consortium for Longitudinal Studies. (1983). *As the twig is bent . . . lasting effects of preschool programs.* Hillsdale, NJ: Erlbaum.

Gersten, R., & White, W. (1986). Castles in the sand: Response to Schweinhart and Weikart. *Educational Leadership, 43,* 19–21.

Gold, M. (1970). *Delinquent behavior in an American city.* Belmont, CA: Brooks/Cole.

Hohmann, M., Banet, B., & Weikart, D. P. (1979). *Young children in action: A manual for preschool educators.* Ypsilanti, MI: High/Scope Press.

Karnes, M. B., Schwedel, A. M., & Williams, M. B. (1983). A comparison of five approaches for educating young children from low-income homes. In Consortium for Longitudinal Studies, *As the twig is bent . . . lasting effects of preschool programs* (pp. 133–170). Hillsdale, NJ: Erlbaum.

Kohlberg, L., & Mayer, R. (1972). Development as the aim of education. *Harvard Educational Review, 42,* 449–496.

McKey, R. H., Condelli, L., Ganson, H., Barrett, B., McConkey, C., & Plantz, M. (1985). *The impact of Head Start on children, families and communities.* Final Report of the Head Start Evaluation, Synthesis and Utilization Project. Washington, DC: CSR, Inc.

Miller, L. B., & Bizzell, R. P. (1983). The Louisville Experiment: A comparison of four programs. In Consortium for Longitudinal Studies, *As the twig is bent . . . lasting effects of preschool programs* (pp. 171–200). Hillsdale, NJ: Erlbaum.

Murray, C. (1984). *Losing ground: American social policy 1950–80.* New York: Basic Books.

Ruopp, R., Travers, J., Glantz, F., & Coelen, C. (1979). *Children at the center: Summary findings and their implications.* Final Report of the National Day Care Study, Vol. 1. Cambridge, MA: Abt Associates.

Schweinhart, L. J. (1987). Can preschool programs help prevent delinquency? In J. Q. Wilson & G. C. Loury (Eds.), *From children to citizens: Families, schools, and delinquency prevention* (pp. 13–153). New York: Springer-Verlag.

Schweinhart, L. J., & Weikart, D. P. (1980). Young children grow up: The effects of the Perry Preschool program on youths through age 15. *Monographs of the High/Scope Educational Research Foundation, 7.* Ypsilanti, MI: High/Scope Press.

Schweinhart, L. J., Weikart, D. P., & Larner, M. B. (1986). Consequences of three preschool curriculum models through age 15. *Early Childhood Research Quarterly, 1,* 15–45.

Terman, L. M., & Merrill, M. A. (1970). *Stanford-Binet Intelligence Scale, Form L-M: Manual for the third revision.* Boston: Houghton Mifflin.

Tiegs, E. W., & Clark, W. W. (1963). *California Achievement Tests: 1957 edition with 1963 norms.* Monterey, CA: California Test Bureau.

U.S. Bureau of the Census. (1980). [October Current Population Survey]. Unpublished data.

Weikart, D. P. (1972). Relationship of curriculum, teaching, and learning in preschool education. In J. C. Stanley (Ed.), *Preschool programs for the disadvantaged* (pp. 22–66). Baltimore: Johns Hopkins University Press.

Weikart, D. P., Epstein, A. S., Schweinhart, L. J., & Bond, J. T. (1978). The Ypsilanti Preschool Curriculum Demonstration Project: Preschool years and longitudinal results. *Monographs of the High/Scope Educational Research Foundation, 4.* Ypsilanti, MI: High/Scope Press.

Weikart, D. P., Rogers, L., Adcock, C., & McClelland, D. (1971). *The Cognitively Oriented Curriculum: A framework for preschool teachers*. Urbana: University of Illinois Press.

Westinghouse Learning Corporation. (1969). *The impact of Head Start: An evaluation of the effects of Head Start on children's cognitive and affective development* (2 vols.). Athens, OH: Ohio University Press.

Whitebook, M., Howes, C., & Phillips, D. (1989). *Who cares? Child care teachers and the quality of care in America* (Executive Summary, National Child Care Staffing Study). Oakland, CA: Child Care Employee Project.

PART III

◆ —— ◆

PREVENTION EXPERIMENTS DURING THE MIDDLE YEARS

◆ ——— ◆

CHAPTER 5

Social Interactions of Children with Attention Deficit Hyperactivity Disorder: Effects of Methylphenidate

GEORGE J. DUPAUL
RUSSELL A. BARKLEY

Children displaying significant problems with inattention, impulsivity, and hyperactivity are often referred to mental health professionals and may be diagnosed as having an Attention Deficit-Hyperactivity Disorder (ADHD) (American Psychiatric Association, 1987).[1] ADHD is found among 3% to 10% of the school-aged population in the United States (Barkley, 1990). Thus there are approximately 1 to 3 children with ADHD in every classroom. In addition to describing the core characteristics of ADHD, numerous studies have reported associated behavioral characteristics including poor tolerance of frustration (Rapport, Tucker, DuPaul, Merlo, & Stoner, 1986), problematic family interactions (Tallmadge & Barkley, 1983), noncompliance with commands of authority figures (Barkley, 1985a; Whalen, Henker, & Dotemoto, 1980), and difficult peer relationships (Pelham & Bender, 1982). Children with ADHD do not necessarily outgrow this disorder (Weiss & Hechtman, 1986) and are at high risk for developing antisocial behavior in adolescence (Barkley, Fischer, Edelbrock, & Smallish, 1990; Gittelman, Mannuzza, Shenker, & Bonagura, 1985), psycho-

1. The diagnostic terms ADHD, ADDH (Attention Deficit Disorder with Hyperactivity), and hyperactivity are used synonymously.

pathology as adults (Weiss & Hechtman, 1986), poor peer relationships and low self-esteem as adolescents and adults (Minde, Weiss, & Mendelson, 1972), and underachievement in school and work (Lambert & Sandoval, 1980). These results provide a strong rationale for implementing multimodal intervention strategies for this disorder across settings.

The prescription of psychostimulant medication is the most common treatment for children with ADHD. More children receive medication (primarily Ritalin or its generic form, methylphenidate) to manage ADHD than medication for any other childhood disorder, with 1% to 2% of the school-aged population in the United States receiving these drugs (Safer & Krager, 1988). Approximately 75% of children with ADHD treated with methylphenidate exhibit a positive behavioral response with primary effects including enhanced attention span, improved impulse control, diminished fidgetiness, increased academic productivity, and a higher probability of compliance with commands by authority figures (Barkley, 1977; DuPaul & Barkley, 1990; Rapport, 1987). Despite the possibility of relatively mild side effects (e.g., insomnia, appetite reduction), methylphenidate and similar central nervous system stimulants remain the treatment of choice for ADHD, particularly when prescribed in the context of a multimodal intervention program incorporating behavior modification procedures (Barkley, 1990; Pelham & Murphy, 1986; Whalen & Henker, 1991).

Given that children with ADHD often exhibit difficulties functioning across home, school, and social settings, the overriding goal in designing an effective intervention program is to engineer a "best fit" between the child and his or her social environment (Barkley, 1990). This view holds that the response of the social environment to a child's ADHD symptoms is a critical determinant of the degree to which he or she will be handicapped by these symptoms and of the relative risk for future antisocial conduct and general maladjustment (Weiss & Hechtman, 1986; Whalen & Henker, 1980). In particular, the social reactions of others toward the child with ADHD and their efforts at managing the child's behavior are known to be critical to the early formation of aggressive response classes. The latter greatly increase the child's risk for antisocial conduct and its attendant academic failure and social rejection (Dumas & Wahler, 1985; Loeber, 1990; Patterson, 1982, 1986). Interventions that address these social exchanges may serve to lower this risk and increase the probability of a positive response to other treatments that do so.

The purpose of the present chapter is to review the effects of methylphenidate (MPH) on the interactions between children with

ADHD and their parents, teachers, and peers. First, research documenting the nature of interactions between children with ADHD and others in their environment will be examined in the context of three theories of family interaction. Next, studies explicating the dose-response effects of MPH on the mother–child, teacher–student, and peer interactions of children with ADHD will be reviewed. This review is intended to demonstrate that MPH helps to promote a "better fit" between child and environment by enhancing the child's behavioral control, resulting in concomitant improvements in the social responses of parents, teachers, and peers when they interact with the ADHD child. Further, we will show that treatment-related changes in the transactional exchanges between the child and his or her environment are a function of a variety of factors, including medication dosage, age of the child, and the setting where the interaction occurs.

THEORIES OF PROBLEMATIC FAMILY INTERACTION

Several theories have been proposed to account for the disturbed relationships between aggressive, noncompliant children and their parents and siblings. Gerald Patterson (1982) views families with such children as participating in a coercive process wherein aggression between family members is negatively reinforced. Specifically, the coercive behavior (e.g., defiance, negative reprimands) of one family member is reinforced when it results in the removal of an aversive event (e.g., task command) being exhibited by another family member. As these interchanges are repeated over the course of time, the rate and intensity of coercive behaviors displayed by family members are significantly increased. Deviant child behavior is also encouraged to flourish since the parent often models an aggressive, coercive response style both with the child and with other family members. Patterson and his colleagues have repeatedly documented the empirical validity of this theory in large samples of aggressive children (Patterson, 1982, 1986). Further, there is an apparent developmental progression in deviant child behavior from "basic training" in coercive parent–child interaction to more generalized maladjustment in self-concept, peer relationships, and academic achievement (Patterson, 1986).

A competing view to Patterson's that also relies on negative reinforcement mechanisms has been proposed by Wahler (1980) and Dumas and Wahler (1985). These theorists assert that child coercive behaviors function to reduce parent inconsistency and unpredictability in exchanges with the child. They argue that children find this inconsistency aversive and act to reduce its frequency by using counteraggressive behavior that is likely to elicit predictable, albeit negative, parental reactions.

A model complementary to both of these views of parent–child interactions has been proposed by Bell and Harper (1977). Parent and child behaviors are posited to be contingently related to and elicited by each other in the ongoing stream of parent–child social exchanges. Hence, causal influences on the behavior of both parent and child are bidirectional and reciprocal. The behavior of each participant in the interaction is seen to be contingent upon and elicited by the antecedent behavior of the other participant as well as an antecedent event for subsequent responses by the other member of the dyad. While the behavior of each participant is assumed to play an equivalent causal role in determining the nature of the interaction, various factors (e.g., context of the interaction, task demands, characteristics of the parent or child) may result in child behaviors (or parental actions) serving a greater controlling function. For example, the presence of ADHD symptoms in the child may alter the balance of the parent–child interaction in certain situations, as discussed below (Mash & Johnston, 1990).

Bell's theory, unlike Patterson's, makes no effort to delineate what specific functions may be served by each person's conduct in the social exchange, other than in very broad terms. For instance, Bell and Harper (1977) note that excessive child behavior may elicit control responses from parents that seem to be emitted to reduce the child's behavior to more tolerable levels. Alternatively, low rates of child behavior (e.g., withdrawn or shy conduct) may elicit "lower limit" controls by parents that seem designed to increase child participation in the social exchange. Why these child behaviors are emitted, how and why they change in response to parental reactions, and why parents use the tactics they do with a child are left unspecified. In contrast, Patterson (1982) relies on a functional analysis and reinforcement theory when addressing these issues, whereas Dumas and Wahler (1985) focus more on the reduction of inconsistencies in the dyadic exchanges.

In the next section, we will briefly discuss the interactions of children with ADHD with their parents, teachers, and peers in the absence of treatment to demonstrate the value of the theoretical models outlined above in explaining some of the social difficulties of these children. While these models were not originally proposed to account for the development of social interaction difficulties in children with ADHD, they do demonstrate a number of factors that must be considered when examining the family, school, and peer relation-ships of this population (Barkley 1985a, 1985b). First, the reciprocal influences of the child and others in his or her environment must be assessed to provide a comprehensive picture of the child's behavioral difficulties. Specific parent, teacher, and peer responses to the child's deviant social behavior may actually promote an increase in negative interactions over time. Second, the nature of interactions between the child with ADHD and others in his or her environment may vary as a function of the age of the child and the setting where the interaction occurs. For example, negative social interchanges may increase in frequency with age as a function of repeated trials of negative rein-forcement for aggressive, noncompliant behavior. Third, to compre-hensively document the impact of any treatment approach, not only should its direct effects on the child's behavior be assessed, but changes in the responses of significant people in the child's environment must also be evaluated. Such changes, or their absence, could encourage or retard the initial treatment effects induced by medication or other therapies.

SOCIAL INTERACTIONS OF CHILDREN WITH ADHD

Parent-Child Interactions

Initial studies using direct observations of the behavior of mothers with their ADHD children found that boys with this disorder initiated more interactions with their mothers during task completion than did their normal counterparts (Campbell, 1973, 1975). In addition, chil-dren spoke more frequently and requested more assistance with the task from their mothers. In turn, mothers of children with ADHD showed higher levels of involvement with their children while giving more suggestions, approval, and disapproval, as well as more direc-tions regarding impulse control. Further studies have extended these results by demonstrating that children with ADHD were less com-pliant, more negative and off-task, and less able to sustain compliance to maternal directives than were normal children (Cunningham & Barkley, 1979). Mothers of these children were more commanding and negative, and less responsive to positive or neutral communications from their children. Similar interaction patterns emerge between chil-dren with ADHD and their fathers, although the former are less negative and off-task with their fathers than with their mothers (Tallmadge & Barkley, 1983). Sex of the child appears to matter little in these exchanges, as girls with ADHD receive as much controlling reactions from parents as boys with this disorder (Barkley, 1989;

Befera & Barkley, 1985). Boys, however, were likely to receive more praise from mothers than girls. Similarly, same-sex siblings who are not ADHD seem to receive nearly as much control from parents as their siblings with ADHD (Mash & Johnston, 1983a; Tarver-Behring, Barkley, & Karlsson, 1985).

Several factors appear to moderate the severity of parent–child conflicts associated with ADHD. The intensity of these interaction conflicts vary as a function of age, with younger children exhibiting greater mother–child conflicts than older children in both ADHD and normal families (Barkley, Karlsson, & Pollard, 1985; Barkley, Karlsson, Strzelecki, & Murphy, 1984). For children in both groups, as the children's ability to comply increased with age, the degree to which mothers issued commands declined (Mash & Johnston, 1982). At all age levels studied, however, more maternal commands and child negative or noncompliant behaviors are found in ADHD families than in normal families (Barkley, Fischer, Edelbrock, & Smallish, 1991; Barkley et al., 1985; Campbell, Breaux, Ewing, Szumowski, & Pierce, 1986; Cohen, Sullivan, Minde, Novak, & Keene, 1983). Despite improvements in ADHD behavior and parent–child conflicts with age, children with ADHD continue to evidence more problematic parent–child interactions than their normal peers well into adolescence (Barkley, Anastopoulos, Guevremont, & Fletcher, in press). Another factor that is important in determining the severity of parent–child conflicts in ADHD families is the setting in which the interaction takes place. Specifically, greater frequencies of conflict occur in task situations than in free play, with negative interactions increasing in intensity as the task demands become more difficult (Campbell, 1973, 1975; Cunningham & Barkley, 1979). Finally, recent studies suggest that the association of Oppositional Defiant Disorder (ODD; American Psychiatric Association, 1987) with ADHD may account for the greater degree of parent–child conflict than the presence of ADHD symptoms alone (Barkley et al., in press; Barkley et al., 1991; Tallmadge, Paternite, & Gordon, 1989).

Teacher–Child Interactions

Relative to the literature documenting parent–child interactions of children with ADHD, surprisingly few studies have investigated the nature of relationships between such children and their teachers. The research that is available would suggest that similar conflicts and negative behaviors are exhibited by children with ADHD and authority figures across home and school settings. Children with ADHD emit a higher frequency of off-task behavior, task-irrelevant activity, talking, and social disruption than do their normal classmates (Whalen, Henker, Collins, Finck, & Dotemoto, 1979). In response, teachers of such children exhibit higher levels of commands and high-intensity contacts toward them relative to their peers (Whalen, Henker, & Dotemoto, 1980, 1981). This result is not unexpected given that teachers observe children primarily in structured task rather than free-play situations, and structured tasks are more likely to elicit conflicts between children with ADHD and authority figures, as summarized above.

Interactions with Peers

Children with ADHD display negative, disruptive behaviors not only with authority figures, but also with their same-aged peers. A number of studies have documented that these children exhibit greater levels of off-task behavior, aggressiveness, and activity level during both structured task and free-play situations than their normal counterparts (Cunningham & Siegel, 1987; Milich & Landau, 1982). In situations that require communication with peers, children with ADHD have evidenced difficulties shifting roles from sender to receiver, and have exhibited a higher rate of ignoring peer questions and greater frequencies of talkativeness relative to normal children (Whalen, Henker, Collins, McAuliffe, & Vaux, 1979). As a result, peers tend to emit more commands and negative responses toward children with ADHD (Cunningham & Siegel, 1987; Madan-Swain & Zentall, 1990; Whalen, Henker, Collins, McAuliffe, & Vaux, 1979). Their disruptiveness may also increase levels of negative, off-task behavior exhibited by their normal peers in classroom settings (Campbell, Endman, & Bernfeld, 1977). Given the potential for social conflict, it is no surprise that children with ADHD are at an increased risk for rejection by peers (Milich & Landau, 1982; Pelham & Bender, 1982).

Summary

The inattentive, impulsive, and overactive behavior patterns of children with ADHD often conflict with the expectations and demands of their parents, teachers, and peers, especially in situations where the task demands exceed behavioral capacities in their deficit areas (Barkley, 1990). These deficits predispose children with ADHD to exhibit greater noncompliance with instructions, to have increased problems inhibiting impulses, and to behave in an intrusive, disruptive manner even in free-play settings. There is no doubt that such behavior is viewed as aversive by others in the child's environment (Fischer, 1990;

Mash & Johnston, 1983b). Greater frequencies of controlling, direct-ing, and potentially angry responses may be exhibited by parents, teachers, siblings, and peers in an attempt to lessen the level of noise, disruption, and noncompliance of children with ADHD (Barkley, 1985a, 1985b). Thus, a reciprocal, coercive interactional process may develop between children with ADHD, especially those with comor-bid ODD, and others who come into contact with such children in a fashion similar to those found in families of aggressive children (Bell & Harper, 1977; Patterson, 1982). Such findings implicate the need to study the effects of interventions designed to address ADHD not only on the behavior of the treated child, but on the concomitant responses of members of the child's interpersonal network as well (Whalen, Henker, & Dotemoto, 1981). If ADHD is to be viewed within the context of a child-by-situation matrix (Barkley, 1990; Henker & Whalen, 1989), then a comprehensive understanding of treatment status would require documenting effects on all components of the matrix.

METHYLPHENIDATE EFFECTS ON SOCIAL INTERACTIONS OF CHILDREN WITH ADHD

Parent-Child Interactions

Numerous studies have been conducted over the past 15 years demon-strating the salutary properties of MPH on the mother–child interac-tions of children with ADHD (Barkley & Cunningham, 1979; Barkley, Karlsson, Strzelecki, & Murphy, 1984; Cunningham & Barkley, 1978; Humphries, Kinsbourne, & Swanson, 1978). Such studies provide a means of teasing apart the direction of effects in parent–child interac-tions (Barkley, 1981a) as well as document the social ecological effects of medication (Whalen & Henker, 1980). Further, such studies provide critical tests of the previously discussed theories of parent–child inter-actions. In this section, we will summarize the most important find-ings emanating from the work of Russell Barkley, Charles Cun-ningham, and colleagues in this area as these investigations share similar subject selection procedures and experimental methodology.

Subjects participating in these investigations were diagnosed as hyperactive or ADHD by their pediatricians, received Conners Parent Rating Scale–Revised (Goyette, Conners, & Ulrich, 1978), Werry-Weiss-Peters Activity Rating Scale (Werry & Sprague, 1970), and Home Situations Questionnaire (Barkley, 1981b) scores placing them two standard deviations above the mean, and were of at least low-average intelligence. Observations of mother–child interactions took place on four occasions: pretreatment baseline, placebo, low-dose of MPH, high-dose of MPH. The latter three conditions occurred in a randomly determined sequence under double-blind conditions. The specific MPH dosages employed varied among studies and ranged between 0.15 mg/kg to 0.50 mg/kg. Mother–child interactions were typically observed during 15 to 20 minutes of free play and an equivalent amount of time engaged in a structured task. The latter involved the mother issuing a standard series of chore commands (e.g., "Pick up the toys and place them on the bookshelf") to the child. Parent and child behavior was unobtrusively coded by trained observers using the Response Class Matrix developed by Mash, Terdal, and Anderson (1973; Mash & Barkley, 1986). The sequence of the parent–child response chain was recorded as the behavior of each participant was coded as an antecedent event for a subsequent response as well as contingent upon the previous action of the other member of the dyad. As such, this observational system is designed to capture the reciprocal and bidirectional nature of these interactions. Interobserver reliabilities for most behavioral categories were reported to be uniformly high across experiments (Mash & Barkley, 1986).

Experimental results have been remarkably consistent across studies and indicate that stimulant medication may "normalize" the mother–child interactions of children with ADHD (Barkley, 1988, 1989, 1990; Barkley et al., 1984). Specifically, children were observed to comply with a greater frequency of maternal commands and to sustain task compliance for longer time intervals during active medication conditions relative to placebo (Barkley, 1989; Barkley & Cunningham, 1979; Barkley et al., 1984; Cunningham & Barkley, 1978). Children were also found to exhibit lower frequencies of "competing" or off-task behaviors following maternal commands as a function of receiving MPH. In turn, their mothers emitted significantly fewer task commands and lower frequencies of negative responses to child behavior following MPH administration. Mothers were also more responsive to initiations of interactions by their children and more likely to pay positive attention to or passively observe child behavior and compliance (Barkley, 1989; Barkley & Cunningham, 1979; Barkley et al., 1984; Cunningham & Barkley, 1978). These findings did not vary as a function of the sex of the child (Barkley, 1989). MPH effects on the behavior of a mother and her hyperactive, identical twin boys across settings are depicted in Figure 5.1 from Cunningham and Barkley (1978). The reciprocal improvements and declines in their interactional behaviors are clearly evident across placebo and active drug conditions.

MPH effects on the behaviors of parents and children participating in these investigations vary as a function of the setting for the

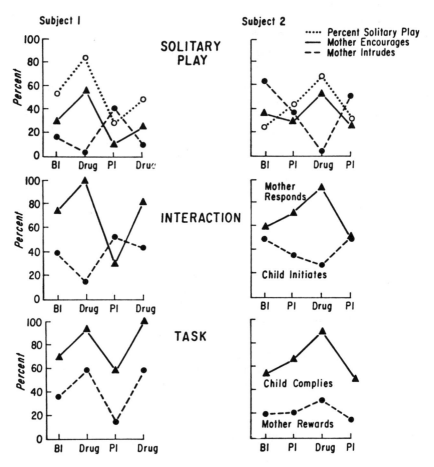

FIGURE 5.1. Selected behavioral measures for twin boys with ADHD and their mother during baseline (Bl), MPH (drug), and placebo (Pl) sessions. Solitary play and interaction measures were derived from free-play periods. Task measures were calculated from the structured task situations. From "The effects of Methylphenidate on the Mother–Child Interactions of Hyperactive Identical Twins" by C. E. Cunningham, & R. A. Barkley, 1978. *Developmental Medicine and Child Neurology, 20*, p. 638. Copyright 1978 by Spastics International Medical Publications. Reprinted by permission.

interaction, medication dosage, and, to a certain extent, the age of the child (Barkley, 1990). For instance, most significant changes in parent and child behavior associated with medication are found to occur during structured tasks rather than free-play conditions. Given that the behaviors of unmedicated children with ADHD and their mothers typically do not differ significantly from normal family interactions under free-play conditions, MPH effects would not be expected in such settings (Barkley, 1990). Higher doses (i.e., 0.35–0.50 mg/kg) of MPH bring about the greatest levels of improvement in child compliance and concomitant decreases in maternal controlling behaviors. Linear dose–response functions favoring higher doses of MPH have been uniformly obtained in group-level analyses across a number of dependent measures (Douglas, Barr, O'Neill, & Britton, 1986; Pelham, Bender, Caddell, Booth, & Moorer, 1985; Rapport, DuPaul, Stoner, & Jones, 1986). While MPH-induced changes in parent–child interactions are found to occur across all age ranges studied, treatment effects are less pronounced among groups of preschool children (Barkley, 1988).

Since the behavior of only one participant (i.e., the child) in the parent–child interaction was *directly* affected by medication, the results of these experiments permit tentative conclusions regarding the relative influence of child and parent behavior in determining the tenor of familial interactions. It appears that the behavior of the mothers during nonmedication conditions in these studies are, in large part, a *reaction* to their children's inability to sustain attention and maintain compliance to commands. As MPH led to enhancement of children's attention to and compliance with maternal commands, mothers' controlling behaviors diminished and more nondirective, passive management responses were displayed (Barkley, 1989). Rather than negative parent–child interactions being caused by poor maternal management skills, mothers of children with ADHD appear to possess effective behavioral monitoring abilities but resort to more coercive, directive strategies when children are unmedicated because a positive management style seems less successful (Cunningham & Barkley, 1978). Thus, at least under structured task conditions, the behavior of the child with ADHD is a more important determinant of parent–child conflicts than is maternal behavior or management style (Barkley, 1989; Mash & Johnston, 1990).

While these studies did not directly examine the effects of the combination of medication and parent training in child management skills, their results do have implications for a multimodal treatment approach. First, parents of children receiving stimulant medication may be more amenable to parent training in child management skills given the adoption of a more positive, less coercive disciplinary style (Barkley, 1988). In turn, training in behavior modification techniques may serve to enhance the child's drug–response as changes in maternal response style could maintain or further improve child behavior changes mediated by MPH (Barkley & Cunningham, 1979; Cunningham & Barkley, 1978). In fact, a positive MPH response over the long term may depend, in part, on contemporaneous changes in the behaviors of those interacting with the child (Cunningham & Barkley, 1978).

Teacher-Child Interactions

A large number of research studies have been conducted documenting the positive effects of MPH on the classroom behavior of children with ADHD (DuPaul & Barkley, 1990). At the group level of analysis, MPH leads to significant improvements in task-related attention, impulse control, and academic productivity, with the greatest effects associated with higher dosages (Douglas et al., 1986; Pelham et al., 1985; Rapport et al., 1986). Despite the voluminous literature documenting treatment-related changes in child behavior associated with MPH, surprisingly few studies have examined the interactions between children with ADHD and their teachers during medication therapy. Those experiments that have been conducted indicate MPH-related increases in both teacher-initiated positive attention toward the child and child-initiated positive attention toward the teacher (Sprague, Barnes, & Werry, 1970; Whalen, Henker, & Dotemoto, 1981). Since the research of Whalen and colleagues is most representative of work in this area, their experiment will be reviewed in detail.

Twenty-two boys with ADHD between the ages of 7 and 11 were recruited to participate in this study based on physician diagnosis of hyperactivity, absence of intellectual deficits or severe behavioral deficits, and a previously established positive response to MPH. A group of 39 normal comparison boys in a similar age range was also recruited to participate. All boys attended the summer school research program coordinated by Whalen and colleagues, under the supervision of an experienced, female teacher who was blind to the diagnostic and medication status of her students.

The study was divided into four experiments wherein several dimensions of classroom structure and procedure were systematically varied across experiments to contrast "provocation" and "rarefaction" ecologies (i.e., settings designed to promote or to diminish ADHD-related behaviors). For example, these dimensions included the presence or absence of teacher supervision and task difficulty of classroom activities. The boys with ADHD received either their regular dosage of MPH (range = 5 to 40 mg; $M = 12.3$ mg) or an inert placebo during two of the experiments, with medication conditions switching within subjects for the remaining two experiments. The sequence of medication conditions was randomly determined across subjects such that half of the ADHD group received MPH and the other half ingested placebo during each experiment.

Individual teacher–student contacts were coded as to function (i.e., controlling vs. regular) and modality (e.g., verbal, nonverbal, physical). The intensity of the contact, whether the child initiated the interaction, and whether the child's name was used by the teacher were also coded. Raters were blind to the purpose of the experiment and medication status of the students with ADHD. The level of interrater agreement was at a satisfactory level across observation categories.

No differences between normal and ADHD groups in the frequency of regular teacher contacts (e.g., small talk, information-giving statements) were obtained across experiments nor were there any changes in this variable associated with MPH. Alternatively, the teacher initiated more controlling, guiding, or disciplinary interactions with students receiving placebo than with those in either the medicated or normal comparison groups. No significant differences were obtained between medicated and normal comparison children. These results were found consistently across experiments (i.e., classroom dimensions) and are graphically displayed in Figure 5.2. Further, boys on placebo were named more frequently by the teacher and

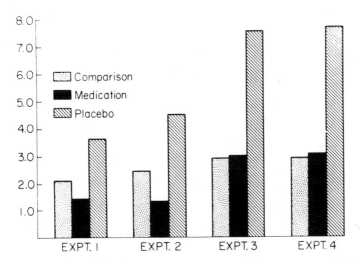

FIGURE 5.2. Frequency of control contacts by teacher toward comparison boys, boys with ADHD on MPH, and boys with ADHD on placebo. From "Teacher Response to the Methylphenidate (Ritalin) versus Placebo Status of Hyperactive Boys in the Classroom" by C. K. Whalen, B. Henker, & S. Dotemoto, 1981. *Child Development, 52,* p. 1009. Copyright 1981 by the Society for Research in Child Development. Reprinted by permission.

received more verbal contacts in the context of controlling statements than students in the other two groups. When the results were examined within individual subjects, the same pattern of findings were obtained. Both control contacts and control naming initiated by the teacher occurred more frequently under placebo than during MPH conditions for 18 of the 22 boys.

The intensity of teacher contacts toward students also varied as function of medication status. Intensity was defined as the teacher displaying an atypical degree of energy, strain, or effort based on speech rate, loudness, bodily tension, and emotionality. The frequency of intense contacts was significantly higher during interactions with students receiving placebo than with medicated and normal comparison subjects (see Figure 5.3). This finding was replicated across all four experiments. Some significant interactions between group and classroom dimensions were obtained across experiments, indicating that changes in classroom variables had more impact on the teacher-student contacts of boys receiving placebo than those in the medication or normal control groups.

The results of this series of experiments indicate that teacher-student interactions vary as a function of MPH among boys with ADHD. The frequency and intensity of controlling behaviors (i.e., commands and reprimands) emitted by the teacher were significantly

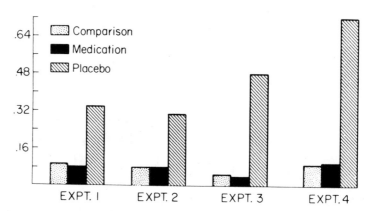

FIGURE 5.3. Frequency of teacher intensity toward comparison boys, boys with ADHD on MPH, and boys with ADHD on placebo. From Whalen, C. K., Henker, B., & Dotemoto, S. (1981). From "Teacher Response to the Methylphenidate (Ritalin) versus Placebo Status of Hyperactive Boys in the Classroom" by C. K. Whalen, B. Henker, & S. Dotemoto, 1981. *Child Development, 52,* p. 1009. Copyright 1981 by the Society for Research in Child Development. Reprinted by permission.

reduced by MPH relative to nonmedication conditions. Further, the teacher–student interactions of medicated children with ADHD appeared to be "normalized," as there were no significant differences in teacher behaviors toward children receiving MPH relative to those in the normal comparison group. Thus, these findings are quite similar to those obtained in studies of MPH effects on parent–child interactions as the management style of the teacher became less controlling as a function of the children's medication status. Alternatively, regular teacher contacts, including positive attention toward students, did not vary across experimental conditions. This finding is in direct contrast to those studies finding an increase in positive attention displayed by mothers of medicated children with ADHD (Barkley & Cunningham, 1979). This discrepancy in results may be a function of the use of different methodologies (e.g., observational coding systems) and experimental settings (school vs. clinic playroom). It is also likely that teachers generally do not use positive attention to compliance frequently as a management strategy (White, 1975).

When combined with the findings of the parent–child interaction literature, the results of the above study lend additional credence to the assumption that the behavior of children with ADHD plays a larger role in determining the nature of their social interactions than do the actions of significant others (e.g., parents, teachers). It is noteworthy that teacher behaviors toward the vast majority of boys with ADHD varied reliably with changes in medication status of treated students. During placebo conditions, teachers exhibited higher rates of controlling, negative statements toward these boys, presumably in reaction to the off-task and disruptive behaviors they evidenced. When MPH resulted in an increase in on-task, compliant behaviors among treated children, teacher-initiated controlling interchanges were reduced to within normal limits. This reliable covariation in teacher and student behavior is directly analogous to those seen in the mother–child interactions of children with ADHD.

Interactions with Peers

A small but growing research literature documents that stimulant medications, including MPH, affect the social interactions of children with ADHD and their normal counterparts. For example, Pelham and Bender (1982) obtained mixed results regarding the effects of stimulant medication on social interactions. Their findings suggested that MPH may have little effect on a child's peer relations, per se, except for reducing high levels of aggression. More recent studies, however, have documented a number of positive MPH effects on peer interactions. Specifically, MPH leads to reduced levels of noncompliance and verbal and physical aggression exhibited by children with ADHD, with higher doses associated with the greatest changes (Hinshaw, Henker, Whalen, Erhardt, & Dunnington, 1989; Whalen, Henker, Swanson, Granger, Kliewer, & Spencer, 1987; Wallander, Schroeder, Michelli, & Gualtieri, 1987). Levels of negative social behavior were brought to within the range of contemporaneously studied peers. MPH has not been found to alter the frequency of prosocial or nonsocial behaviors (Hinshaw et al., 1989; Whalen, Henker, Swanson, Granger, Kliewer, & Spencer, 1987; Wallander et al., 1987). Since children with ADHD were not found to differ from their normal peers in the frequencies of the latter social behaviors during placebo conditions, one would not expect an increase in prosocial behavior to be associated with MPH.

Normal peers are able to discern behavioral differences in children with ADHD between medication and nonmedication conditions. A sample of normal children viewing videotapes of social interactions rated boys with ADHD taking placebo to exhibit greater frequencies of externalizing problem behaviors than ratings of boys with ADHD taking MPH or normal comparison boys (Whalen, Henker, Castro, & Granger, 1987). Peer sensitivity to medication effects may also alter judgments of the sociometric status of children with ADHD. MPH has been found to enhance sociometric ratings, as well as to increase peer nominations of treated boys as best friends, cooperative, and fun to be with (Whalen, Henker, Buhrmester, Hinshaw, Huber, & Laski, 1989). Peer judgments of boys with ADHD were not completely "normalized" by treatment, however, and MPH effects on peer appraisals were highly subject to interindividual variability.

While positive MPH effects on the social behavior of children with ADHD and resultant changes in peer judgments have been explicated across a number of studies, relatively few experiments have examined alterations in peer social responses as a function of stimulant medication. For example, Cunningham, Siegel, and Offord (1985) studied the dyadic interactions of 42 boys with ADHD and an equal number of normal comparison peers. Boys were divided into three subgroups by age (i.e., 4–6, 7–9, and 10–12 years old). Subjects in the ADHD group had to have received a physician diagnosis of this disorder, parental ratings on the Hyperactivity Index of the Conners Parent Rating Scale–Revised at least two standard deviations above the mean, and to have an onset of symptoms before the age of 4 years. Normal comparison subjects were within one standard deviation of the mean on the Hyperactivity Index.

Dyads of ADHD and normal control boys were videotaped interacting in three situations (e.g., free play, cooperative task, simulated classroom) in a clinic playroom. Each of the three situations lasted 15 minutes. Observations were conducted on four separate occasions. During the latter three observation conditions, boys with ADHD received either an inert placebo, 0.15 mg/kg, or 0.50 mg/kg of MPH in a randomly determined sequence. Dyadic interactions were coded by trained observers using a modified version of the Response Class Matrix. In addition, the frequency of on-task behavior of both participants was coded and actometer readings were collected to measure wrist and ankle activity levels.

As found in the parent–child studies, no MPH effects on the interactions of children with ADHD and their peers were obtained in the free-play situation. It should be noted that although there were group differences in attention and activity level during free play, these discrepancies were not as great as were evidenced during the other two conditions. Not surprisingly, therefore, the strongest MPH effects on dyadic interactions were obtained during the cooperative task and simulated classroom situations. In the cooperative task condition, MPH increased the percentage of controlling antecedents children with ADHD either ignored or responded to positively. Meanwhile, normal children exhibited a decrease in ignoring or responding positively to the controlling antecedents of the boys with ADHD who had received MPH.

The greatest number of MPH effects on dyadic social interactions were found in the simulated classroom setting. MPH led to decreased actometer scores and increased on-task frequencies among treated children. Reduced activity level and enhanced attention to task were also obtained for the normal boys during active medication conditions. Further, MPH significantly reduced the overall frequency of controlling and dominating interactions while also diminishing the number of controlling responses to both positive and controlling initiations. Reductions in the controlling behavior of children with ADHD were associated with reciprocal changes in the same behaviors among normal peers.

There are a number of parallels between the above findings and the results of studies examining the mother–child interactions of children with ADHD. Group differences in social behavior between ADHD and normal children were primarily found during structured situations that presumably require sustained concentration, impulse control, and compliance. During structured situations, normal children, like parents, were less likely to respond positively to interactions initiated by boys with ADHD. Changes mediated by MPH in the social behaviors of ADHD and normal children were found solely during structured situations where the greatest room for improvement existed.

The results of the Cunningham et al. (1985) study provide additional evidence of the relative importance of the behavior of children with ADHD in determining the nature of their interactions with others and the reactions they receive in turn. Specifically, the high rate of controlling and dominating behaviors exhibited by such children may lead to increased rates of similar negative responses among their normal peers. The latter were found to be two to five times more likely to exhibit controlling responses following controlling antecedents than following interactional or play antecedents emitted by children with ADHD (Cunningham et al., 1985). Further, MPH-induced reductions in the controlling behavior of children with ADHD were strongly associated with reciprocal decreases in the frequencies of the controlling responses of normal peers.

While the responses of normal peers to the behavior of children with ADHD are largely determined by the latter, they also serve to elicit and maintain further behaviors in keeping with the bidirectional nature of the social interaction chain (Bell & Harper, 1977). The social performance difficulties of children with ADHD may be compounded and maintained by the negative reactions exhibited by their classmates and peers (Cunningham et al., 1985). Alternatively, the medication-response of children with ADHD could be further enhanced by reciprocal changes in the social behaviors of normal peers. Peer behaviors (e.g., controlling responses) that could elicit or maintain inappropriate behavior among children with ADHD are reduced when the latter are treated with MPH. The treatment-related enhancement of the on-task behavior and activity level of normal peers may also help to sustain a positive medication response in children with ADHD (Cunningham et al., 1985). Presumably, peer social responses that could reinforce or maintain the positive social behavior of children with ADHD are increased with treatment, although the latter was not found to occur in the Cunningham et al. (1985) study.

SUMMARY AND FUTURE DIRECTIONS

The social interactions of children with ADHD and their parents, teachers, and peers are bidirectional and reciprocal, in keeping with Bell and Harper's (1977) theory. In the absence of treatment, these interactions are characterized by high frequencies of negative, controlling behaviors exhibited not only by those with ADHD but also by significant people in their lives. A coercive interaction pattern develops over time similar to that described by Patterson (1982), particularly among children with ADHD and comorbid ODD. It is not clear, however, whether this mechanism relates to escape behavior as hypothesized by Patterson or to increased consistency as argued by Wahler (1980). For those children with ADHD who respond positively to stimulant medication treatment, MPH diminishes the coercive nature of their social interactions with parents, teachers, and peers. This is accomplished, in part, by a reduction in the frequency of noncompliant and/or controlling responses emitted by the child with ADHD. In response to these changes in the child's behavior, parents, teachers, and peers reduce their levels of controlling, negative behaviors toward the child with ADHD and adopt a "softer," more facilitative management style. In general, the effects of MPH are strongest at higher dosages and for those interactions that occur in the context of structured task situations rather than unstructured, free-play settings, since the former are more likely to elicit difficulties with sustained attention, impulse control, and compliance with the directives of others. As with other behavioral domains, MPH dose and setting effects are highly subject to interindividual variability (DuPaul & Barkley, 1990).

The research studies reviewed in the present chapter provide strong evidence that the behavior of children with ADHD plays a primary role in determining the nature of their interactions with others. MPH effects on the behavior of children with ADHD have been found to alter the social responses of mothers, teachers, and peers to such children. Treatment-related reductions in negative, controlling responses to the behavior of children with ADHD are remarkably consistent across settings and studies. The change in response pattern of both members of the social dyad after one member of the interaction receives treatment indicates that the latter (i.e., the child with ADHD) plays the predominant role in determining whether the interaction will be positive or negative (Barkley, 1981a).

Studies of MPH effects on the social interactions of children with ADHD have several implications for the treatment of this population. For example, changes in the response patterns of parents, teachers, and peers may help to maintain the positive behavioral effects of stimulant medication (Cunningham et al., 1985). Reductions in negative, controlling social responses exhibited by others in the child's environment may reinforce and maintain MPH-induced behavioral improvements exhibited by the latter. Alternatively, behavioral changes that are not reinforced by others may not be maintained over long time periods, although this possibility has not been addressed in studies conducted to date. The "softening" of parent and teacher management styles as a reaction to MPH-related improvements in child behavior may provide an impetus for greater levels of involvement and success with training in behavior management strategies (Barkley, 1988). There is a growing consensus in the ADHD literature that stimulant medication and behavior therapy are complementary treatments that, when combined, could provide synergistic results (Barkley, 1990; Pelham & Murphy, 1986; Whalen & Henker, 1991).

While the effects of stimulant medication on the interactions of children with ADHD have been consistently documented across settings and significant others, further research is necessary to provide a comprehensive picture of this complex phenomenon. First, most of the studies conducted in this area have examined MPH-related changes in mother–child interactions. Only a handful of experiments have assessed treatment effects on teacher–child and peer social interchanges and none have evaluated changes in father–child interactions. Further, we know little about factors, such as age, gender, or dosage, that could impact upon MPH effects in these relatively unstudied social domains. Second, increases in positive attention to the MPH-treated child have been found to occur only with mothers and not with teachers or peers. This may be a result of differing methodologies (e.g., observational coding systems) across studies or could be representative of discrepant response styles between parents and others interacting with the child secondary to different social roles played by these individuals. Certainly, future studies of teacher–child and peer interactions should employ observational systems that allow positive attention/behavior to be coded separately for each participant in the dyad. Third, recent investigations have documented that the impaired relations between children with ADHD and their parents continues into adolescence (Barkley et al., 1991, in press). Yet, we do not know whether MPH alters negative interaction patterns among this older age group. It is possible that positive effects on parent–teen interactions are absent or milder than those obtained with younger children since there is a longer history of coercive interchanges for adolescents with ADHD. Since ADHD is potentially a chronic and socially debilitating disorder, elucidation of stimulant medication effects on the social interactions of these children remains an important objective for future research.

A significant paradox in the literature on stimulant medications and ADHD is the contrast between the findings reviewed above and those from long-term follow-up studies. As already noted, the short-term studies demonstrate significant effects of stimulants on noncompliant, off-task, and negative or defiant child behavior which, in turn, results in a diminution of control responses by caregivers and peers toward the child with ADHD. Long-term follow-up studies, however, have found that protracted use of stimulant medication may not alter the risks for later antisocial behavior, substance abuse, academic failure, or emotional psychopathology *in adolescence* (Fischer, Barkley, Edelbrock, & Smallish, 1990; Loney, Kramer, & Milich, 1981; Weiss, Kruger, Danielson, & Elman, 1975). In fact, in some studies (Barkley et al., 1991; Lambert, 1988), duration of treatment with stimulants is actually negatively related to outcome in that the more treatment subjects received, the more antisocial behaviors displayed at adolescent follow-up. In such cases, treatment is serving as a marker variable for severity of the children's disorder. One study, in contrast, found that children with ADHD receiving stimulants for at least 3 years and followed into *adulthood* had fewer car accidents, were less aggressive, had fewer episodes of stealing in elementary school (but not high school), and had better self-images than untreated children with ADHD (Hechtman, Weiss, & Perlman, 1984). The groups did not differ, however, in rates of antisocial acts, educational attainment, work adjustment, or substance use and abuse. Another adult outcome study (Loney, Whaley-Klahn, Kosier, & Conboy, 1981) found that duration of stimulant medication use was associated only with a reduction in later substance use and abuse in hyperactive children.

If stimulants produce such dramatic improvements in social interactions, thought to be the arena from which later aggression and antisocial behavior may originate, then why are the results of the long-term follow-up studies not more consistent in demonstrating the positive benefits of stimulant use in reducing the risks for antisocial outcomes? There are several possible reasons. First, the stimulant drugs produce their peak effects during school hours due to their short half-life and predominant use for school-related behavior problems. Drug effects on parent–child and peer–child interactions outside of school are therefore weak to nonexistent unless the child is taking medications several times per day throughout the entire week with little interruption. Such has not been the common clinical practice until very recently (DuPaul & Barkley, 1990). Even under such ideal circumstances, these medications are typically not given in the afternoons or later in the day, leaving the major part of the weekday unaffected by medication. In short, the time-limited manner in which the stimulants are used could preclude their producing significant and sustained benefits on family and peer interactions for the majority of children with ADHD.

A second and related reason may be that the stimulants are simply not employed over sufficient developmental time spans to dramatically affect the risks for later antisocial behavior. Until recently, it has been common practice for physicians to cease a child's stimulant medication at puberty in the belief that the drugs would no longer be beneficial and might even be detrimental to the adolescent's adjustment (e.g., increase hyperactive behavior). Research now suggests that adolescents with ADHD respond positively to the stimulants (Klorman, Coons, & Borgstedt, 1987). Yet, this traditional approach to stimulant drug therapy could have resulted in children with ADHD being off medication during those critical early adolescent years when they are more mobile, less supervised by adults, and more susceptible to antisocial peer influences than at earlier times in their development. Although speculative, if correct this approach would argue for maintaining medication treatment well into the adolescent years, particularly for those children with early aggressive behavior patterns.

A third reason for the failure of short-term medication effects on social behavior to translate into longer-term positive outcomes may pertain to the possibility that stimulants do not directly affect aggressive behavior in children with ADHD (Loney, 1980). Alternatively, this explanation has been refuted by a substantial body of recent research (Barkley, McMurray, Edelbrock, & Robbins, 1989; Hinshaw, 1991) that finds the stimulants to produce a reduction in aggressive behavior in children with comorbid ADHD. Again these findings lead to the question of why such acute reductions in childhood aggression fail to reliably result in reduced adolescent and young adult antisocial conduct.

Perhaps a fourth reason may be operative in this area. It is possible that early aggressive behavior in children with ADHD may not be the causal mechanism by which the risk of later aggressive or antisocial behavior is increased, but rather serves as a marker variable for other factors that may be associated with this risk (Barkley, 1990). Aggressive child behavior is strongly associated with family adversity, low social class, and parental psychopathology, especially maternal depression and paternal antisocial personality (Loeber, 1990; Patterson, 1982). Perhaps it is these factors that play a stronger causal role in later antisocial behavior rather than simply child aggression alone. This would imply that childhood aggression is a necessary but not sufficient condition for elevating the risk of later antisocial conduct. If so, then it is clear why stimulant medications might produce short-term acute or even sustained effects on childhood ADHD and aggressive symptoms while in use, yet have minimal impact on risk for later antisocial behavior. The stimulants simply cannot address the family and parental contributors to this multivariate model of adolescent and young adult antisocial conduct.

REFERENCES

American Psychiatric Association. (1987). *Diagnostic and statistical manual of mental disorders* (3rd ed., revised). Washington, DC: Author.

Barkley, R. A. (1977). The effects of methylphenidate on various measures of activity level and attention in hyperkinetic children. *Journal of Abnormal Child Psychology, 5*, 351–369.

Barkley, R. A. (1981a). The use of psychopharmacology to study reciprocal influences in parent–child interaction. *Journal of Abnormal Child Psychology, 9*, 303–310.

Barkley, R. A. (1981b). *Hyperactive children: A handbook for diagnosis and treatment.* New York: Guilford Press.

Barkley, R. A. (1985a). The social interactions of hyperactive children: Developmental changes, drug effects, and situational variation. In R. McMahon & R. Peters (Eds.), *Childhood disorders: Behavioral-developmental approaches* (pp. 218–243). New York: Brunner/Mazel.

Barkley, R. A. (1985b). The family interactions of hyperactive children: Precursors to aggressive behavior? In D. Routh & M. Wolraich (Eds.), *Advances in behavioral pediatrics* (Vol. 2, pp. 117–150). Greenwich, CT: JAI Press.

Barkley, R. A. (1988). The effects of methylphenidate on the interactions of pre-school ADHD children with their mothers. *Journal of the American Academy of Child and Adolescent Psychiatry, 27*, 336–341.

Barkley, R. A. (1989). Hyperactive girls and boys: Stimulant drug effects on mother–child interactions. *Journal of Child Psychology and Psychiatry, 30*, 379–390.

Barkley, R. A. (1990). *Attention deficit-hyperactivity disorder: A handbook for diagnosis and treatment.* New York: Guilford Press.

Barkley, R. A., Anastopoulos, A. D., Guevremont, D. C., & Fletcher, K. (in press). Adolescents with attention deficit hyperactivity disorder: Mother-adolescent interactions, family beliefs, and conflicts, and maternal psychopathology. *Journal of Abnormal Child Psychology.*

Barkley, R. A., & Cunningham, C. E. (1979). The effects of methylphenidate on the mother–child interactions of hyperactive children. *Archives of General Psychiatry, 36*, 201–208.

Barkley, R. A., Fischer, M., Edelbrock, C. S., & Smallish, L. (1990). The adolescent outcome of hyperactive children diagnosed by research criteria: 1. An 8 year prospective follow-up study. *Journal of the American Academy of Child and Adolescent Psychiatry, 29*, 546–557.

Barkley, R. A., Fischer, M., Edelbrock, C. S., & Smallish, L. (1991). The adolescent outcome of hyperactive children diagnosed by research criteria: 3. Mother–child interactions, family conflicts, and maternal psychopathology. *Journal of Child Psychology and Psychiatry, 32*, 233–256.

Barkley, R. A., Karlsson, J., & Pollard, S. (1985). Effects of age on the mother–child interactions of hyperactive children. *Journal of Abnormal Child Psychology, 13*, 631–638.

Barkley, R. A., Karlsson, J., Strzelecki, E., & Murphy, J. (1984). Effects of age and Ritalin dosage on the mother–child interactions of hyperactive children. *Journal of Consulting and Clinical Psychology, 52,* 750–758.

Barkley, R. A., McMurray, M. B., Edelbrock, C. S., & Robbins, K. (1989). The response of aggressive and non-aggressive ADHD children to two doses of methylphenidate. *Journal of the American Academy of Child and Adolescent Psychiatry, 28,* 873–881.

Befera, M., & Barkley, R. A. (1985). Hyperactive and normal boys and girls: Mother–child interaction, parent psychiatric status, and child psychopathology. *Journal of Child Psychology and Psychiatry, 26,* 439–452.

Bell, R. Q., & Harper, L. (1977). *Child effects on adults.* New York: Wiley.

Campbell, S. B. (1973). Mother–child interaction in reflective, impulsive, and hyperactive children. *Developmental Psychology, 8,* 341–349.

Campbell, S. B. (1975). Mother–child interactions: A comparison of hyperactive, learning disabled, and normal boys. *American Journal of Orthopsychiatry, 45,* 51–57.

Campbell, S. B., Breaux, A. M., Ewing, L. J., Szumowski, E. K., & Pierce, E. W. (1986). Parent-identified problem preschoolers: Mother–child interaction during play at intake and 1 year follow-up. *Journal of Abnormal Child Psychology, 14,* 425–440.

Campbell, S. B., Endman, M., & Bernfield, G. (1977). A three year follow-up of hyperactive preschoolers into elementary school. *Journal of Child Psychology and Psychiatry, 18,* 239–249.

Cohen, N. J., Sullivan, J., Minde, K., Novak, C., & Keene, S. (1983). Mother–child interaction in hyperactive and normal kindergarten-aged children and the effect of treatment. *Child Psychiatry and Human Development, 13,* 213–224.

Cunningham, C. E., & Barkley, R. A. (1978). The effects of methylphenidate on the mother–child interactions of hyperactive twin boys. *Developmental Medicine and Child Neurology, 20,* 634–642.

Cunningham, C. E., & Barkley, R. A. (1979). The interactions of hyperactive and normal children with their mothers during free play and structured task. *Child Development, 50,* 217–224.

Cunningham, C. E., & Siegel, L. S. (1987). Peer interactions of normal and attention-deficit disordered boys during free-play, cooperative task, and simulated classroom situations. *Journal of Abnormal Child Psychology, 15,* 247–268.

Cunningham, C. E., Siegel, L. S., & Offord, D. R. (1985). A developmental dose response analysis of the effects of methylphenidate on the peer interactions of attention deficit disordered boys. *Journal of Child Psychology and Psychiatry, 26,* 955–971.

Douglas, V. I., Barr, R. G., O'Neill, M. E., & Britton, B. G. (1986). Short term effects of methylphenidate on the cognitive, learning, and academic performance of children with attention deficit disorder in the laboratory and the classroom. *Journal of Child Psychology and Psychiatry, 27,* 191–211.

Dumas, J. E., & Wahler, R. G. (1985). Indiscriminate mothering as a contextual factor in aggressive-opposition child behavior: "Damned if you do and damned if you don't." *Journal of Abnormal Child Psychology, 13,* 1–17.

DuPaul, G. J., & Barkley, R. A. (1990). Medication therapy. In R. A. Barkley, *Attention deficit hyperactivity disorder: A handbook for diagnosis and treatment* (pp. 573–612). New York: Guilford Press.

Fischer, M. (1990). Parenting stress and the child with attention deficit hyperactivity disorder. *Journal of Clinical Child Psychology, 19,* 337–346.

Fischer, M., Barkley, R. A., Edelbrock, C. S., & Smallish, L. (1990). The adolescent outcome of hyperactive children diagnosed by research criteria: 2. Academic, attentional, and neuropsychological status. *Journal of Consulting and Clinical Psychology, 58,* 580–588.

Gittelman, R., Mannuzza, S., Shenker, R., & Bonagura, N. (1985). Hyperactive boys almost grown up. *Archives of General Psychiatry, 42,* 937–947.

Goyette, C. H., Conners, C. K., & Ulrich, R. F. (1978). Normative data on Revised Conners Parent and Teacher Rating Scales. *Journal of Abnormal Child Psychology, 6,* 221–236.

Hechtman, L., Weiss, G., & Perlman, R. (1984). Young adult outcome of hyperactive children who received long-term stimulant treatment. *Journal of the American Academy of Child Psychiatry, 23,* 261–269.

Henker, B., & Whalen, C. K. (1989). Hyperactivity and attention deficits. *American Psychologist, 44,* 216–223.

Hinshaw, S. P. (1991). *Stimulant medication and the treatment of aggression in children with attentional deficits.* Manuscript submitted for publication.

Hinshaw, S. P., Henker, B., Whalen, C. K., Erhardt, D., & Dunnington, R. E., Jr. (1989). Aggressive, prosocial, and nonsocial behavior in hyperactive boys: Dose effects of methylphenidate in naturalistic settings. *Journal of Consulting and Clinical Psychology, 57,* 636–643.

Humphries, T., Kinsbourne, M., & Swanson, J. (1978). Stimulant effects on cooperation and social interaction between hyperactive children and their mothers. *Journal of Child Psychology and Psychiatry, 19,* 13–22.

Klorman, R., Coons, H. W., & Borgstedt, A. D. (1987). Effects of methylphenidate on adolescents with a childhood history of attention deficit disorder: 1. Clinical findings. *Journal of the American Academy of Child and Adolescent Psychiatry, 26,* 363–367.

Lambert, N. M. (1988). Adolescent outcomes of hyperactive children: Perspectives on general and specific patterns of childhood risk for adolescent educational, social, and mental health problems. *American Psychologist, 43,* 786–799.

Lambert, N. M., & Sandoval, J. (1980). The prevalence of learning disabilities in a sample of children considered hyperactive. *Journal of Abnormal Child Psychology, 8,* 33–50.

Loeber, R. (1990). Development and risk factors of juvenile antisocial behavior and delinquency. *Clinical Psychology Review, 10,* 1–41.

Loney, J. (1980). The Iowa theory of substance abuse among hyperactive adolescents. In D. J. Lettieri, M. Sayers, & H. W. Pearson (Eds.), *Theories on drug abuse: Selected contemporary perspectives* (National Institute on Drug Abuse Research Monograph No. 30, DHHS Pub. No. ADM 80-967). Washington, DC: U.S. Government Printing Office.

Loney, J., Kramer, J., & Milich, R. (1981). The hyperkinetic child grows up: Predictors of symptoms, delinquency, and achievement at follow-up. In K. D. Gadow & J. Loney (Eds.), *Psychosocial aspects of drug treatment for hyperactivity* (pp. 381–415). Boulder, CO: Westview Press.

Loney, J., Whaley-Klahn, M. A., Kosier, T., & Conboy, J. (1981, November). *Hyperactive boys and their brothers at 21: Predictors of aggressive and antisocial outcomes.* Paper presented at the annual meeting of the Society for Life History Research, Monterey, CA.

Madan-Swain, A., & Zentall, S. S. (1990). Behavioral comparisons of liked and disliked hyperactive children in play contexts and the behavioral accommodations by their classmates. *Journal of Consulting and Clinical Psychology, 58,* 197–209.

Mash, E. J., & Barkley, R. A. (1986). Assessment of family interaction with the Response Class Matrix. In R. Prinz (Ed.), *Advances in behavioral assessment in children and families* (Vol. 2, pp. 29–67). Greenwich, CT: JAI Press.

Mash, E. J., & Johnston, C. (1982). A comparison of the mother–child interactions of younger and older hyperactive and normal children. *Child Development, 53,* 1371–1381.

Mash, E. J., & Johnston, C. (1983a). Sibling interactions of hyperactive and normal children and their relationship to reports of maternal stress and self-esteem. *Journal of Clinical Child Psychology, 12,* 91–99.

Mash, E. J., & Johnston, C. (1983b). The prediction of mother's behavior with their hyperactive children during play and task situations. *Child and Family Behavior Therapy, 5,* 1–14.

Mash, E. J., & Johnston, C. (1990). Determinants of parenting stress: Illustrations from families of hyperactive children and families of physically abused children. *Journal of Clinical Child Psychology, 19,* 313–328.

Mash, E. J., Terdal, L., & Anderson, K. (1973). The Response Class Matrix: A procedure for recording parent–child interactions. *Journal of Consulting and Clinical Psychology, 40,* 163–164.

Milich, R., & Landau, S. (1982). Socialization and peer relations in hyperactive children. In K. D. Gadow & I. Bialer (Eds.), *Advances in learning and behavioral disabilities* (Vol. 1, pp. 283–339). Greenwich, CT: JAI Press.

Minde, K. K., Weiss, G., & Mendelson, N. (1972). A 5-year follow-up study of 91 hyperactive school children. *Journal of the American Academy of Child Psychiatry, 11,* 595–610.

Patterson, G. R. (1982). *Coercive family process.* Eugene, OR: Castalia.

Patterson, G. R. (1986). Performance models for antisocial boys. *American Psychologist, 41,* 432–444.

Pelham, W. E., & Bender, M. E. (1982). Peer relationships in hyperactive children: Description and treatment. In K. D. Gadow & I. Bialer (Eds.), *Advances in learning and behavioral disabilities* (Vol. 1, pp. 365–436). Greenwich, CT: JAI Press.

Pelham, W. E., Bender, M. E., Caddell, J., Booth, S., & Moorer, S. H. (1985). Methylphenidate and children with attention deficit disorder. *Archives of General Psychiatry, 42,* 948–952.

Pelham, W. E., & Murphy, H. A. (1986). Attention deficit and conduct disorders. In M. Hersen (Ed.), *Pharmacological and behavioral treatment: An integrative approach* (pp. 108–148). New York: Wiley.

Rapport, M. D. (1987). Attention deficit disorder with hyperactivity. In M. Hersen & V. B. Van Hasselt (Eds.), *Behavior therapy with children and adolescents: A clinical approach* (pp. 325–361). New York: Wiley.

Rapport, M. D., DuPaul, G. J., Stoner, G., & Jones, J. T. (1986). Comparing classroom and clinic measures of attention deficit disorder: Differential, idiosyncratic, and dose-response effects of methylphenidate. *Journal of Consulting and Clinical Psychology, 54,* 334–341.

Rapport, M. D., Tucker, S. B., DuPaul, G. J., Merlo, M., & Stoner, G. (1986). Hyperactivity and frustration: The influence of control over and size of rewards in delaying gratification. *Journal of Abnormal Child Psychology, 14,* 191–204.

Safer, D. J., & Krager, J. M. (1988). A survey of medication treatment for hyperactive/inattentive students. *Journal of the American Medical Association, 260,* 2256–2258.

Sprague, R. L., Barnes, K. R., & Werry, J. S. (1970). Methylphenidate and thioridazine: Learning, activity, and behavior in emotionally disturbed boys. *American Journal of Orthopsychiatry, 40,* 615–628.

Tallmadge, J., & Barkley, R. A. (1983). The interactions of hyperactive and normal boys with their mothers and fathers. *Journal of Abnormal Child Psychology, 11,* 565–579.

Tallmadge, J., Paternite, C., & Gordon, M. (1989, April). *Hyperactivity and aggression in parent–child interactions: Test of a two-factor theory.* Paper presented at the annual meeting of the Society for Research in Child Development, Kansas City, MO.

Tarver-Behring, S., Barkley, R. A., & Karlsson, J. (1985). The mother–child interactions of hyperactive boys and their normal siblings. *American Journal of Orthopsychiatry, 55,* 202–209.

Wahler, R. G. (1980). The insular mother: Her problems in parent–child treatment. *Journal of Applied Behavior Analysis, 13,* 207–219.

Wallander, J. L., Schroeder, S. R., Michelli, J. A., & Gualtieri, C. T. (1987). Classroom social interactions of attention deficit disorder with hyperactivity children as a function of stimulant medication. *Journal of Pediatric Psychology, 12,* 61–76.

Weiss, G., & Hechtman, L. (1986). *Hyperactive children grown up: Empirical findings and theoretical considerations.* New York: Guilford Press.

Weiss, G., Kruger, E., Danielson, U., & Elman, M. (1975). Effect of long-term treatment of hyperactive children with methylphenidate. *Canadian Medical Association Journal, 112*, 159–164.

Werry, J. S., & Sprague, R. L. (1970). Hyperactivity. In C. G. Costello (Ed.), *Symptoms of psychopathology* (pp. 397–417). New York: Wiley.

Whalen, C. K., & Henker, B. (Eds.). (1980). *Hyperactive children: The social ecology of identification and treatment.* New York: Academic Press.

Whalen, C. K., & Henker, B. (1991). Therapies of hyperactive children: Comparisons, combinations, and compromises. *Journal of Consulting and Clinical Psychology, 59*, 126–137.

Whalen, C. K., Henker, B., Buhrmester, D., Hinshaw, S. P., Huber, A., & Laski, K. (1989). Does stimulant medication improve the peer status of hyperactive children? *Journal of Consulting and Clinical Psychology, 57*, 545–549.

Whalen, C. K., Henker, B., Castro, J., & Granger, D. (1987). Peer perceptions of hyperactivity and medication effects. *Child Development, 58*, 816–828.

Whalen, C. K., Henker, B., Collins, B. E., Finck, D., & Dotemoto, S. (1979). A social ecology of hyperactive boys: Medication effects in systematically structured classroom environments. *Journal of Applied Behavior Analysis, 12*, 65–81.

Whalen, C.K., Henker, B., Collins, B. E., McAuliffe, S., & Vaux, A. (1979). Peer interaction in structured communication task: Comparisons of normal and hyperactive boys and of methylphenidate (Ritalin) and placebo effects. *Child Development, 50*, 388–401.

Whalen, C. K., Henker, B., & Dotemoto, S. (1980). Methylphenidate and hyperactivity: Effects on teacher behaviors. *Science, 208*, 1280–1282.

Whalen, C. K., Henker, B., & Dotemoto, S. (1981). Teacher response to methylphenidate (Ritalin) versus placebo status of hyperactive boys in the classroom. *Child Development, 52*, 1005–1014.

Whalen, C. K., Henker, B., Swanson, J. M., Granger, D., Kliewer, W., & Spencer, J. (1987). Natural social behaviors in hyperactive children: Dose effects of methylphenidate. *Journal of Consulting and Clinical Psychology, 55*, 187–193.

White, M. A. (1975). Natural rates of teacher approval and disapproval in the classroom. *Journal of Applied Behavior Analysis, 8*, 367–372.

CHAPTER 6

◆ ——— ◆

Parent and Child Training to Prevent Early Onset of Delinquency:
The Montréal Longitudinal-Experimental Study

RICHARD E. TREMBLAY
FRANK VITARO
LUCIE BERTRAND
MARC LEBLANC
HÉLÈNE BEAUCHESNE
HÉLÈNE BOILEAU
LUCILLE DAVID

The power of longitudinal studies to test causal hypotheses is relatively weak, especially when the onset of causal factors cannot be clearly identified in time. Experimental studies will reveal causal effects only if the subjects are followed until the effects are manifested. If a preschool intervention aims at preventing delinquency, the impact of the intervention must obviously be measured when delinquent behavior usually appears, that is, no earlier than preadolescence. Clearly, we must expect interventions that aim to change the course of human development will have long-term effects. In fact, there may be more long-term effects than short-term effects (McCord, 1978). Unfortunately, most experimental studies concerned with changing children's or parents' behavior have had very short follow-ups. By nesting an experimental study in a longitudinal study, the long-term effects of the experiment can become part of the routine assessments of the longitudinal study. The latter gives a broader perspective to the experimental study by showing how the experimental group develops compared to the whole cohort. The experimental study also permits the test of causal hypotheses that the longitudinal study itself cannot test (Farrington, Ohlin, & Wilson, 1986; Tonry et al., 1991).

The results from longitudinal studies of large samples from childhood to adolescence and adulthood suggest that poor parenting may lead to disruptive and antisocial behavior (Loeber & Stouthamer-Loeber, 1986). It must be noted, however, that parents' poor parenting has been shown to be antecedent to delinquent behavior only because a distinction has been made between *disruptive* behavior and *delinquent* behavior. Longitudinal studies that have measured both parenting skills and disruptive behavior in childhood have shown that they are highly concurrently correlated (Campbell, 1990; Eron, Huesmann, & Zelli, 1991). Because disruptive behavior in childhood is also highly correlated with later delinquent behavior, it has been suggested that they are both the expression of an underlying continuum (Rowe & Osgood, 1990). Thus, poor parenting may be antecedent to delinquent behavior, but it may not be antecedent to disruptive behavior (Bates, Bayles, Bennett, Ridge, & Brown, 1991).

In a review of research on parent and child effects leading to boys' conduct disorder, Lytton (1990) has argued that the boys' characteristics are generally more important as a cause of conduct disorder than their parents' parenting behavior. Indeed, some evidence indicates that genetic and/or perinatal factors can lead to disruptive behaviors (Cloninger & Gottesman, 1987; Mednick, Gabrielli, & Hutchings, 1987), and that children's disruptive behavior has an impact on the quality of parenting behaviors (Bell & Chapman, 1986). However, both parenting skills and the child's inherited behavioral dispositions are related to the parents' behavioral characteristics before the birth of the child (Huesmann, Eron, Lefkowitz, & Walder, 1984; Plomin, DeFries, & Fulker, 1988). Thus, the search for "The" cause of antisocial behavior can lead to a neverending search for antecedents to the antecedents.

These genetic-intergenerational-developmental studies do make sense if we want to understand the ontogenesis as well as the intergenerational basis of deviant behavior. However, the problem of causation can be addressed from a more circumscribed perspective. For example, if we start with a group of disruptive 6 year olds, we can ask the question "Will the future quality of parenting behavior have an effect on their social development?" A longitudinal study would enable us to monitor the variation in disruptive behavior and parenting behavior to verify the extent to which they covary over time. If amelioration in parenting behavior is followed by less disruptive behavior and lower levels of delinquent behavior, these results would be an indication that parenting has a causal effect on deviant behavior. If, conversely, decreasing disruptive behavior is followed by better parenting, this would indicate that children's behavior has an effect on parenting.

However, we know that disruptive behavior is quite stable, and we expect that parenting behavior will also be relatively stable. In such a stable world we will observe high correlations between variables both cross-sectionally and longitudinally. This argument has been used by Gottfredson and Hirschi (1987) to justify cross-sectional studies and to critize longitudinal studies. Experimental studies are probably the only way to solve these causal questions (Farrington et al., 1986; Gottfredson & Hirschi, 1987). *If* good parenting can prevent antisocial behavior in boys who are disruptive, and *if* we can change parenting behavior from inadequate to adequate, *then* we should observe the causal effect of better parenting behavior on antisocial behavior.

A number of parent-management training programs have been devised in the past 20 years, based on the hypothesis that parenting skills have an impact on children's disruptive behaviors. Dumas (1989) and Kazdin (1987) reviewed studies of the effects of these programs and both concluded that they were the most promising forms of intervention. If we are interested in verifying the hypothesis that parenting has an effect on the social development of disruptive boys, we must continue to ameliorate parent-management training programs so that they will be more successful in changing the parents' behavior, and then verify if a change in the child's behavior will occur.

But we are asking a lot from these training programs and from parents. Since the boys are already disruptive, training programs for parents appear to be based on the idea that parenting skills should succeed independently from the child's behavior. The child effect studies (Bell & Chapman, 1986) have shown that adults' behaviors toward children are strongly affected by the children's behaviors. If children's behavior could be changed *at the same time* as parents' behavior, we would expect that such concurrent changes would have a greater impact on preventing delinquency than if change occured only in the parents' behavior. Such a strategy for intervention, from a theory-based, causal perspective, confounds parents' and child behavior as "The" cause for future antisocial behavior. But it replaces the single-cause model by an interactive model that can be formulated as follows: the social development of a child is dependent on the interaction of his or her parents' parenting skills and the behavioral dispositions of the child himself or herself. Most studies of mother–infant interactions have indeed shown that they form an interactive system in which both partners are constantly affecting each other (Trevarthen, 1980; Tronick, Ricks, & Cohn, 1982). It would be surprising if this were not also the case when the infants have grown up to become cognitively and behaviorally more sophisticated. This truth appears to have been recognized for a number of centuries. Gouge (1627), in a volume on "domestical duties," outlines in detail the duties of the child toward his parents as well as the duties of the parents toward the child. There is no reason to believe that a one-sided approach, in a situation which is interactional, would change these interactions.

Evidence shows that poor peer relations are preceded by poor parent-child relationships (Putallaz & Heflin, 1990). One would not expect a child with significant behavior problems to have positive peer relations. The basics of positive communication between parent and child must be closely related to the basics of positive communication with other adults and peers. Thus, one would expect that social skills learned to interact with parents would generalize to peer relationships. Inversely, learning of interpersonal skills through social skills training would improve peer and parent relationships. Together, parent training and social skills training could prove successful in reducing disruptive behaviors and improving parent child interaction, whereas only one component could prove insufficient.

We have conducted a longitudinal–experimental study to describe the social interactions of disruptive boys during the primary school years, and also to verify the effects of both parent training and children's social skills training for the prevention of delinquent behavior. The aim of the experimental intervention was clearly pragmatic (see Schwartz, Flamant, & Lellouch, 1981). We were interested in the preventive impact of the intervention, but both forms of interventions were aimed at variables that have been postulated to be causes of delinquent behavior; poor parenting skills and poor social skills. Thus, if a change in these behaviors leads to lower delinquency involvement, these results could be interpreted as confirming the hypothesis that parenting skills *and* social skills are causally related to delinquent behavior. We did not have control groups that received *only* parent training or *only* social skills training. Thus the design did not enable us to see the extent to which both types of interventions are needed to prevent delinquent behavior. However, there are enough studies of each type of intervention to indicate the low level of their effectiveness when used individually (Dumas, 1989; Kazdin, 1987).

SUBJECTS AND RANDOMIZATION PROCEDURE

The study's population consisted of kindergarten boys from low socioeconomic areas of Montréal, a large metropolitan city with a 70% French population. To control for cultural effects, boys were included in the study only if both their biological parents were born in Canada and the parents' mother tongue was French. These criteria created a culturally homogeneous, white, francophone sample. To ensure that the sample would consist of boys from families of low socioeconomic background, we also eliminated each family in which either of the parents had more than 14 years of schooling. This criterion eliminated families in which a parent had completed postsecondary technical training (a 3-year program after high school), or had completed more than 2 years of college education.

Boys were assessed by their kindergarten teachers at the end of the school year, in May. Two questionnaires, the Preschool Behavior Questionnaire (Behar & Stringfield, 1974; Tremblay, Desmarais-Gervais, Gagnon, & Charlebois, 1987) and the Prosocial Behavior Questionnaire (Weir & Duveen, 1981), were mixed to form one containing 38 items. The resulting Social Behavior Questionnaire yields four components: disruptive (13 items), anxious (5 items), inattentive (4 items), and prosocial (10 items) (Tremblay, Loeber, Gagnon, Charlebois, Larivée, & LeBlanc, 1991). The disruptive factor was subdivided into three a priori categories of behavior (Loeber, Tremblay, Gagnon, & Charlebois, 1989): fighting (3 items), oppositional behavior (5 items), and hyperactivity (2 items). We obtained an 87% response rate from the kindergarten teachers. Questionnaires were received from 53 schools and 1161 boys were evaluated. After having eliminated subjects who did not meet the ethnic criteria or could not be reached to obtain the information, 1034 subjects were retained for the longitudinal study. This total sample has been followed yearly from age 10 onward (Tremblay, 1992). For example, teachers rated 96% of the boys at age 9, 90% at age 11, and 85% at age 12.

A random subsample ($n = 118$) of the 1161 boys was first created to obtain a small normative sample. For purposes of comparison with the disruptive boys, 43 nondisruptive boys were identified from among the randomly selected normative sample. All boys who had a disruptive score above the 70th percentile were considered to be "at risk."

These disruptive boys ($n = 319$) were randomly allocated to three groups. For each boy selected, a brief telephone interview with the mother verified whether the family met the criteria for ethnicity and education. If the family did not meet the criteria, or if it could not be found or refused to answer the relevant questions, the boy was excluded from the study. Altogether, 248 (78%) of the disruptive boys met the selection criteria.

The first of the at-risk groups was created for the experimental study of prevention. This treatment group, originally composed of 96 subjects, was reduced to 68 (71%) through the criterial screening. Among these, 46 families (68%) agreed to participate in the treatment program. The second of the three at-risk groups is called the observation group. This group is providing information for a longitudinal observational study of disruptive boys' social interactions (Tremblay, Gagnon, Vitaro, Boileau, & Charlebois, 1991). This group is equivalent to a no-treatment contact control group. In all, 152 boys were allocated to this group. After elimination of cases that failed to meet criteria and cases lost because the family had moved to an unknown address or could not be reached by telephone, 123 families (81%) remained. Each of these families was invited to participate in the study and 84 (68%) accepted. The last group of at-risk boys was created to act as a no-treatment, no-contact control group for assessing effects of the prevention experiment, and also for evaluating effects of the longitudinal follow-up. The control group consisted of 71 subjects when it was created and was reduced to 58 (80%) after considering the qualifying variables described above. In order to ensure that the control group was equivalent to the other two groups, each of which required consent, those assigned to the control group were asked if they would participate in the activities required for the observational group if the research team was able to include them. Among the control group, 42 families (72.4%) agreed to participate in the study. Consent from the control group not only contributed to making the three groups equivalent but also permitted the outcome assessments.

We compared the groups on kindergarten teacher ratings (evaluating disruptiveness, oppositional behavior, hyperactivity, fighting, anxiety, prosocial behavior, and inattentiveness) to see whether the randomization process had successfully created equivalent groups on the outcome variables we intended to measure, and whether the consent requirement had operated differently among the groups. No main effect was found for consent, but an interaction effect indicated that more families of boys who were frequent fighters consented among the treatment group than among the control or observation groups. A post hoc comparison of the consenters among the three groups showed that in no case did the treatment group differ significantly from the other two (Tremblay, McCord, Boileau, Charlebois, Gagnon, LeBlanc, & Larivée, 1991). The same type of analysis was done for family characteristics. There were no significant differences in number of children in the families, for family structure (intact, single-mother, other), for number of years mothers and fathers went to school, or for age of parents at birth of first child. The socioeconomic status of the treatment group mothers, based on last occupation, was significantly lower than that of the other two groups, but no significant differences were observed for the fathers' SES. There was also a significant difference in ages of parents at birth of subject. Mothers of the observational group were younger than the control group mothers, while fathers of the observational group were younger than fathers of the treated group.

TREATMENT

During the planning phase of the study in 1982–83, the Oregon Social Learning Center's work with parents (Patterson, 1982; Patterson, Reid, Jones, & Conger, 1975) appeared to us to be one of the most innovative training programs for parents with aggressive children. It was decided that techniques developed at the Oregon Social Learning Center would be a major component of the treatment program. Accordingly, the program coordinator was trained at the Center. In brief, the procedure involved: (1) giving parents a reading program; (2) training parents to monitor their children's behavior; (3) training parents to give positive reinforcement for prosocial behavior; (4) training parents to punish effectively without being abusive; (5) training parents to manage family crises; and (6) helping parents to generalize what they have learned. The parent training component was supplemented by eliciting cooperation from the teacher. Work with parents and teachers was carried out by two university-trained child-care workers, one psychologist, and one social worker, all working full-time. Each of these professionals had a caseload of 12 families. The team was coordinated by a fifth professional who worked on the project half-time. Work with the parents was planned to last for 2 school years with one session every 2 weeks. The professionals were, however, free to decide that a given family needed more or fewer sessions at any given time. The maximum number of sessions given to any family was 46 and the mean number of sessions over the 2 years was 17.4, counting families that refused to continue.

For the social skills training component of our intervention, two types of training were given to the disruptive boys within a small group of prosocial peers in school. During the first year a prosocial skills program was devised based on other programs (Cartledge & Milburn, 1980; Michelson, Sugai, Wood, & Kazdin, 1983; Schneider & Byrne, 1987). Nine sessions were given on themes such as "How to make contact," "How to help," "How to ask 'why?'," and "How to invite someone in a group." Coaching, peer modeling, role playing, and reinforcement contingencies were used during these sessions. During the second year the program aimed at self-control. Using material from previous studies (Camp, Blom, Hebert, & Van Doorminck, 1977; Goldstein, Sprafkin, Gershaw, & Klein, 1980; Kettlewell & Kausch, 1983; Meichenbaum, 1977), 10 sessions were developed on themes such as "Look and listen," "Following rules," "What to do when I am angry," "What to do when they do not want me to play with them," and "How to react to teasing." Coaching, peer modeling, self-instructions, behavior rehearsal, and reinforcement contingencies were also used during these sessions. This treatment too was offered by the professionals who provided parental training, although different workers assisted the parents and the child.

We also experimented with stimulating fantasy play and teaching the boys to be critical of television. However, because of lack of funds, only half the treated group ($n = 25$) received the fantasy play training and one fifth ($n = 9$) received the television intervention.

FOLLOW-UP ASSESSMENTS

After an assessment period of 4 months, the treatment lasted 2 school years (September 1985 to June 1987). The boys were in treatment from an average age of 7 to an average age of 9. Behavior ratings were obtained from teachers, peers, mothers, and subjects themselves each year since the spring of 1987.

Teacher and mother ratings were obtained with the Social Behavior Questionnaire that had been used for the original assessments in kindergarten. This questionnaire yielded main factor scores for disruptive behavior, anxiety, inattentiveness, and prosocial behavior. Additionally, the disruptive factor was subdivided into fighting, oppositional behavior, and hyperactivity.

Subject and peer assessments were obtained with the Pupil Evaluation Inventory (PEI; Pekarik, Prinz, Liebert, Weintraub, & Neale, 1976). The PEI contains 34 short behavior descriptors. Each child in the class of at least one of our subjects was asked to identify four children in his class who were best described by each of the items. Children responded to the PEI in a group format. The PEI yields three factors: disruptive behavior,[1] containing 20 items (e.g., Those who can't sit still; Those who start a fight over nothing; Those who are rude to the teacher); withdrawal, with 9 items (e.g., Those who are too shy to make friends easily; Those whose feelings are easily hurt; Those who are unhappy or sad); and likability, with 5 items (e.g., Those who are liked by everyone; Those who help others; Those who are especially nice). Each rater can nominate himself for each item, so the instrument provides both a self-rating and a peer rating for each scale.

At age 10 (spring 1988), the boys answered a 27-item self-report antisocial behavior questionnaire asking them to report if they had ever been involved in antisocial behavior (LeBlanc & Fréchette, 1989). The questions enabled measurement both of frequency and of range of involvement. The questions asked about misbehavior in the home (including fighting, theft, and vandalism) and outside the home (including fighting, theft, vandalism, and trespassing), and about drinking alcohol and using illegal drugs. In the following years the same questions were modified to obtain answers about involvement in antisocial behavior during the past 12 months.

To measure achievement in school, grade point average in mathematics and French were obtained from the files of the schoolboard. However, grade point average is related to the school level, so a boy who was held back could have a relatively high grade point average compared to another at his age-appropriate level. We thus decided that being in a regular classroom appropriate for their age provided a better measure of school achievement.

To provide a *global assessment of adjustment*, children were classified as *well adjusted* if they were in a regular classroom at the appropriate level for their age and were also rated by teachers and peers below the 70th percentile in disruptive behavior. Children were classified as having *few difficulties* if they were in a regular classroom appropriate for their age but were rated above the 70th percentile by peers or teachers; or were not disruptive (i.e., were rated below the 70th percentile in disruptive behavior by peers and teachers), and were in a regular classroom but not at the level appropriate for their age. Children classified as having *serious difficulties* were both not in a regular classroom at the level appropriate for their age and rated by peers or teachers above the 70th percentile on disruptive behavior. Children who were placed in a special environment be-

---

1. This factor was originally labeled "Aggression," but it contains only two clear physical aggression items. The content is similar to the disruptive factor of the SBQ.

cause of their adjustment problems in school (special class, special school, residential institution) were automatically classified as having serious difficulties.

RESULTS

Achievement in School

To obtain a general estimate of achievement in school we charted the percentage of boys who were in an age-appropriate regular grade. That is, at age 7 they should have been in grade 1, at age 9 they should have been in grade 3, and so on. Results are presented in Figure 6.1. It can be seen that at age 12 only 62% of the whole sample were in a regular sixth grade. This is a good indication that our original sample was taken from a population that is at high risk for psychosocial adjustment problems. We can observe that there were no significant

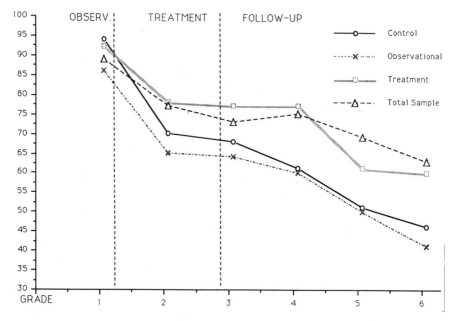

FIGURE 6.1 Percent in age-appropriate regular grade from grade 1 to 6. For grade 1: age = 7, $\chi^2 = 0.36$, $p = .55$. For grade 2: age = 8, $\chi^2 = 1.87$, $p = .17$. For grade 3: age = 9, $\chi^2 = 2.14$, $p = .14$. For grade 4: age = 10, $\chi^2 = 4.15$, $p = .04$. For grade 5: age = 11, $\chi^2 = 1.43$, $p = .23$. For grade 6: age = 12, $\chi^2 = 3.95$, $p = .05$. χ^2 compares the treatment group to both the observational and control groups.

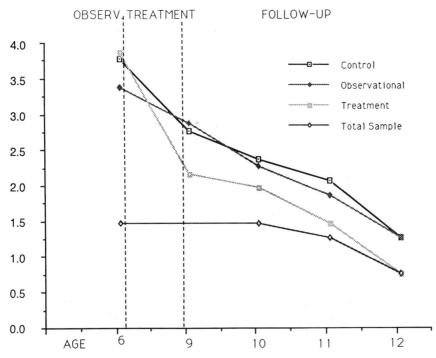

FIGURE 6.2 Teacher-rated fighting from age 6 to 12 (adjusted scores at age 9–12). For age 6: $F = 1.67$; $p = .19$. For age 9: $F = 3.33$; $p = .07$. For age 10: $F = 1.06$; $p = .31$. For age 11: $F = 1.55$; $p = .22$. For age 12: $F = 4.69$; $p = .03$. F is based on a comparison of the treatment group with the observational and control groups combined.

differences at age 6, before treatment.[2] During treatment, at age 8 and 9 the treated group started to differentiate itself from the control and observational group. The year after the end of treatment the difference was significant. There was some form of relapse at age 11. But at age 12, the last year of primary school, we still had a significant difference between the treated and not treated high-risk boys.

Teacher-Rated Fighting

One of the major aims of our treatment was to reduce the boys' aggressive behavior. Teacher ratings of the boys' fighting behavior from the end of kindergarten at age 6 to the end of primary school at age 12 are presented in Figure 6.2. These results show that the

2. The χ^2 compares the treatment group to the combined observational and control groups. There were no significant differences between the observational and control groups at any age.

treatment achieved its aim to a certain extent. We can see that at age 6, in kindergarten, the treatment group had the highest fighting score. At age 9, when treatment ended, the treated group mean fighting score was lower than the control and observational group. At age 12, three years after treatment, the treatment group had a mean fighting score identical to the mean of the total sample, whereas the control and observational group had a significantly higher mean fighting score. Note that the scores from age 9 to age 12 were adjusted with a covariance procedure, using age 6 fighting scores in order to correct for differences among the groups before treatment started. The difference at age 12 remained significant when the groups were compared without the introduction of the covariate ($t = 2.02$, $p = .04$).

Global School Adjustment

We created an index to take into account both school behavior problems and school performance. To be classified as having serious school adjustment problems, a boy needed to be rated among the 30% most disruptive by his teacher or his peers and not be in his age-appropriate regular grade or be placed in a special environment. We first computed this index at the end of treatment, when the boys were age 9. The treatment group tended to have fewer boys with serious adjustment problems than the nontreatment groups, although the difference was not significant. We computed the same index 3 years later, when the boys were age 12. The mean disruptive scores at ages 11 and 12 was used with the grade status at age 12. Mean scores of 2 school years for behavior problems are probably a better reflection of the subjects' adjustment level, since it captures ratings from two different teachers and two somewhat different sets of peers over 2 years. Results presented in Figure 6.3 clearly show that the treated group had proportionally more well-adjusted boys (29% vs. 19%), and fewer boys with serious difficulties. There were twice as many boys with serious difficulties in the nontreatment groups (44%) as there were in the treatment group (22%). When the comparison between the treated and not-treated boys was made using the dichotomy "serious difficulties versus others," the chi-square test indicated that there was only 1% chance of making an error in rejecting the null hypothesis ($\chi^2 = 6.40$, $df = 1$) concerning the interaction between treatment status and adjustment.

In order to test if these differences could be due to differences already present in kindergarten, we did a discriminant function analysis, where the two groups to be predicted were the boys with serious difficulties and those without these serious difficulties, as defined in

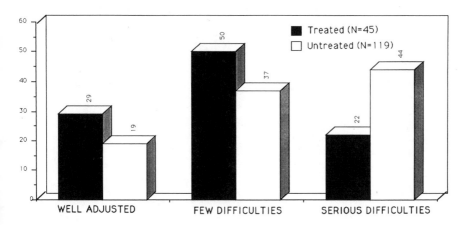

FIGURE 6.3 Percent of treated and untreated boys in different school adjustment groups at age 11–12. $\chi^2 = 6.49$; $p = .04$; $df = 2$.

the previous analysis. It should be noted here that the groups were created without reference to the fact that they were treated or not. Treatment, in this analysis, was considered a predictor that would discriminate between the groups created on the basis of their adjustment level at age 11–12. The predictors where (1) the kindergarten behaviors: fighting, hyperactivity, inattentiveness, anxiety, prosociality; (2) an index of family adversity, created with family structure, parents' education, parents' age at birth of first child, and parents occupational status (Tremblay, Loeber, Gagnon, Charlebois, Larivée, & LeBlanc, 1991); (3) having received the treatment or not. It was expected that if treatment had an effect on adjustment level at age 11–12, over and above behavioral problems and family adversity, which were present before treatment started, it would be a significant predictor in the discriminant function analysis.

Table 6.1 shows the results of the discriminant function analysis. Family adversity in kindergarten had the highest standardized canonical discriminant function coefficient (.70), followed by the presence or absence of treatment (.54), disruptive behavior in kindergarten (.49), and anxiety in kindergarten (.33). From these results it is clear that treatment explains part of the outcome in adjustment problems at the end of primary school after the level of family adversity before treatment has been taken into account. Treatment is also a better predictor of outcome than differences in behavior before the treatment started. The discriminant function correctly classified 69% of

TABLE 6.1. Results of discriminant Function Analysis to Predict Boys with Serious School Adjustment Problems at Age 11-12

Predictors	SCDF coefficients	Wilks lambda
Family adversity in kindergarten	.70	.91
Treatment (Y-N)	.54	.85
Disruptive in kindergarten	.49	.84
Anxiety in kindergarten	−.33	.83
Hyperactivity in kindergarten	−.28	.82
Inattentiveness in kindergarten	.21	.82
Total cases correctly classified	69% (112/162)	
True positives cases	69% (42/61)	
True negatives cases	69% (70/101)	

Note. Canonical correlations = .43; $p = .000$.

the subjects, including 69% of the true positives and 69% of the true negatives.

Onset of Delinquent Behavior

One of the important aims of our intervention was to prevent delinquent behavior. The boys in our study have not yet reached the age of intense delinquency involvement, but early onset of delinquent behavior is a predictor of later serious delinquency (Farrington et al., 1990). We have data on self-reported delinquent behavior form age 10 to age 12. Results indicating the preventive effects of the experiment on early onset of self-reported delinquency are presented in Table 6.2. At age 10 (1 year after treatment) the boys were given a list of 27 delinquent acts and asked how often they had ever been involved in

TABLE 6.2. Percentage of Boys Ever Involved in Selected Delinquent Behaviors Up to Age 12

	Treated ($n = 42$)	Untreated ($n = 118$)	χ^2
Trespassing	40%	62%	5.76**
Taking objects worth < $10	19%	45%	9.01***
Taking objects worth > $10	7%	20%	3.85*
Stealing bicycles	5%	19%	5.10**

*$p < .05$
**$p < .03$
***$p < .003$

such acts. Then at ages 11 and 12 they were given the same list and asked how often they were involved in the acts during the past 12 months. The percentage of boys from the treated and not-treated groups who reported to have ever been involved in a given delinquent behavior up to age 12 are reported for each item for which there was a significant difference. It can be observed that for all four behaviors where there was a significant difference, a smaller percentage of the treated group were involved: fewer treated boys reported trespassing, stealing objects worth less and more than $10, and stealing bicycles.

Mothers' Perception of Antisocial Behavior

All the results presented above indicate that the treatment has had beneficial effects. These results were based on teacher and peer ratings as well as self-reports. Our intervention was focused on parent training and social skills training. We expected that both parent training and social skills training would have an impact on the boys' social adjustment. This appears to have been the case with regard to school adjustment and general delinquency. How about home adjustment? One would expect that if parent training has had an impact on school adjustment and general delinquency, it would also have an impact on social adjustment at home. Mothers rated the behavior of their sons each year in the spring at the same time as did teachers and peers.

Results from mother ratings indicate that treatment had a short-term paradoxical effect on mother's perceptions, but no long-term effects were observed. Indeed, at the end of treatment, when the boys were age 9, the treated boys' mothers reported that their sons were more disruptive compared to mothers of the nontreated boys ($M_1 = 13.11$; $M_2 = 10.87$; $t = 2.48$, $p = .02$), fought more ($M_1 = 2.78$; $M_2 = 1.85$; $t = 3.08$; $p = .003$), and were more inattentive ($M_1 = 5.19$, $M_2 = 4.52$; $t = 1.99$, $p = .05$). These significant differences had disappeared by age 10 and were not observed again at age 11 or 12. Since part of the parent training program was focused on helping parents monitor their boys' behavior, mothers of the treated group could be expected to report more accurately their child's behavior. If this were the case, we would have to conclude that mothers who did not receive the parent training underreport their sons' disruptive behavior. There was an indication that this was indeed the case when we compared mothers' report of their sons' stealing to the sons' self-report of stealing. Table 6.2 indicates that 45% of the untreated boys reported having stolen objects worth less than $10, compared to 19% of the treated boys. Mothers were asked if their son ever steals, and how often. The percentage of mothers, from both treated and untreated groups, who reported their son between ages 9 and 12 to "sometime or often" steal varied between 20% and 25%; there was never more than a 4% difference between the two groups in any given year. Thus, the reports of the mothers from the treated group appears to be close to their sons' reports, while mothers from the nontreated groups clearly underestimated their sons' stealing behavior.

Parent Behavior

If parent training had an impact on a boys' behavior, we expect that this will be because it modified parents' behaviors meant to be changed by the training. Our research program did not include direct observation of parenting behaviors for the treated group during or after treatment. This is clearly a necessary procedure if we want to establish a causal link between changes in parent behavior and changes in the child's behavior. But there is an indirect way to measure changes in parents' behavior: through the sons' perceptions of their parents' behavior. There is a possibility that the changes in a parent's behavior that have the greatest impact on a boy's behavior would be those that the boy himself has perceived. This idea is somewhat speculative since one could argue that children are far from being conscious of parent behaviors having an effect on them. But, since part of our knowledge of the relationship between parenting behavior and antisocial behavior comes from the child's report of his parent's behavior (Hirschi, 1969), the former should help understand the causal links between parent training and antisocial behavior.

Each year, from age 10 onward, the boys were asked a series of questions on their relationship with their fathers and their mothers. Some of these questions referred to parental monitoring and discipline, the basis of the parent training program. Of 15 questions asked each year for 3 years, such as "Do your parents physically punish you," "Do your parents praise you when you have behaved well," "Is there a rule about how late you can stay out at night," "Do your parents know where you are when you are out of the house," "Do your parents know with whom you are when you are out of the house," there was only one significant difference between the treated and untreated groups: at age 12 the boys from the untreated group reported more often than those from the treated group that there was a rule at home concerning the friends with whom they could play ($M_1 = 21\%$; $M_2 = 38\%$; $\chi^2 = 3.95$, $df = 1$, $p = .05$).[3] Clearly, there

---

3. No significant differences when the items were grouped into scales for monitoring and disciplining.

was no indication from the boys' perception of their parents' behavior that the treatment had an effect on the parents' monitoring and disciplining behavior. One could argue that the lack of significant differences between the treated and untreated subjects could be due to a lack of sensitivity of the measures. However, developmental changes within groups appears to rule out this hypothesis. For example, reports of physical punishment by parents were made by 70% of the boys at age 10 and only 42% at age 12.

DISCUSSION

The aim of our experimental study was to help prevent the antisocial behavior of boys who were disruptive in kindergarten. Although this aim was clearly pragmatic, it offered the opportunity to test the hypothesis that poor parental management of disruptive boys contributes to the development of antisocial behavior.

The results from 3 years of follow-up (from ages 9 to 12), after 2 years of treatment (at ages 7 and 8) indicated that the treated disruptive boys were less physically aggressive in school, that they were more often in an age-appropriate regular classroom, that they had less serious school adjustment problems, and that they reported fewer delinquent behaviors. A discriminant function analysis indicated that treatment helped discriminate between the well-adjusted and not-well-adjusted boys, after having controlled for family adversity.

Thus, there are relatively strong indications that the intervention was successful in helping some of the kindergarten disruptive boys. It is still too early to confirm that treatment has helped prevent juvenile delinquency. Although the treated group was better adjusted on a number of important indicators, there were no significant differences on other indicators (e.g., hyperactivity, prosociality, vandalism). If fighting, stealing, and poor school adjustment between age 9 and 12 are important precursors of later delinquency (Farrington et al., 1990), there is a chance that our intervention succeeded in breaking the path between childhood disruptive behavior and juvenile delinquency (Tremblay, 1992). Eron (1990) has suggested that aggressive antisocial behavior crystallizes around age 8. Our intervention between age 7 and age 9 may have hit a sensitive period in some of these boys' social development. Other experiments will have to show if these results can be replicated. Still others should aim at younger boys to see if the effects can be greater at an earlier age. There is a possibility that in the worst of cases antisocial behavior crystallizes much before age 8.

Although our treatment program, which included parent management training and social skills training, appears to have had an impact on the course of disruptive boys' development, we need further evidence to attribute the changes in the boys' behavior to changes in parent management, and thus confirm the theory that parent management is an important cause of antisocial behavior. An attempt was made to obtain such evidence by analyzing the boys' perceptions of their parents' monitoring and disciplining strategies. We did not observe any differences between the treated and untreated group that would indicate that the group of parents who received training had better management strategies. Although these results do not prove that parent training did not change parent monitoring and disciplining techniques in the long run, they do show that disruptive boys' behavior can be changed without changing their perception of their parents' monitoring and disciplining techniques. This is an indication that we should not attribute a causal effect to the correlation between self-reported delinquency and perceptions of parental management. Parent training may have indirect effects on their children's disruptive behavior. For example, parent training may have a general impact on parents' attitudes toward child rearing without changing their "style" of interaction with the child. They may, for instance, meet teachers more often, be more receptive to teachers' comments, and thus change teachers' attitudes toward the parents and the child. In turn, parents may adopt more positive attitudes toward school and foster positive expectancies towards school for their son. In this way parent training would have an effect on the type of environment parents create for their child, without necessarily changing their behavioral style with the child.

Few investigators disagree with the statement that experimental studies are better than longitudinal studies to verify causal effects. However, causal effects are extremely hard to clearly demonstrate in the field of human development. A large number of experimental studies with long-term follow-ups will have to be undertaken before we start really understanding the complexity of child rearing and child development. This could be a discouraging statement for those who want to help at-risk children *now*. They should find comfort in the results from this experiment and others presented in this book. Experiments are useful not only to test theories but also to show that a given intervention achieves its aim. In most of these cases we cannot demonstrate that the cause-effect mechanism works exactly the way it was planned. We still do not know exactly how aspirin relieves pain or how certain drugs reduce hallucinations. But we know that a particular medication for a particular syndrome generally has a beneficial effect. We are starting to obtain evidence that particular deviant behaviors can be prevented by a particular set of interventions. What we urgently need are experimental replications that will show that these positive effects are not the product of a unique set of circumstances.

ACKNOWLEDGMENTS

This study was funded by the following agencies: National Welfare Grants Program of the Canadian Ministry of Health and Welfare, Conseil Québécois de la Recherche Sociale, Conseil de la Santé et des Services Sociaux Régional du Montréal Métropolitain, Fondation Cité des Prairies, Fonds FCAR-Centre et Équipes, Institut de la Recherche en Psycho-Éducation de Monréal, and Centre d'Accueil le Mainbourg. Lucie Bertrand, Rita Béland, Michel Bouillon, Raymond Labelle, Hélène O'Reilly, and Daniel Reclus-Prince performed the intervention. Pierre Charlebois, Claude Gagnon, and Serge Larivée collaborated on the planning and execution of the longitudinal study. Danièle Royal and Minh T. Trinh provided the documentation, and Chantal Bruneau typed the manuscript.

REFERENCES

Bates, J. E., Bayles, K., Bennett, D. S., Ridge, B., & Brown, M.M. (1991). Origins of externalizing behavior problems at eight years of age. In D. J. Pepler & K. H. Rubin (Eds.), *The development and treatment of childhood aggression* (pp. 93–120). Hillsdale, NJ: Erlbaum.

Behar, L. B., & Stringfield, S. (1974). A behavior rating scale for the preschool child. *Developmental Psychology, 10*, 601–610.

Bell, R. O., & Chapman, M. (1986). Child effects in studies using experimental or brief longitudinal approaches to socialization. *Developmental Psychology, 22*, 595–603.

Camp, B. W., Blom, G. E., Hebert, F., & Van Doorminck, W. J. (1977). Think Aloud: A program for developing self-control in young aggressive boys. *Journal of Abnormal Child Psychology, 5*(2), 157–169.

Campbell, S. B. (1990). The socialization and social development of hyperactive children. In M. Lewis & S. M. Miller (Eds.), *Handbook of developmental psychopathology* (pp. 77–91). New York: Plenum Press.

Cartledge, G., & Milburn, J. F. (1980). *Teaching social skills to children. Innovative approaches* (pp. 92–109). New York: Pergamon Press.

Cloninger, C. R., & Gottesman, I. I. (1987). Genetic and environmental factors in antisocial behavior disorders. In S. A. Mednick, T. E. Moffitt, & S. A. Stack (Eds.), *The causes of crime: New biological approaches* (pp. 92–109). New York: Cambridge University Press.

Dumas, J. E. (1989). Treating antisocial behavior in children: Child and family approaches. *Clinical Psychology Review, 9*, 197–222.

Eron, L. D. (1990). Understanding aggression. *Bulletin of the International Society for Research on Aggression, 12,* 5–9.

Eron, L. D., Huesmann, L. R., & Zelli, A. (1991). The role of parental variables in the learning of aggression. In D. J. Pepler & K. H. Rubin (Eds.), *The development and treatment of childhood aggression* (pp. 169–188). Hillsdale, NJ: Erlbaum.

Farrington, D. P., Loeber, R., Elliott, D. S., Hawkins, J. D., Kandel, D. B., Klein, M. W., McCord, J., Rowe, D. C., & Tremblay, R. E. (1990). Advancing knowledge about the onset of delinquency and crime. In B. B. Lahey & A. E. Kazdin (Eds.), *Advances in clinical child psychology* (pp. 283–342). New York: Plenum Press.

Farrington, D. P., Ohlin, L. E., & Wilson, J. Q. (1986). *Understanding and controlling crime: Towards a new research strategy.* New York: Springer-Verlag.

Goldstein, A. P., Sprafkin, R. P., Gershaw, N. J., & Klein, P. (1980). The adolescent: Social skills training through structured learning. In G. Cartledge & J. F. Milburn, (Eds.), *Teaching social skills to children: Innovative approaches* (pp. 249–277). New York: Pergamon Press.

Gottfredson, M., & Hirschi, T. (1987). The methodological adequacy of longitudinal research on crime. *Criminology, 25,* 581–614.

Gouge, W. (1627). *The workes of William Gouge: Vol. 1. Domesticall duties.* London.

Hirschi, T. (1969). *Causes of delinquency.* Berkeley and Los Angeles: University of California Press.

Huesmann, L. R., Eron, L. D., Lefkowitz, M. M., & Walder, L. O. (1984). Stability of aggression over time and generations. *Developmental Psychology, 20,* 1120–1134.

Kazdin, A. E. (1987). Treatment of antisocial behavior in children: Current status and future directions. *Psychological Bulletin, 102,* 187–203.

Kettlewell, P. W., & Kausch, D. F. (1983). The generalization of the effects of a cognitive behavioral treatment program for aggressive children. *Journal of Abnormal Child Psychology, 11,* 101–114.

LeBlanc, M., & Fréchette, M. (1989). *Male criminal activity from childhood through youth.* New York: Springer-Verlag.

Loeber, R., & Stouthamer-Loeber, M. (1986). Family factors as correlates and predictors of juvenile conduct problems and delinquency. In M. Tonry & N. Morris (Eds.), *Crime and justice: An annual review* (pp. 29–149). Chicago: University of Chicago Press.

Loeber, R., Tremblay, R. E., Gagnon, C., & Charlebois, P. (1989). Continuity and desistance in boys' early fighting at school. *Development and Psychopathology, 1,* 39–50.

Lytton, H. (1990). Child and parent effects in boys' conduct disorder: A reinterpretation. *Developmental Psychology, 26,* 683–697.

McCord, J. (1978). A thirty-year follow-up of treatment effects. *American Psychologist, 33,* 284–289.

Mednick, S. A., Gabrielli, W. F., & Hutchings, B. (1987). Genetic factors in the etiology of criminal behavior. In S. A. Mednick, T. E. Moffitt, &

S. A. Stack (Eds.), *The causes of crime: New biological approaches* (pp. 74–91). New York: Cambridge University Press.

Meichenbaum, D. (1977). *Cognitive-behavior modification: An integrative approach.* New York: Plenum Press.

Michelson, L., Sugai, D., Wood, R., & Kazdin, A. E. (1983). *Social skills assessment and training with children.* New York: Plenum Press.

Patterson, G. R. (1982). *Coercive family process.* Eugene, OR: Castalia.

Patterson, G. R., Reid, J. B., Jones, R. R., & Conger, R. E. (1975). *A social learning approach to family intervention: Vol. 1. Families with aggressive children.* Eugene, OR: Castalia.

Pekarik, E. G., Prinz, R. J., Liebert, D. E., Weintraub, S., & Neale, J. M. (1976). The Pupil Evaluation Inventory: A sociometric technique for assessing children's social behavior. *Journal of Abnormal Child Psychology, 4,* 83–97.

Plomin, R., DeFries, J. C., & Fulker, D. W. (1988). *Nature and nurture during infancy and early childhood.* New York: Cambridge University Press.

Putallaz, M., & Heflin, A. H. (1990). Parent-child interaction. In S. R. Asher & J. D. Coie (Eds.), *Peer rejection in childhood* (pp. 189–216). New York: Cambridge University Press.

Rowe, D., & Osgood, D. W. (1990). A latent trait approach to unifying criminal careers. *Criminology, 28,* 237–270.

Schwartz, D., Flamant, R., & Lellouch, J. (1981). *Clinical trials.* New York: Academic Press.

Schneider, B. H., & Byrne, B. M. (1987). Individualizing social skills training for behavior-disordered children. *Journal of Consulting and Clinical Psychology, 55*(3), 444–445.

Tonry, M., Ohlin, L. E., Farrington, D. P., Adams, K., Earls, F., Rowe, D. C., Sampson, R. J., & Tremblay, R. E. (1991). *Human development and criminal behavior: New ways of advancing knowledge.* New York: Springer-Verlag.

Tremblay, R. E. (1992). The prediction of delinquent behavior from childhood behavior: Personality theory revisited. In J. McCord (Ed.), *Advances in criminological theory: Vol. 3. Facts, frameworks, and forecasts* (pp. 193–230). New Brunswick, NJ: Transactions.

Tremblay, R. E., Desmarais-Gervais, L., Gagnon, C., & Charlebois, P. (1987). The Preschool Behavior Questionnaire: Stability of its factor structure between cultures, sexes, ages and socioeconomic classes. *International Journal of Behavioral Development, 10,* 467–484.

Tremblay, R. E., Gagnon, C., Vitaro, F., Boileau, H., & Charlebois, P. (1991). *The prediction of conduct disorder in early adolescence from childhood laboratory observations of parent–child interactions.* Paper presented at the Third Annual Meeting of the Society for Research in Child and Adolescent Psychopathology, Zandvoort, The Netherlands.

Tremblay, R. E., Loeber, R., Gagnon, C., Charlebois, P., Larivée, S., & LeBlanc, M. (1991). Disruptive boys with stable and unstable high fighting behavior patterns during junior elementary school. *Journal of Abnormal Child Psychology, 19,* 285–300.

Tremblay, R. E., McCord, J., Boileau, H., Charlebois, P., Gagnon, C., LeBlanc, M., & Larivée, S. (1991). Can disruptive boys be helped to become competent? *Psychiatry, 54,* 148-161.

Trevarthen, C. (1980). The foundations of intersubjectivity: Development of interpersonal and cooperative understanding in infants. In D. R. Olson (Eds.), *The foundations of language and thought* (pp. 316-342). New York: Norton.

Tronick, E. Z., Ricks, M., & Cohn, J. F. (1982). Maternal and infant affective exchange: Patterns of adaptation. In T. Field & A. Fogel (Eds.), *Emotion and early interaction* (pp. 83-100). Hillsdale, NJ: Erlbaum.

Weir, K., & Duveen, G. (1981). Further development and validation of the prosocial behaviour questionnaire for use by teachers. *Journal of Child Psychology and Psychiatry, 22*(4), 357-374.

CHAPTER 7

◆ ─────── ◆

The Seattle Social Development Project:
Effects of the First Four Years on Protective Factors and Problem Behaviors

J. DAVID HAWKINS
RICHARD F. CATALANO
DIANE M. MORRISON
JULIE O'DONNELL
ROBERT D. ABBOTT
L. EDWARD DAY

Adolescent health and behavior problems including drug abuse and delinquency remain major concerns. Importantly, an early onset of delinquent behavior or of drug use has been shown to be predictive of prolonged involvement in serious crime (Farrington et al., 1990) and drug abuse (Robins & Przybeck, 1985). Moreover, patterned serious delinquent behavior and chronic drug abuse often co-occur (Elliott, Huizinga, & Menard, 1989). There is evidence that these behaviors are predicted by a common set of risk factors observable in childhood (Hawkins, Jenson, Catalano, & Lishner, 1988). It also appears that the greater the number of risk factors to which an individual is exposed, the greater is that individual's risk of developing drug abuse problems (Bry, McKeon, & Pandina, 1982; Newcomb, Maddahian, & Bentler, 1986) and delinquency (Kolvin, Miller, Fleeting, & Kolvin, 1988). These findings suggest the importance of preventing the early initia-

139

tion of alcohol and other drug use and delinquent behavior in childhood and early adolescence, well before detection and legal intervention or treatment are likely (Ellickson & Bell, 1990). Thus, effective strategies for preventing the onset of delinquent behavior and drug use are required.

Most substance-abuse prevention studies have focused on the prevention of tobacco, alcohol, and marijuana use among children in grades 6 through 9. The most promising of these interventions have sought to help young adolescents to develop strong norms against drug use and skills to refuse drug offers (Ellickson & Bell, 1990; Pentz et al., 1989). They have shown modest, significant effects on tobacco and marijuana initiation rates in general population samples (Botvin & Wills, 1985; Ellickson & Bell, 1990; Flay, 1985; Hansen, Johnson, Flay, Graham, & Sobel, 1988; Pentz et al., 1989) as well as in specific communities of color (Botvin et al., 1989; Schinke, Bebel, Orlandi, & Botvin, 1988; Schinke, Botvin, Trimble, Orlandi, Gilchrist, & Locklear, 1988). However, these interventions have not proven effective with early initiators of tobacco use characterized by childhood experiences of early conduct problems, low academic achievement, low commitment to school, and high levels of family conflict (Ellickson & Bell, 1990). These factors have all been identified as childhood antecedents of both early drug use and delinquency (Farrington & Hawkins, 1991; Loeber, 1988; Rutter & Giller, 1983; Shedler & Block, 1990). Their discovery has focused interest on efforts to reduce shared childhood risk factors for health and behavior problems.

Even when broadened to include family, school, and community levels of intervention (Pentz et al., 1989), recently reported drug abuse prevention efforts have confined their focus largely to risk factors that become salient at the point of drug-use initiation, specifically norms regarding drug use and social influences to use drugs. Alcohol and other drug abuse preventive interventions typically have not sought to address risk factors that appear earlier in childhood and that characterize those who initiate drug use early. These childhood risk factors for drug abuse include poor and inconsistent family management practices, high levels of family conflict, low bonding to family, early conduct disorders, academic failure, low commitment to school, early peer rejection, association with antisocial peers, alienation and rebelliousness, attitudes favorable to drug use, and an early onset of drug use itself (Hawkins, Catalano, & Miller, 1992). Typically, alcohol is the drug first used by children.

Interventions in related fields have addressed some of the childhood risk factors for delinquency and drug abuse. Early childhood education has been found to be a cost-effective intervention to improve academic and social competence and to reduce rates of crime in adolescence (Berrueta-Clement, Schweinhart, Barnett, Epstein, & Weikhart, 1984), though effects on drug use have not been investigated. Separately, parent training programs and teacher training programs have shown positive effects on conduct problems and school performance of elementary-aged children (Bank, Patterson, & Reid, 1987; Comer, 1988; Dumas, 1989; Hawkins & Lam, 1987; Michelson, 1987; Slavin, 1991; Tremblay et al., 1990). However, with some exceptions (Tremblay et al., 1991), these interventions have focused on changing either family risk factors *or* school risk factors, not both. If exposure to a greater number of risk factors during childhood increases risk exponentially, as suggested by Rutter (1980) and Newcomb, Maddahian, Skager, and Bentler (1987), then interventions that target multiple childhood risk factors in both family and school domains appear worthy of exploration. Few controlled studies have reported on the effects of simultaneous intervention in family and school contexts as a preventive intervention for delinquency and drug abuse. Little is known about the effectiveness of interventions focused on multiple risk factors in family and school contexts in the elementary grades. In fact, few previous studies have sought to prevent both delinquency and drug abuse by addressing childhood precursors or risk factors common to both types of behavior.

This chapter reports the results of 4 years of experimental intervention with teachers and parents of a multiethnic panel of children as they passed from grades 1 through 4 in eight schools of an urban school district. The Seattle Social Development Project sought to reduce shared childhood risk factors for delinquency and drug abuse by enhancing factors hypothesized by the social development model to protect against both types of behavior.

The intervention was guided theoretically by the social development model (Farrington & Hawkins, 1991; Hawkins & Lam, 1987; Hawkins & Weis, 1985), an integration of social control (Hirschi, 1969) and social learning (Akers, Krohn, Lanza-Kaduce, & Radosevich, 1979; Bandura, 1977) theories. Following control theory (Hirschi, 1969), the social development model hypothesizes that strong bonds to family and school serve as protective factors against delinquency and drug abuse. In the social development model, bonding consists of three elements: *attachment*, a positive emotional or affective feeling toward others; *commitment*, a sense of investment in a social unit; and *belief* in the general morals or values held by a social unit. Such bonds are hypothesized to moderate the effects of social norms regarding specific behaviors such as drug use or delinquent acts. To the extent that children are bonded to family and/or school, the social norms prevalent in these social units are expected to influence their behaviors. Thus, both bonding and clear norms proscribing delinquent or drug-using behavior are hypothesized as protective factors against delinquency and drug use in the model.

In designing the intervention reported here, we reasoned that during the early elementary grades prevention intervention should focus on promoting the development of strong bonds to family and school so that children would be motivated to adhere to the behavioral standards advanced by those social units. We assumed that the levels of bonding to family and school established in childhood influence the extent to which individuals will subscribe to norms against drug use promoted by family members, school personnel, or peers enlisted in classroom drug abuse prevention programs. We also assumed that levels of bonding would influence the extent to which children exposed to training in resistance or refusal skills would actually use those skills when confronted with an opportunity to participate in delinquency or drug use. We hypothesized that, as a protective factor, bonding to family and school is a necessary precondition for the endorsement of antidrug norms and for the use of refusal skills included in widely tested and disseminated school-based drug abuse prevention interventions. The experimental intervention during grades 1 through 4 did not teach skills to resist influences to use drugs and did not seek to directly affect children's norms regarding delinquent behavior or drug use in these early elementary grades. In this respect, the intervention is distinct from most previously tested drug abuse prevention interventions.

Instead, the intervention sought to affect the processes by which bonding to family and school are hypothesized to develop. The model hypothesizes that an individual's level of bonding to a social unit is determined by the amount of opportunity for involvement available to the individual in that social unit; by the skills that the individual applies in participating in the social unit; and by the reinforcements provided by the unit for the individual's behavior. The social development model's focus on skills and reinforcements is derived from social learning theory. In the present study, we sought to intervene in families and school classrooms to increase the levels of opportunity for prosocial involvement, to increase the levels of children's skills for successful participation in those social units, and to increase the reinforcements forthcoming from those social units for prosocial participation. We hypothesized that interventions that achieved these goals would lead to stronger bonding to family and to school, and in turn to lower rates of early initiation of drug use and delinquent behavior. The intervention sought explicitly to reduce identified risk factors for drug abuse and delinquency of poor and inconsistent family management practices, early conduct disorders, peer rejection, and academic failure, by introducing multiple interventions in families and schools. All of the component interventions were selected or designed for consistency with the social development model and were aimed at promoting conditions conducive to the development of strong bonds to family, school, and prosocial peers, namely opportunities, skills, and reinforcements for prosocial involvement in family and in the school classroom.

METHODS

The Seattle Social Development Project is a longitudinal field experiment following a group of multiethnic urban students who entered the first grade in eight Seattle Public Schools in 1981. At that time, two schools were assigned to be full control or full experimental intervention sites. In the remaining six schools, entering first grade students were assigned to intervention and control classrooms randomly (see Hawkins, Von Cleve, & Catalano, 1991). During grades 1–4, newly entering students to project schools were assigned randomly to experimental and control classrooms and added to the panel. In 1985, when the initial subjects entered the fifth grade, the panel was expanded to include all fifth grade students in 18 Seattle elementary schools, which resulted in the recapture of some intervention students and the addition of more control children to the study.[1] The project tested an intervention combining modified teaching practices in mainstream classrooms and parent training designed to be developmentally appropriate as students progressed through grades 1, 2, 3, and 4. These strategies were chosen and designed to enhance opportunities, skills, and rewards for children's prosocial involvement in both the classroom and family settings. This chapter reports the effects of exposure to these interventions for at least 1 semester in grades 1 to 4. Positive effects on students' attitudes, achievement, and behavior were hypothesized.

Experimental Interventions

In grades 1 to 4, teachers of children in the intervention condition were trained in a package of instructional methods that included three

---

1. A complete description of the study design may be obtained from J. David Hawkins.

major components: proactive classroom management, interactive teaching, and cooperative learning (Hawkins, Doueck, & Lishner, 1988; Hawkins & Lam, 1987). First grade teachers were also trained to provide cognitive problem-solving instruction to their first grade students using a curriculum developed by Shure and Spivack (1988). Parent training classes were offered to the adult caretakers of intervention students on a voluntary basis when students were in the first, second, and third grades. Project professional staff of mixed ethnicity provided parenting workshops in collaboration with local school and parent councils. Project staff and school principals were trained to observe intervention teachers in the classroom and to provide feedback on use of the project teaching techniques. Intervention teachers were observed and given feedback approximately once every 3 weeks. Control teachers and parents did not receive training in instructional or parenting skills from the project. However, control teachers were observed for a series of 4 class periods on different days in the fall and spring each year to document teaching practices in the control condition. The components of classroom teaching practices, child skills training, and parent training are described more fully below.

Classroom Teaching Practices

Proactive classroom management (Brophy, 1986; Brophy & Good, 1986; Cummings, 1983; Emmer & Everston, 1980; Martin, 1977) is aimed at establishing an environment that is conducive to learning and that promotes appropriate student behavior while minimizing disruption of classroom activities. In this intervention, teachers established classroom routines at the beginning of the year to create a consistent pattern of expectations. Prior to the beginning of each year, intervention teachers were taught to give clear expectations and explicit instructions about attendance, classroom procedures, and student behavior, and to recognize and reward attempts to comply. Teachers were also taught methods to maintain classroom order that minimize interruptions to instruction and learning. Teachers were taught to provide frequent, specific, and contingent encouragement and praise for student effort and progress that identified the student behavior being rewarded.

Interactive teaching (Block, 1971, 1974; Bloom, 1976; Brophy, 1987; Brophy & Good, 1986; Hawkins & Lam, 1987; Peterson, 1972; Stallings, 1980) is based on the premise that virtually all students can develop the skills necessary to succeed in the classroom under appropriate instructional conditions. The components of interactive teaching used in this project were assessment, mental set, objectives, input, modeling, and checking for understanding and remediation (Hawkins & Lam, 1987). Interactive teaching requires the mastery of specified learning objectives before proceeding to more advanced work. Demonstration of mastery and improvement over past performance are considered in determining students' grades. The training in interactive teaching taught methods for frequent monitoring of all students to assess their comprehension of material as it is presented.

Cooperative learning involves teachers' use of small groups of students as learning partners (Slavin, 1983, 1989, 1990, 1991; Slavin & Karweit, 1984). Students of differing abilities and backgrounds are provided the opportunity to work together in teams to master curriculum material and receive recognition as a team for their group's academic performance. Students are dependent on one another for positive rewards and team scores are based on the individual student's academic improvement over past performance, allowing each student to contribute to the team's overall achievement. Research has shown that cooperative learning methods that incorporate team rewards, individual accountability, and equal opportunity for success are more effective than traditional instructional methods in terms of increasing student achievement, encouraging positive attitudes toward school, and developing mutual concern among students across racial groups (Slavin, 1990, 1991). The cooperative learning techniques used in this experiment were Student Teams Achievement Divisions (STAD) and Teams-Games-Tournaments (TGT). Teachers of second, third, and fourth grade intervention classrooms were trained in the use of cooperative learning methods in February of each academic year and were expected to use these methods in their classrooms for the remainder of the school year.

Introduction of the teacher training interventions was sequenced across the academic year beginning with proactive classroom management training and introduction to interactive teaching in August before school began, interactive teaching training in October, and training in cooperative learning methods in February. This schedule of training was designed to allow sufficient guided and independent practice in each method before introduction of new methods. Further, it was our impression that introduction of cooperative learning in midwinter introduced an atmosphere of change and innovation in the classroom helpful in keeping the focus on learning during an educational season that some teachers describe as the "winter doldrums."

These classroom interventions sought to reduce academic failure, early conduct disorders, and peer rejection as risk factors for delinquency and drug use. The theoretical base for their inclusion was the hypothesis that the methods would provide increased opportunities for classroom involvement as well as increased skills and rewards for classroom involvement. Through these changes, this set of teaching practices was expected to strengthen the protective factor of bonding (e.g., attachment and commitment) to school.

Child Skills Training

Children in the intervention group received cognitive-based social competence training in the first grade. The training program, *Interpersonal Cognitive Problem Solving* (Shure & Spivack, 1988), teaches communication, decision-making, negotiation, and conflict-resolution skills. It seeks to increase students' problem-solving ability as a means of improving social adjustment (Spivack & Shure, 1974). First grade teachers were instructed in the use of this curriculum to teach children how to think through alternative solutions to problems.

The child skills training component targeted the risk factors of early conduct disorders, peer rejection, and involvement with antisocial others. This intervention sought to develop skills for conventional involvement so that children could accomplish their goals without resorting to problem behavior. Skillful problem solving was also hypothesized to strengthen bonding to school.

Parent Training

Two parent training components developmentally adjusted for the age of the children in the study were offered to families in the intervention condition on a voluntary basis. The first component, *Catch 'Em Being Good*, is a seven-session curriculum offered to parents when intervention students were in first grade and again when they were in second grade. The curriculum teaches parents how to: (1) monitor and pinpoint desirable and undesirable behaviors in their children; (2) teach expectations for behavior; and (3) provide positive reinforcement for desired behaviors and moderate negative consequences for undesired behaviors in a consistent and contingent fashion. To increase involvement in the family, parents also were encouraged to create age-appropriate family roles for their children and to increase shared family activities and time together (Hawkins, Catalano, Jones, & Fine, 1987). The curriculum uses a standard skills training format including demonstration and modeling of skills, role play, feedback, and homework practice assignments.

The second component of parent training was an academic support curriculum, *How to Help Your Child Succeed in School*, offered to parents during the spring of second grade and again when children in the intervention group were in the third grade. This four-session curriculum is designed to improve positive parent–child communication and involvement by teaching parents to provide a positive learning environment at home, to help their children develop reading and math skills, to communicate effectively with their children's teachers, and to support their childrens' progress (Hawkins et al., 1987).

These parent training interventions focused on reducing the risk factors of poor and inconsistent family management practices, family conflict, academic failure, and low commitment to school. The parent training classes sought to increase the level of bonding to the family and school as a protective mechanism.

During the first 3 years of the project, parents of approximately 43% of the intervention students attended at least 1 of the parenting classes. The mean class attendance among attenders at *Catch 'Em Being Good* was 5.5 (78%) sessions. The mean attendance for *How to Help Your Child Succeed in School* was 3.6 (90%) sessions. Forty percent of those attending the classes were single parents, 46% were from low-income families, and the majority (52%) were members of ethnic minorities.

Data Collection Methods

Data reported here were collected from students during the fall of 1985 when those normally progressing entered the fifth grade. A self-report survey administered to all consenting study participants measured perceived opportunities, skills, and rewards in the family and classroom, peer interactions, and problem behavior including substance use and delinquent behavior. Questionnaires were administered in classrooms. Project personnel read each question and its response categories aloud and then instructed students to record their answers. Students were told that their responses were completely confidential and they were monitored to ensure independent response.

Treatment Status

The independent measure in the present analyses was treatment status. For these analyses, students were divided into two conditions: (1) full intervention group—students exposed to at least one semester of the combined intervention in grades 1 to 4 ($n = 199$); and (2) control group—students who were enrolled in control classrooms and received no intervention during grades 1 to 4 plus unexposed students who were added to the project in the fall of fifth grade when the panel was expanded to include 10 additional schools ($n = 709$). It should be noted that the additional control students consisted of students already attending the Seattle public schools who joined the research project in 1985. Students enrolled in either intervention or control classrooms for less than a semester prior to the fifth grade were classified as not having been fully exposed during this period and were excluded from these analyses.

Sample

In the fall of 1985, 919 (87%) of the 1,053 fifth grade students enrolled in 18 participating Seattle elementary schools completed usable surveys. Forty-six percent of the sample were white, 25% were African-American, and 21% were Asian-American. Fifty-two percent of respondents were male and 48% were female. Ninety-three percent of the sample were 10 or 11 years of age. Thirty-eight percent of the students qualified for the National School Lunch/School Breakfast Program in the fall of the fifth grade. No significant differences were found between intervention students and students in the control group on the demographic variables of ethnicity, gender, age, or socioeconomic status. The demographic characteristics of this sample are shown in Table 7.1.

Measures

TEACHER INSTRUCTIONAL PRACTICES

Teacher use of the intervention instructional practices was assessed annually through structured observations of both intervention and

TABLE 7.1. Sample Characteristics

	Intervention group		Control group	
	Boys $n = 102$ (51.3%)	Girls $n = 97$ (48.7%)	Boys $n = 365$ (51.5%)	Girls $n = 344$ (48.5%)
Ethnicity				
White	50 (49.0%)	41 (42.3%)	169 (46.3%)	162 (47.1%)
African American	23 (22.5%)	24 (24.7%)	86 (23.6%)	86 (25.0%)
Asian American	25 (24.5%)	22 (22.7%)	79 (21.6%)	66 (19.2%)
Other	4 (3.9%)	10 (10.3%)	31 (8.5%)	30 (8.7%)
Socioeconomic status				
Eligible for free lunch	37 (36.3%)	49 (50.5%)	127 (34.8%)	133 (38.7%)
Not eligible for free lunch	62 (60.8%)	45 (46.4%)	221 (60.5%)	191 (55.5%)
Unknown	3 (2.9%)	3 (3.1%)	17 (4.7%)	20 (5.8%)

control teachers using an observational recording system developed specifically to measure the teaching practices tested in this study (Kerr, Kent, & Lam, 1985). Each classroom was observed for one 50-minute observation period on 2 successive days during the fall and again in the spring of each academic year from grade 2 through grade 4. Separate observations of students and teachers were made and recorded every 60 seconds during each observation period. The observations were then computed into summary scores as an objective implementation check of teaching practices in classrooms. As predicted, intervention teachers utilized intervention teaching strategies significantly more than control teachers (Hawkins, Von Cleve, & Catalano, 1991). These findings support the use of the treatment classification measure in this study by demonstrating that the project teaching practices differed significantly between intervention and control conditions. Future analyses will focus on issues of dose response, seeking to link degree of implementation of and exposure to the intervention to student outcomes. The present analysis asks simply whether students exposed to the intervention for at least one semester in grades 1 through 4 differ significantly from students not exposed to the intervention. This is a conservative test of the intervention's overall effects.

DEPENDENT MEASURES

Social development constructs and outcome measures were assessed in the family, school, norms, substance use, and delinquency domains. The scales were composed of conceptually grouped items. Reliability estimates were determined for all composite indexes using Cronbach's alpha. All scales were judged to have acceptable psychometric properties.[2]

Family Constructs. Two Likert-type scales measured student perceptions of family management practices. The first scale, proactive family management, was composed of six items coded so that higher mean scores correspond with greater use of proactive management practices. Four response categories were offered. One item was "The rules in my family are clear." The alpha reliability is .66. The second scale, parents use restrained punishment, was the mean of three reverse-coded items including "When you have misbehaved, do your parents spank you?" The alpha reliability is .65.

2. For a complete description of each scale used in these analyses, contact J. David Hawkins.

Two scales were utilized to measure family involvement and interaction. The first scale, good family communication, was the mean rating on two frequency and four Likert items measuring the extent of family communication. One item was "I find it easy to discuss problems with my mother or father." The alpha reliability is .68. The second scale, involvement in family work and play, was constructed from the mean rating on two frequency and nine Likert items that measured level of involvement. One item was "Last week did you read a book or story with your mom or dad?" The alpha reliability is .56.

Attachment to family was measured by a scale combining the mean rating on two frequency and three Likert items. One item was "Our family members get along well with each other." In single-parent families, the index consisted of an average of responses to how well family members get along and those items referring to the parent with whom the child lives.

School Constructs. Three scales were used to examine school risk and protective factors. The first scale, school rewards, was the mean rating of four items measuring student perceptions of rewards for conventional school involvement. One item was "My teacher is fair in dealing with students." The alpha reliability is .57. The second scale, attachment to school, was the average of four student survey items including "I like my teacher this year." The alpha reliability is .70. The third scale, commitment to school, was the average of two standardized Likert items that measured student commitment to school. "I do extra work on my own in class" was one of the items included in the scale. The alpha reliability for this two-item scale is .47.

The fourth school scale, academic performance, was the mean of the reading, math, and language subscales of the California Achievement Test. The alpha reliability is .88. The final school scale, school misbehavior, was constructed from the mean rating on four items. One item was "Have you ever hit a teacher?" The alpha reliability is .50.

Beliefs and Norms. Four scales were used to measure students' general beliefs and values and their specific norms regarding drug use. Responses on each of the scales were measured on a 4-point Likert-type scale. The first scale, belief in the moral order, was intended as a general measure of belief as a dimension of social bonding. It was constructed from the average of six items on the student survey that were coded so that higher mean scores represent greater belief in conventional moral values. One item on the scale was: "To get ahead, you have to do some things that are not right." The alpha reliability is .69.

The experimental interventions in grades 1 to 4 did not specifically seek to alter norms or expectations regarding drug use or delinquent behavior. It was not hypothesized that norms specific to drug use would be affected by this intervention. Nevertheless, measures of norms regarding drug use were included, in part to help rule out possible threats to internal validity. Any differences between intervention and control subjects detected on these measures could be taken to indicate an effect of factors other than the experimental interventions. Three scales were created to measure expectations and norms regarding drug use. A scale measuring the perceived risk of substance use for the respondent was constructed from five student survey items that were coded and averaged so that higher scores indicate greater perceived risk. One item was "Do you think it hurts people if they smoke marijuana regularly?" The alpha reliability is .90.

The respondent's expectation of whether they would be caught and punished for drug use was measured by the mean of two combined student survey items. One item was "If you smoked marijuana, would you be caught and punished?" The alpha reliability is .72.

The final measure of expectations and norms regarding drug use was a three-item scale measuring respondents' perceptions of the acceptability of drug use at their current age. The items were coded so that higher scores mean greater acceptance of use. One item was "Do you think it is okay for someone your age to smoke cigarettes?" The alpha reliability is .80.

Early Substance Use and Delinquency. Two measures of early involvement in substance use and delinquency were included in these analyses. The substance use item was a dichotomous single question, "Have you ever drunk beer, wine, whiskey, gin, or other liquor?" Measures of smoking and marijuana use were not included in the analyses since few students had initiated use of these substances by fifth grade entry. Delinquency initiation was measured by a scale composed of six dichotomous questions including "Have you ever thrown objects such as rocks or bottles at cars or people?"

Analyses

Continuous measures were analyzed using analysis of covariance (ANCOVA). These analyses controlled for ethnicity (whether students were African-American or of other ethnicity), socioeconomic status (eligibility for the free and reduced-price school lunch program), and mobility (whether student had been out of the Seattle school district for one semester or more). Categorical and dichotomous measures were analyzed using the chi-square statistic.

Of particular concern in this study is sample accretion. Accretion occurs when new participants enter after the initial cohort has been established (Tebes, Snow, Arthur, & Tapasak, 1991). Accretion may pose a potential threat to internal validity. Internal validity would be threatened and spurious treatment effects could be asserted when, for example, "worse" students are added to the control group. Given the addition of control students in the fall of the fifth grade, an accretion analysis was conducted to explore for possible differences between control students who had been in the project prior to the fifth grade and the controls who entered the study when their schools joined the experiment. Analysis of variance was used to compare the initial control group with the additional available control students on each of the intervening and outcome variables assessed in Table 7.2. No significant overall differences were found between the two groups, and they

TABLE 7.2. Cumulative Effects of Intervention on Fifth-Grade Constructs: Controlling for Race, Socioeconomic Status, and Mobility

| Variable | Intervention | | | Control | | | |
	Adjusted mean	SD	n	Adjusted mean	SD	n	F
Family constructs							
Family Management	3.54	0.44	182	3.41	0.46	660	9.97**
Restrained Punishment	3.14	0.78	164	3.08	0.73	594	0.88
Family Communication	2.97	0.57	185	2.83	0.58	665	6.96**
Family Involvement	0.06	0.49	189	−0.01	0.45	664	3.55*
Attachment to Family	3.04	0.63	181	2.92	0.62	649	4.57**
School constructs							
School Reward	3.17	0.60	187	2.95	0.68	660	16.87**
School Attachment	3.36	0.63	189	3.13	0.71	661	15.27**
School Commitment	0.12	0.80	188	−0.04	0.86	662	5.29**
Achievement Tests	499	48	185	508	48	644	5.73**
School Trouble	0.05	0.66	161	−0.03	0.64	570	0.13
Norms							
Belief in Moral Order	3.63	0.49	185	3.60	0.47	642	0.46
Drug Use Risk	1.83	1.04	75	1.73	0.88	640	2.01
Drug Use Punishment	1.25	0.62	173	1.25	0.57	615	0.00
Drug Use Acceptability	3.90	0.29	180	3.88	0.39	644	0.19

*$p < .05$
**$p < .025$

TABLE 7.3. Cumulative Effects of Intervention on Alcohol and Delinquency Initiation

| | Percent initiated use by fifth grade | |
Variable	Intervention	Control
Alcohol use*		
No	138 (79.3%)	460 (72.1%)
Yes	36 (20.7%)	173 (27.3%)
Delinquency**		
No	102 (54.5%)	318 (47.8%)
Yes	85 (45.5%)	347 (52.2%)

*$p < .05$; $\chi^2 = 3.14$
**$p < .05$; $\chi^2 = 2.64$

were combined in these analyses to enhance statistical power. However, it is noteworthy that, when analyzed separately by gender, the added control girls had significantly higher mean standardized achievement test scores ($\bar{x} = 515$) than did the girls from the initial control group ($\bar{x} = 508$), suggesting a possible accretion effect on this variable for girls. No similar accretion effect was observed for control boys. Since the social development model makes specific directional hypotheses regarding intervention effects, all reported p-values are one-tailed.

RESULTS

A number of statistically significant differences were found between the intervention group and the control group in the fall of the fifth grade. A summary of the findings is included on Tables 7.2 and 7.3. Table 7.2 reports results of the continuous variables. Table 7.3 reports results on dichotomous variables.

Family Constructs

As hypothesized, intervention students reported significantly more proactive family management by their parents ($F_{1,837} = 9.97, p < .025$) as well as greater family communication ($F_{1,845} = 6.96 \ p < .025$) and involvement ($F_{1,848} = 3.55, p < .05$) than their control counterparts. In addition, intervention students reported greater bonding to family ($F_{1,825} = 4.57, p < .025$) than control students. While these differences are statistically significant, the effect sizes on these family variables are all small. The mean differences between groups do not exceed .30

standard deviations. Nevertheless, these significant differences are noteworthy given the fact that this is a conservative test of the effects of the parenting intervention in which all subjects in the intervention condition were included though less than half of their parents actually attended parenting training.

School Constructs

As predicted, intervention students perceived school as more reward-ing ($F_{1,842} = 16.87$, $p < .025$) than did controls. Further, intervention students were significantly more attached ($F_{1,845} = 15.27$, $p < .025$) and committed ($F_{1,845} = 5.73$, $p < .025$) to school than control students. The effects on perceived school rewards and attachment to school are larger than the effects observed on family variables.

Contrary to hypothesized expectations, control students scored significantly higher than intervention students on the California Achievement Test (CAT) ($F_{1,824} = 5.73$, $p < .025$). Analyses revealed that this difference reflected a difference in CAT scores for female students only. No significant difference in CAT scores was observed for male students. Moreover, the overall difference in CAT scores for females appears to reflect the effects of accretion, specifically the addition of new control girls whose mean CAT score was 515, compared with a mean CAT score for girls from the initial control group of 508. Subsequent analyses of CAT scores for this sample at grades 6 and 7 currently in preparation for publication show no evidence of significantly lower CAT scores among students exposed to the full social development intervention. These results suggest that the present CAT findings are anomalous, reflecting the addition of a group of more high achieving girls to the study who serve as controls in the present analyses.

Norms

As expected, no significant differences on drug-related norms were found between the intervention and control groups in the fall of the fifth grade. The groups did not differ with respect to their degree of belief in the moral order. It should be noted that the mean scores on all these variables were generally extreme and prosocial, indicating that at fifth grade entry, the great majority of students in this study held socially conventional beliefs about behavior and perceptions of drug use as risky and unacceptable. These results are consistent with hypotheses that at this age, children generally share the normative consensus of the dominant social order.

In spite of this apparent normative consensus, as hypothesized, intervention students reported significantly lower rates of alcohol initiation than their control counterparts ($\chi^2 = 3.13$, $p < .05$). Intervention students also reported significantly less delinquency initiation than controls ($\chi^2 = 2.64$, $p < .05$).

DISCUSSION

These results generally appear promising. This conservative test suggests that the family interventions have slightly improved family management, communication, and involvement at home in the intervention group, and as hypothesized, these changes have been accompanied by higher levels of bonding to family. Similarly, intervention students report that their school experiences have been more rewarding, and, as predicted, they are more attached to school and committed to getting an education than controls. In summary, the interventions appear to have been implemented with sufficient fidelity to achieve significant difference in social bonding to family and school during the early elementary grades. This result is important from a theoretical perspective. The social development model hypothesizes that higher levels of bonding to family and school are associated with lower levels of drug and delinquency initiation. Thus, higher levels of bonding to family and school should be accompanied by lower rates of drug use and initiation in the experimental group in this study.

In this study, the classroom teaching interventions were more completely and consistently implemented by experimental teachers than were the parenting interventions. Less than half of all eligible parents attended training but all teachers of intervention classrooms were trained in the project's classroom management and teaching methods. It is not surprising that the largest effect sizes are observed for school constructs. Exposure to the intervention as implemented in this study appears to have had its greatest effects on students' perceptions of schools as rewarding environments and on their attachment to school.

Though the teaching interventions were expected to significantly enhance students' academic as well as social and behavioral skills, at the end of grade 4 students exposed to the intervention did not have higher standardized achievement test scores than controls. The small (i.e., less than 0.20 standard deviations) observed difference in CAT scores favoring the control group appears to reflect the effects of the addition of girls with higher mean CAT scores to the study's control group when the panel was expanded. The likelihood that this is an anomalous effect reflective of sample accretion is supported by earlier research. A previous study in which experimental teachers were trained in the teaching practices tested here found a positive correlation between the use of these practices and student scores on math achievement tests at grade 7 (Hawkins & Lam, 1987). Further, analyses of California Achievement Test data from the present panel at grades 6 and 7, which are in preparation for publication, have found only positive significant differences in the hypothesized direction for boys and no significant differences for girls, again suggesting that the present finding is an anomaly.

A finding worthy of note is the absence of difference between intervention and control students with respect to social norms and attitudes toward drugs. This finding is important in at least three respects. First, this result helps to rule out "halo" and Hawthorne effects as threats to the validity of the conclusion that the interventions produced the observed effects on bonding and behavior. Norms regarding drug use were not a focus of this intervention, and interventions and controls did not differ at the end of 4 years of intervention in this respect. This suggests that intervention students did not simply subscribe to more socially desirable responses across the board. They expressed no greater perception that drug use is risky or unacceptable. However, they were more strongly bonded to family and school and fewer had initiated either delinquent behavior or alcohol use by fifth grade than controls.

Another finding suggests that increasing bonds to family and school can reduce delinquency and drug use initiation as hypothesized by the social development model. Both delinquency and drug use initiation were less prevalent in the experimental than in the control group. This appears to have occurred even in the absence of intervention focused on ensuring the development of antidrug norms in the early elementary grades. Strong bonding to family and school may help to reduce the early initiation of delinquent and drug-using behaviors during a developmental period when there is a normative consensus that such behaviors are generally not accepted, as is the case in this sample.

Finally, in spite of these positive effects on early delinquency and alcohol use initiation, it is plausible that even greater effects might be produced if the intervention promoted norms against alcohol and other drug use by children. This suggestion is worthy of investigation in future prevention trials.

These global analyses of cross-sectional differences in outcome between experimental and control groups after 4 years of intervention show promising results. However, they underscore for us the importance of more closely linking measures of intervention strength or fidelity with theoretically endogenous variables and outcomes in seeking to empirically test hypothesized causal sequences hypothesized to prevent delinquency and drug abuse (Hawkins, Abbott, Catalano, & Gillmore, 1991). These findings suggest the importance of modeling the relationships between parent and teacher training, the use of the teaching practices, classroom opportunities and rewards, achievement, school bonding, and delinquency and drug use developmentally. Subsequent investigations will look at consistency and change in these constructs over time as well as interrelationships among them longitudinally.

ACKNOWLEDGMENTS

This research was supported by grants from the Prevention Research Branch, National Institute on Drug Abuse, the Office of Juvenile Justice and Delinquency Prevention, and the Burlington Northern Foundation. An earlier version of this paper was presented at Society for Research in Child Development, Kansas City, Missouri, April 1989.

REFERENCES

Akers, R. L., Krohn, M. D., Lanza-Kaduce, L., & Radosevich, M. (1979). Social learning and deviant behavior: A specific test of a general theory. *American Sociological Review, 44*, 636–655.

Bandura, A. (1977). Self-efficacy: Toward a unifying theory of behavioral change. *Psychological Review, 84*, 191–215.

Bank, L., Patterson, G. R., & Reid, J. B. (1987). Delinquency prevention through training parents in family management. *Behavior Analyst, 10*(1), 75–82.

Berrueta-Clement, J. R., Schweinhart, L. J., Barnett, W. S., Epstein, A. S., & Weikhart, D. P. (1984). *Changed lives: The effects of the Perry Preschool Program on youth through age 19*. Ypsilanti, MI: High/Scope Press.

Block, J. H. (1971). *Mastery learning: Theory and practice*. New York: Holt Rinehart and Winston.

Block, J. H. (1974). *Schools, society and mastery learning*. New York: Holt Rinehart and Winston.

Bloom, B. S. (1976). *Human characteristics and school learning*. New York: McGraw-Hill.

Botvin, G. J., Batson, H. W., Witts-Vitale, S., Bess, V., Baker, E., & Dusenbury, L. (1989). A psychosocial approach to smoking prevention for urban black youth. *Public Health Reports, 104*(6), 573–582.

Botvin, G. J., & Wills, T. A. (1985). Personal and social skills training:

Cognitive-behavioral approaches to substance abuse prevention. In C. Bell & R. J. Battjes (Eds.), *Prevention research: Deterring drug abuse among children and adolescents* (NIDA Research Monograph No. 63, pp. 8–49), Washington, DC: U.S. Government Printing Office.

Brophy, J. (1986). Classroom management techniques. *Education and Urban Society, 18*(2), 182–194.

Brophy, J. (1987). Synthesis of research on strategies for motivating students to learn. *Educational Leadership, 45*(2), 40–48.

Brophy, J., & Good, T. L. (1986). Teacher behavior and achievement. In M. C. Wittrock (Ed.), *Handbook of research on teaching* (3rd ed., pp. 328–375). New York: Macmillan.

Bry, B. H., McKeon, P., & Pandina, R. J. (1982). Extent of drug use as a function of number of risk factors. *Journal of Abnormal Psychology, 91,* 273–279.

Comer, J. P. (1988). Educating poor minority children. *Scientific American, 259,* 42–48.

Cummings, C. (1983). *Managing to teach.* Snohomish, WA: Snohomish Publishing.

Dumas, J. E. (1989). Treating antisocial behavior in children: Child and family approaches. *Clinical Psychology Review, 9,* 197–222.

Ellickson, P. L., & Bell, R. M. (1990). Drug prevention in junior high: A multi-site longitudinal test. *Science, 247*(16), 1299–1305.

Elliott, D. S., Huizinga, D., & Menard, S. (1989). *Multiple problem youth: Delinquency, substance use and mental health problems.* New York: Springer-Verlag.

Emmer, E. T., & Everson, C. M. (1980). *Effective management at the beginning of the school year in junior high classes* (R & D Report #6107). Austin: University of Texas at Austin, Research and Development Center for Teacher Education.

Farrington, D. P., & Hawkins, J. D. (1991) Predicting participation, early onset, and later persistence in officially recorded offending. *Criminal Behaviour and Mental Health, 1,* 1–33.

Farringtron, D. P., Loeber, R., Elliott, D. S., Hawkins, J.D., Kandel, D. B., Klein, M. W., McCord, J., Rowe, D. C., & Tremblay, R. E. (1990). Advancing knowledge about the onset of delinquency and crime. In B. B. Lahey & A. E. Kazdin, (Eds.), *Advances in clinical child psychology* (Vol. 13, pp. 283–342). New York: Plenum Press.

Flay, B. R. (1985). Psychosocial approaches to smoking prevention: A review of findings. *Health Psychology, 5,* 449–488.

Hansen, W. B., Johnson, C. A., Flay, B. R., Graham, J. D., & Sobel, J. (1988). Affective and social influences approaches to the prevention of multiple substance abuse among seventh grade students: Results from Project SMART. *Preventive Medicine, 17,* 135–154.

Hawkins, J. D., Abbott, R., Catalano, R. F., & Gillmore, M. R. (1991). Assessing effectiveness of drug abuse prevention: Long-term effects and replication. In C. Leukfeld & W. J. Bukoski (Eds), *Drug abuse prevention research: Methodological issues* (pp. 195–212). Washington DC: National Institute on Drug Abuse.

Hawkins, J. D., Catalano, R. F., Jones G., & Fine, D. (1987). Delinquency prevention through parent training: Results and issues from work in progress. In J. Q. Wilson & G. C. Lowry (Eds.), *From children to citizens: Families, schools, and delinquency prevention* (Vol. 3, pp. 186–204). New York: Springer-Verlag.

Hawkins, J. D., Catalano, R. F., & Miller, J. Y. (1992). Risk and protective factors for alcohol and other drug problems in adolescence and early adulthood: Implications for substance abuse prevention. *Psychological Bulletin, 112*(1).

Hawkins, J. D., Doueck, H. J., & Lishner, D. M. (1988). Changing teaching practices in mainstream classrooms to reduce discipline problems among low achievers. *American Educational Research Journal, 25*, 31–50.

Hawkins, J. D., Jenson, J. M., Catalano, R. F., & Lishner, D. M. (1988). Delinquency and drug abuse: Implications for social services. *Social Service Review, 62*, 258–284.

Hawkins, J. D., & Lam, T. C. (1987). Teacher practices, social development and delinquency. In J. D. Burchard (Ed.), *The prevention of delinquent behavior* (pp. 241–274). Beverly Hills, CA: Sage.

Hawkins, J. D., Von Cleve, E., & Catalano, R. F. (1991). Reducing early childhood aggression: Results of a primary prevention program. *Journal of the American Academy of Child and Adolescent Psychiatry, 30*(2), 208–217.

Hawkins, J. D., & Weis, J. G. (1985). The social development model: An integrated approach to delinquency prevention. *Journal of Primary Prevention, 6*(2), 73–79.

Hirschi, T. (1969). *Causes of delinquency.* Berkeley and Los Angeles: University of California Press.

Kerr, D. M., Kent, L., & Lam, T. C. M. (1985). Measuring program implementation with a classroom observation instrument: The interactive teaching map. *Evaluation Review, 9*, 461–482.

Kolvin, I., Miller, F. J. W., Fleeting, M., & Kolvin, P. A. (1988). Social and parenting factors affecting criminal-offence rates: Findings from the Newcastle Thousand Family Study (1947–1980). *British Journal of Psychiatry, 152*, 80–90.

Loeber, R. (1988). *Development and risk factors of juvenile antisocial behavior and delinquency.* Unpublished manuscript, University of Pittsburgh, Pittsburgh, PA.

Martin, D. L. (1977). Your praise can smother learning. *Learning, 5*, 42–51.

Michelson, L. (1987). Cognitive-behavioral strategies in the prevention and treatment of antisocial disorders in children and adolescents. In J. D. Burchard & S. N. Burchard (Eds.), *The prevention of delinquent behavior* (Vol. 10, pp. 275–310). Newbury Park, CA: Sage.

Newcomb, M. D., Maddahian, E., & Bentler, P. M. (1986). Risk factors for drug use among adolescents: Concurrent and longitudinal analyses. *American Journal of Public Health, 76*, 525–530.

Newcomb, M. D., Maddahian, E., Skager, R., & Bentler, P. M. (1987). Substance abuse and psychosocial risk factors among teenagers: Associations with sex, age, ethnicity and type of school. *American Journal of Drug and Alcohol Abuse, 13*, 413–433.

Pentz, M. A., Dwyer, J. H., Mackinnon, D. P., Flay, B. R., Hansen, W. B., Wang E. Y., & Johnson, C. A. (1989). A multicommunity trial for primary prevention of adolescent drug abuse: Effects on drug use prevalence. *Journal of the American Medical Association, 261*(22), 3259–3266.

Peterson, P. (1972). *A review of research on mastery learning strategies.* Unpublished manuscript, International Association for the Evaluation of Educational Achievement, Stockholm, Sweden.

Robins, L. N., & Przybeck, T. R. (1985). Age of onset of drug use as a factor in drug and other disorders. In C. L. Jones & R. J. Battjes, (Eds.), *Etiology of drug abuse: Implications for prevention* (NIDA Research Monograph No. 56, DHHS Publication ADM 85-1335, pp. 178–192). Washington, DC: U.S. Government Printing Office.

Rutter, M. (1980). *Changing youth in a changing society.* Cambridge: Harvard University Press.

Rutter, M., & Giller, H. (1983). *Juvenile delinquency: Trends and perspectives.* New York: Penguin Books.

Schinke, S. P., Bebel, M. Y., Orlandi, M. A., & Botvin, G. J. (1988). Prevention strategies for vulnerable pupils: School social work practices to prevent substance abuse. *Urban Education, 22*(4), 510–519.

Schinke, S. P., Botvin, G. J., Trimble, J. E., Orlandi, M. A., Gilchrist, L. D., & Locklear, V. S. (1988). Preventing substance abuse among American-Indian adolescents: A bicultural competence skills approach. *Journal of Counseling Psychology, 35*(1), 87–90.

Shedler, J., & Block, J. (1990). Adolescent drug use and psychological health: A longitudinal inquiry. *American Psychologist, 45*, 612–630.

Shure, M. B., & Spivack, G. (1988). Interpersonal cognitive problem solving. In R. H. Price, E. L. Cowen, R. P. Lorion, & J. Ramos-McKay (Eds.), *14 Ounces of Prevention* (pp. 69–82). Hyattsville, MD: American Psychological Association.

Slavin, R. E. (1983). When does cooperative learning increase student achievement? *Psychological Bulletin, 94*, 429–445.

Slavin, R. E. (1989). Students at risk of school failure: The problems and its dimensions. In R. E. Slavin, N. L. Karweit, & N.A. Madden (Eds), *Effective programs for students at risk* (pp. 3–19). Boston: Allyn and Bacon.

Slavin, R. E. (1990). *Cooperative learning: Theory, research, and practice.* Englewood Cliffs, NJ: Prentice Hall.

Slavin, R. E. (1991). Synthesis of research on cooperative learning. *Educational Leadership, 48*(5), 71–82.

Slavin, R. E., & Karweit, N. (1984). Mastery learning and student teams: A factorial experiment in urban general mathematics classes. *American Educational Research Journal, 21,* 725–736.

Spivack, G., & Shure, M. B. (1974). *Social adjustment of young children.* San Francisco: Jossey Bass.

Stallings, J. (1980). Allocated academic learning time revisited, or beyond time on task. *Educational Researcher, 9*(11), 11–16.

Tebes, J. K., Snow, D. L., Arthur, M. W., & Tapasak, R. C. (1991). *Sample accretion and validity in prevention research.* Unpublished manuscript. New Haven: Yale University Consultation Center.

Tremblay, R. E., McCord, J., Boileau, H., Charlebois, P., Gagnon, C., LeBlanc, M., & Larivée, S. (1991). Can disruptive boys be helped to become competent? *Psychiatry, 54,* 148–161.

Tremblay, R. E., McCord, J., Boileau, H., LeBlanc, M., Gagnon, C., Charlebois, P., & Larivée, S. (1990, November). *The Montreal prevention experiment: School adjustment and self-reported delinquency after three years of follow-up.* Paper presented at the annual meeting of the American Society of Criminology, Baltimore, MD.

CHAPTER 8

♦ ——— ♦

Building Developmental and Etiological Theory through Epidemiologically Based Preventive Intervention Trials

SHEPPARD G. KELLAM
GEORGE W. REBOK

The purpose of this chapter is to describe the role of developmental epidemiologically based preventive intervention trials in building and testing developmental and etiological theory in psychopathology. Developmental epidemiology is the result of combining community epidemiology and life-course development. This integration of orientations and methods characterized our earlier Chicago/Woodlawn studies and our current Baltimore prevention intervention research. We will focus on the importance for theory building of mapping developmental paths from early child maladaptive behaviors to later psychopathology and of targeting antecedents along these paths for experimental interventions.

Maladaptive behavioral responses to classroom task demands such as aggressive behavior and poor academic achievement mark children who are at increased risk of specific problem outcomes later in life. An important argument of this chapter is that such antecedents are potential targets for preventive intervention trials that fulfill a double function: they test the developmental roles of the antecedents and, if the interventions are effective, contribute to effective prevention programing. We argue that such preventive trials, when done in epidemiologically clearly defined populations, are indispensable to developing and testing developmental and etiological theory in psychopathology.

Our research in Woodlawn and Baltimore has centered on the interface over the life course between social task demands and adequacy of performance on the one hand, and the individual's psychological well-being on the other. This focus has led us to define mental health from two perspectives. The first is the vantage point of society; we have called it *social adaptational status* to denote the adequacy of social performance in the view of natural raters such as teachers, parents, or work supervisors. The second perspective is internal to the individual and his or her *psychological well-being*. This component includes psychiatric symptoms and disorders, as well as neuropsychological and physiological states. By separating these two conceptually distinct developmental perspectives, we are able to study their interrelations as they evolve from early childhood through adolescence and adulthood.

Preventive mental health trials serve two basic and related purposes. They contribute to the empirical basis for theory construction, particularly in regard to life-course development, socialization, and psychopathogenesis. More specifically, they add an experimental or quasi-experimental capacity to our research in natural settings. For example, maladaptive aggressive responses to classroom social demands (breaking rules, truancy, and fighting) occurring as early as first grade and even in preschool, have repeatedly been shown to predict later antisocial behavior, criminality, and heavy substance use—including I.V. drug use—through adolescence and into adulthood, especially in males (Block, Block, & Keyes, 1988; Ensminger, Kellam, & Rubin, 1983; Farrington, Gallagher, Morley, St. Ledger, & West, 1988; Kellam, Brown, Rubin, & Ensminger, 1983; Robins, 1978; Shedler & Block, 1990; Tomas, Vlahov, & Anthony, 1990; Tremblay et al., 1992). If we are successful in reducing aggressive behavior in elementary school and if the consequences of the early reduction in turn reduce the risk of delinquent behavior later, then the preventive trial supports the hypothesis that early classroom aggressive behavior has a functional role in the developmental path leading to delinquency.

In addition to providing evidence of specific intervention impact and of the developmental significance of early risk behaviors or conditions, preventive trials will inform us about the degree of malleability of the components of the course and interrelationships in the developmental model being studied under specific intervention conditions. Preventive trials that change specific social task demands, contextual conditions, or particular behavioral responses and then have a significant effect on developmental outcomes can provide tests of hypothetical models of development and socialization that attempt to explain outcomes.

Single antecedents can have multiple developmental outcomes and multiple antecedents can have a single developmental outcome (Kellam et al., 1983). For example, in the Woodlawn studies aggressive behavior by males in first grade was an antecedent of heavy drug use 10 years later, but so was higher scoring on the first grade Metropolitan Readiness Test by both genders. These predictors operated independently of each other in analytic models involving drug use as the dependent variable. These results suggest different developmental paths leading to heavy drug use by age 16 or 17. The aggression path hypothetically involves less social control of aggressive behavior and rule breaking; the other path hypothetically involves readiness to explore school in first grade and an enduring interest in exploring later new arenas such as drugs. It is noteworthy that the readiness test scores, unlike the early aggressive behavior ratings, did not predict later delinquency but did predict heavy drug use (Ensminger, Kellam, & Rubin, 1983).

Developmental models testing the mediators and moderators of each path can be examined by experimental preventive interventions aimed at the specific hypothesized mediator, the nature of which guides the choosing of the appropriate intervention. The hypothesized mediator then becomes the proximal target of the intervention trial, the distal target being drug use later in the life course. We will illustrate this by describing the Baltimore trial aiming at reducing early aggressive behavior for this model-testing purpose. The Baltimore trial illustrates another issue, the use of two interventions in a parallel design to test direction of effects of two correlated variables in the same model, both predictors of outcomes.

The kinds of models we refer to in this chapter can be considered partial in the sense that they do not encompass all relevant aspects of the origins and courses leading to a developmental outcome. In models that lend themselves to experimental preventive intervention trials, four or five variables are hypothesized to relate to each other and to the outcome, and the trial or trials are designed to alter one or another specific aspect of the model. Often the model will involve aspects of behavior in response to environmental demand and aspects of psychological well-being, with characteristics of the social field in the model as well. More complete theoretical models can be built on such parsimonious testing of developmental models particularly when the testing is done on carefully defined populations and conditions.

THE DEVELOPMENTAL
EPIDEMIOLOGICAL PERSPECTIVE

In previous writings we have described a research perspective integrating the life-course developmental orientation with community epidemiology (Kellam, 1990; Kellam, Branch, Agrawal, & Ensminger, 1975; Kellam & Ensminger, 1980; Kellam et al., 1983; Kellam & Werthamer-Larsson, 1986; Kellam, Werthamer-Larsson, Dolan, Brown, Mayer, Rebok, Anthony, Laudolff, Edelsohn, & Wheeler, 1991). This *developmental epidemiological* perspective, a phrase coined by the Woodlawn research group, is intended to allow the mapping of developmental paths within representative samples from a defined community population over significant portions of the life course.

A core concept underlying this integrated perspective is the tracking of total populations or of representative samples of populations over time and defined stages of development (Kellam, 1990, 1991). The mapping of developmental paths within defined populations over different periods of the life course has already supplied the target risk behaviors for our preventive trials in Baltimore. It is now providing the basis for periodic follow-up of intervention outcomes along with the identification of targets for further intervention research.

The Community Epidemiological Orientation

In contrast to a more demographic epidemiological perspective concerned with larger population characteristics, here we focus on fairly small populations in their environments such as the neighborhood, community, or a factory and its work force. We hold constant general characteristics such as poverty and ethnicity, and examine processes within the community that explain variation in outcomes. When coupled with the developmental perspective, community epidemiology allows study of the developmental paths of specific cohorts of children who develop toward disorders, compared to those in the same community and cohort who do not. This is accomplished by examining variation in the children and in such social fields as family, classroom, or peer group within the community.

From a developmental epidemiological perspective, our effort is to explain variation in developmental paths including antecedents, moderators, and outcomes within or across neighborhoods or other fairly small populations. By starting with epidemiologically defined populations, we can control selection bias; calculate rates of the antecedents, mediators, moderators, and outcomes; and examine variation in the function of hypothesized mediators or moderators in their relationships to each other and to the outcome. This population-based strategy informs us about development and prevention in a particular community. It then requires direct and systematic replication in similar or different communities to define the variation in the frequency and in the consequences of a developmental model in different and similar community conditions.

Social Adaptation and Psychological Well-Being

While the developmental epidemiological orientation provided a broad framework, a more elaborated and developmentally specified framework was needed. The conceptual framework guiding our previous Woodlawn studies and the current preventive trials in Baltimore provides a basis for choosing early measures and for maintaining the validity of the methods as the life courses of the children evolve. The framework first distinguishes social task performance from *psychological well-being*. The latter concerns internal states such as anxiety, depression, bizarre feelings and thoughts, self-esteem, neuropsychological processes, and physiological status. Social task performance is external to the individual and refers to the social task demands and the adequacy of behavioral responses of the individual in particular social fields at particular stages of life. We have termed this interactive process of demand/response *social adaptation*, and the judgments of adequacy of the individual's performance by powerful people such as parents, teachers, and supervisors *social adaptational status* (Kellam et al., 1975).

At each stage of life individuals are confronted with specific social task demands defined by a person or persons we have termed the *natural rater(s)*, who not only define the tasks but rate the adequacy of performance of the individual. Parents function as natural raters in the family, peers rate their peer group, and teachers rate students in the classroom. Important peers rate the child's accommodation of peer demands, and in the early grades of school, classmates are the most important peer group. In addition to the actual performance of individuals, chance and idiosyncrasy also play roles in the natural rater's judgments of adequacy of performance (Kellam, 1990; Kellam et al., 1975; Kellam & Ensminger, 1980).

By contrast and as noted, psychological well-being refers to the individual's internal state. The distinction here is between the failing math grade as an example of social adaptational status, and the depression the child may feel prior to taking the test or as a consequence of the grade as an example of psychological well-being. Although the two domains may be highly interrelated, they quite clearly represent two different conceptual domains, and problems in each have very different long-term outcomes (Ensminger et al., 1983; Kellam et al., 1983).

It is crucial that research into their developmental interrelationships must measure social adaptational status and psychological well-being separately to avoid confounding one with the other (Bank, Dishion, Skinner, & Patterson, 1990). Throughout our work in Woodlawn and now in Baltimore, the developmental relationships between these two distinct domains—social adaptational status and psychological well-being—have been central to the questions addressed in our prevention research.

The Life-Course Developmental Orientation

Baltes, Reese, and Lipsitt (1980) describe this theoretical orientation as "concerned with the description, explanation, and modification (optimization) of developmental processes in the human life course from conception to death" (p. 66). Development is conceptualized as a lifelong process that occurs as a result of biological and environmental determinants and their interaction. Life-course changes have been found to take many forms in terms of their directionality, time course, degree of intraindividual and interindividual variability, and malleability (Baltes, 1987; Brim & Kagan, 1980; Neugarten, 1969; Uttal & Perlmutter, 1989). From an epidemiological perspective, variation among subgroups in regard to an antecedent's function or outcome is assumed to derive from characteristics of the host, the agent, and the environment, either jointly or separately (Anthony, 1990). The results of our preventive interventions are hypothesized to be moderated by these three sources of variation (Kellam, 1990; Kellam et al., 1991).

In the life-course developmental approach, behavioral development is codetermined by three major systems of influence: (1) normative age-graded (ontogenetic) influences; (2) normative history-graded influences (cohort effects); and (3) nonnormative life events (Baltes, 1987; Baltes, Reese, & Lipsitt, 1980). Age-graded influences refer to events that occur in very similar ways for all individuals in a culture or subculture. This system of influences includes biological maturation and age-determined socialization events, involving aspects of social fields such as the family life cycle, and entrance into and progression through the educational system.

History-graded events also involve biological and environmental determinants, but their influence is associated with historical time. Baltes (1987) has proposed two types of history-graded events: those that define long-term functions (e.g., cultural evolution), and those that are more time- or period-specific (e.g., economic recession). The third type of influence, idiosyncratic or nonnormative life events, refers to a class of developmental influences that vary among individuals. While entrance into elementary school represents a normative influence, serious illness or imprisonment of a parent are examples of influences not shared as a normative event across the population.

From a life-course developmental perspective, the Woodlawn studies served well to illustrate the operation of these multiple influences. There was a clear relationship between family structure, social adaptation to school, and child psychological well-being (Ensminger, 1990; Kellam, Adams, Brown, & Ensminger, 1982; Kellam, Ensminger, & Turner, 1977). These relationships were found in both the 1964–65 and 1966–67 Woodlawn first grade populations, but there was a marked shift in the baseline percentage of maladapting children in these two separate groups (Kellam et al., 1977). This difference in rates is probably a cohort effect which changed the frequency of social maladaptation and psychological well-being but did not affect their interrelationships. Hence, cohort effects must be taken into account as potential influences on the developmental paths leading to long-term child outcomes.

Representative Multistage Sampling and Assessment

Prevention research often requires precise microanalytic interpersonal, diagnostic, or biological assessment of subgroups within specified populations. This can be economically achieved through multistage assessment and sampling. We can assess all individuals in a sample from a population using ecologically valid and reliable measures of such variables as grades or teachers' ratings of student behavior. We can then draw representative smaller numbers of individuals from relevant strata of the total population based on the first-stage measures. These would be called second-stage samples and can be used for more microanalytic studies on selected small populations. Third-stage measures and samples can be drawn in the same fashion for even more intense studies of smaller yet representative samples of the original population. This link between population-based epidemiological research and smaller, but still representative, samples shows great promise for integrating more ecologically valid measures at the first stage with more precise laboratory measures at the second or third stages (Anthony et al., 1985; Kellam, 1990).

DEVELOPMENTAL EPIDEMIOLOGY, PREVENTIVE TRIALS, AND BUILDING AND TESTING THEORY

Both continuities and discontinuities are to be expected across the life course (Bloom, 1964; Brim & Kagan, 1980; Neugarten, 1969; Rutter, 1989). The process of development involves both diverse patterns that may not be preset at birth but appear at later periods of life, and causal processes that may or may not operate throughout the life course. Age-related biological and psychological changes and interactions with new social fields (classroom, peer group, workplace) may alter life course. Particularly the individual's success or failure in each social field, that is, their social adaptational status, will affect the life course. Nevertheless, some continuities will persist because children carry with them the results of earlier learning, successes, and failures (Kellam et al., 1975; Rutter, 1989).

The search for developmental continuities and discontinuities and the mechanisms that underlie them is supported, but not satisfied by the integration of epidemiological and life-course developmental orientations (Kellam, 1990). Aggressive behavior in first grade or earlier, for example, is a significant predictor of criminal or assaultive behavior in adolescence and adulthood. However, its role in etiology remains unclear. Assuming we can reduce early aggressive behavior, we do not know whether we have changed the probability of the criminal outcome. The same question arises in predicting whether improving reading achievement will result in reduced risk of depression later.

These questions require experimentation that is prospective, longitudinal, and epidemiologically based. In fact, such experimental research is at the core of what we mean by prevention research, which tests the etiological and developmental meaning of proximal target antecedents and their relationships to distal outcomes. Such preventive trials can involve biological, psychological, or social interventions and/or targets. Furthermore, the target antecedents need not fall within the same domain as the developmental outcome to be effective (Brown, in press). Thus, an intervention designed to reduce psychiatric symptoms may be less effective in reducing later depression than would an intervention targeting another domain, such as poor achievement test performance.

A related issue here is the differentiation of individuals who would most likely exhibit continuities leading to disorder in adolescence and adulthood. For example, the Woodlawn studies revealed that aggressive behavior of first grade boys was strongly predictive of delinquency and heavy substance use 10 years later. Aggressive behavior interacted with shy behavior to enhance the aggressive effect in later delinquency and substance use. These shy/aggressive children—a group to which we and several other groups have been calling attention—are children who are loners, who do not participate much with others, but who break rules and fight (Block, Block, & Keyes, 1988; Ensminger et al., 1983; Farrington et al., 1988; Farrington & Gunn, 1985; Hans, Marcus, Henson, Auerbach, & Mirsky, 1991; Kellam et al., 1983; McCord, 1988; Schwartzman, Ledingham, & Serbin, 1985).

In Woodlawn, the subpopulation of boys both shy *and* aggressive was only slightly smaller than that of boys who were aggressive, but not shy. Using a level of moderately to severely shy and aggressive behavior as a cutoff point, this subpopulation represented about 10 percent of the Woodlawn first grade males, a sizeable portion of children who, we believe, were at considerably increased risk for major behavioral and psychiatric problem outcomes later.

Universal, Selected, and Indicated Interventions

A useful conceptual organization for the prevention trials described here is derived from Gordon's views on *universal, selected,* and *indicated* preventive interventions (Gordon, 1983).

- *Universal* interventions are applied to total classrooms or other total populations of children without labeling or singling out high-risk children, but with careful assessment of the impact of the interventions on those at increased risk.
- *Selected* interventions are directed at high-risk children who do not respond to the universal interventions and who remain at increased risk of problem outcomes.
- *Indicated* interventions are actually treatment programs for children who do not respond to either of the two levels of preventive interventions cited above.

The interventions used in the Baltimore preventive trials are examples of universal interventions because they are applied to all children in the intervention classrooms. Children who already demonstrate high-risk behavior are a focus in the analysis of impact to determine whether the universal intervention can reduce risk behavior. Children not yet demonstrating the risk behavior but who might do so at some later point are studied to determine whether universal interventions reduce the incidence of risk behavior.

We use universal interventions on broad populations first because they are more integrated into the social context, reflecting the socialization processes more than the somewhat removed and more clinical selected interventions. Effects of universal interventions can be hypothesized to affect not just the target children but future generations of children through changing the context and socialization processes. Universal interventions are by definition less reparative and more socialization enhancing; they are usually more economical and entail less of a labeling effect than selected or indicated interventions. The moderate size of the effects of the universal interventions particularly on the children who appeared more severe in first grade were surprising considering the low cost and fairly low intensity of the interventions. The nonresponders to universal interventions may be the right children to link to selected interventions in any case.

Designating children for selected interventions is a problem when there is no universal intervention as a first stage. The first appearance of a risk behavior such as aggressive behavior extends over months or years in the population. At any one point of selecting high-risk children for a selected intervention, an unknown population of children who are not yet aggressive will be destined to become aggressive later. Because children would not be detectable, they will be missed; and they may even attenuate differences if the design involves comparing high-risk children's developmental paths to those of the general population of children.

Also, selected interventions directed at high-risk children often label them more than do universal interventions, and they generally place greater demands on mental health professionals. Yet they are a necessary part of a child mental health service system.

The selected interventions can be tested within a multistage model. For example, at the system intervention level, prevention research on services for children would include first-stage measures of how each child is doing in terms of social adaptation to classroom, classmates/peers, and family. Universal intervention programs with documented outcomes might be in place in each of these social fields, backed up by selected interventions for those who do not respond to the universal interventions. Those who do not respond to the universal or selected interventions might then require indicated treatments. Indicated interventions are essentially treatment services for those already identifiably ill or with a diagnosable disorder, and are the most costly and demanding for professional training and staffing.

Dual Preventive Trials Testing Developmental Paths in Baltimore

Developmental models can often be tested best by using two interventions in a parallel design, rather than one, thereby attacking alternative parts of a developmental model. Such a dual intervention strategy allows direction of effects among the variables to be tested along with the specificity of effects of the interventions. We will illustrate this point by describing two trials done on defined populations of first grade children in Baltimore in a randomized design, one aimed at raising reading achievement, the other at reducing aggressive and shy behaviors. We defined aggressive behavior as fighting and breaking rules, and shy behavior as not raising your hand, and sitting and playing alone. As we described earlier, children who are shy *and* aggressive are loners who break rules and fight. These two targets have been found to be antecedents of specific later outcomes, depressive symptoms in the case of low achievement, and heavy drug use and delinquency in the case of aggressive (and particularly shy and aggressive) children. Shy behavior by itself has been found to predict anxiety later (Kellam et al., 1983).

The targets are correlated with each other, but the direction of effects has not been clear. In a recent paper we reported on the fall to spring evolution of aggressive and shy behavior and achievement test scores (Kellam et al., 1991), using a cross-lag strategy. These analyses pointed to the central role of concentration problems in the expression of both poor achievement and of shy and aggressive behaviors. At the time of the initiation of the dual trial design these results were not known, however. The trials were designed to allow testing whether improving aggressive or shy behavior would improve achievement or vice versa. The alternative is whether the correlation of poor achievement with shy and aggressive behavior was due to a third source, such as concentration problems (as the later analyses suggest).

Even with the results from the cross-lag analyses, it is still quite possible that an active intervention or interventions could produce effects not visible from longitudinal correlational analyses without the preventive intervention experiment. The two parallel trials allow direct as well as crossover effects to be assessed, thus informing theory about direction of effects of the targets on each other or determining whether other forces, such as concentration problems may be operating on both to account for the intercorrelation.

To use the intervention impact in testing theory, the effect of the intervention must be specific for the mediator variable, rather than just a function of general attention. Only the proximal target must be changed. The other parts should be changed only through changing the hypothesized mediator, which is the proximal target.

The first-stage assessments in Baltimore that enter into the evaluation of the field trials are done periodically before and during interventions and annually thereafter on all children in two cohorts. They include evaluation of both social adaptational status and psychological well-being. The proximal targets of the two preventive trials done thus far are maladaptive behavioral responses to classroom task demands: low achievement on the one hand and aggressive and shy behaviors on the other.

Three social fields and their natural raters are involved in each of our two preventive trials: the classroom in which the teacher is the natural rater; the classmate/peer group in which classmates are the natural raters; and the family in which parents are the natural raters. Two of these three kinds of natural raters in their social fields provide the structure for much of the following descriptions of the measures of social adaptational status and psychological well-being.

Assessing Social Adaptational Status in the Classroom and Peer Group

The first-stage core assessments of children's social adaptational status we will describe here include teacher's ratings of how well each child was meeting classroom task demands and peer nominations of the children's social adaptational status in regard to peer relationships. Using a time sampling method, direct observation of classroom behavior was also employed to inform our analyses of impact as to the meaning of the peer and teacher ratings. Achievement test scores were used to augment the core task demand facing the child in the classroom, namely, learning the subject matter.

A structured teacher interview called the Teacher Observation of Classroom Adaptation–Revised (TOCA-R) was developed by revising the teacher interview used in the Woodlawn studies (Kellam et al., 1975; Werthamer-Larsson, Kellam, & Wheeler, 1991). The updated TOCA-R is administered in a quiet room in the school through a carefully constructed interview that requires about two hours to obtain ratings of how each child in the teacher's class is performing the basic classroom task demands. While the teacher is being interviewed two other staff administer two classroom instruments, the peer nomination method and an instrument used by the children to report their feelings.

Psychometric work on the TOCA-R confirmed three factors that represent the basic social task demands of the teacher (the fourth being achievement). These were found to be: (1) *Social Contact*, consisting of child's social participation in the classroom processes; the maladaptive response to this task was named many years ago in the Woodlawn studies as *shy behavior*; (2) *Authority Acceptance*, consisting of accepting the teacher's and school's rules; the maladaptive response was named *aggressive behavior* and consists of breaking rules, harming property, and fighting; and (3) *Concentration*, consisting of being ready to work and paying attention; the maladaptive response is rated by the teacher as *concentration problems*. The California Achievement Test provided the measure of social adaptational status for the fourth classroom task.

While the TOCA-R provides the teacher's social adaptational status ratings of the children's performance of classroom task demands, a peer nomination measure called the Peer Assessment Inventory provides the children's perspective of each other's social adaptational status in their classmate/peer group. This measure is a classroom-administered, modified version of the Pupil Evaluation Inventory (PEI) (Pekarik, Prinz, Leibert, Weintraub, & Neale, 1976). Ten items were selected from the original PEI on the basis of their relevance to three social adaptational status constructs: aggressive behavior, shy behavior, and likability. Items reflective of rejection and bullying have been added since the first year.

Assessing Child Psychological Well-Being

The measures of child psychological well-being include self-report first-stage measures of depressive and anxious symptoms called the Baltimore How I Feel (BHIF). Children report the frequency of symptoms on a four-point scale: "never," "once in a while," "sometimes," and "most times." Items were keyed for the most part to DSM-III-R (American Psychiatric Association, 1987) criteria for major depression and overanxious and separation anxiety disorders. A number of items were drawn from existing child self-report measures including the Revised Children's Manifest Anxiety Scale (RCMAS) (Reynolds & Richmond, 1985), the Children's Depression Inventory (CDI) (Kovacs, 1983), the Depression Self-Rating Scale (Asarnow & Carlson, 1985), and the Hopelessness Scale for Children (Kazdin, Rodgers, & Colbus, 1986). The remaining items were developed by an expert panel of judges consisting of two child psychiatrists and two clinical psychologists. The revisions were done to improve the psychometric properties of the CDI and RCMAS, particularly the separation of anxiety items from depression items and their integration into a single instrument that allowed developmental study of anxiety and depression without method variance confusing them.

A critical aspect of this work was the initial worry as to whether first graders could understand, let alone rate, their feelings of anxiety and depression. As in many other instances the epidemiological base for this developmental question allowed us to study this issue. We found that children at this grade level could meaningfully report their feelings with considerable psychometric strength (Edelsohn, Ialongo, Werthamer-Larsson, Crockett, & Kellam, 1992).

Assessing the Environments of the Classroom and Peers/Classmates

First-stage measures of social adaptational status and psychological well-being administered in the classroom lend themselves to calculating prevalence rates and variances in the classroom and in those grade levels assessed in school. Classrooms with greater prevalence of poor achievement test scores, greater prevalence of teacher ratings of high aggressive behavior or high shy behavior, or high prevalence of child self-reports of depressed mood may influence the child's responses to the preventive intervention trials in that classroom.

Prevalence rates of social adaptational status measures can indicate schools and classrooms where tracking or ability grouping of students into homogeneous classrooms occurs (Kellam, 1990). Analyses from a recently published study indicate that children in low-achieving classrooms had significantly higher teacher ratings of aggressive and shy behavior than children in higher achieving classrooms, after controlling for potentially confounding child characteristics and classroom behavior environment effects (Werthamer-Larsson et al., 1991). Children in poor-behaving classrooms also had significantly higher teacher ratings of shy behavior than children who were not in poor-behaving classrooms. Results of a hierarchical analysis of variance for both the classroom achievement environment hierarchical model and the classroom behavior environment hierarchical model are shown in Table 8.1.

We are using prevalence rates based on peer nominations of aggressive behavior, shy behavior, and likability, as well as the peer attributions of psychological well-being, to construct similar classifications of classmate/peer groups. In the Baltimore study, the Peer Assessment Inventory described earlier has been used to obtain peer assessments of all children in each classroom of 19 East Baltimore public schools. Figures 8.1 and 8.2 show the percent of the peer-nominated aggressive behavior for males and females across the 19 schools, using a cutoff of peer nominations for aggressive behavior by one third or more of classmates. For males, schools are ordered from

TABLE 8.1. Effect of Classroom Environment on Child Behavior, Controlling for Child Characteristics[a]

Class environment	Social contact		Authority acceptance		Concentration	
	M	F	M	F	M	F
Class achievement		3.45[b]		4.15[b]		1.32
Low achieving	.31		.33		.36	
Mixed achieving	.25		.27		.38	
High achieving	.25		.31		.40	
Class behavior		22.90[c]		0.01		1.62
Satisfactory	.25		.30		.37	
Poor behaving	.35		.30		.40	

[a]Gender, age, kindergarten grades, kindergarten work habit problems, first grade repeater, preschool experience, and between-year change were entered into the model before the Class Environment variable. Means are adjusted for all variables in the model.
[b]$p < .05$. [c]$p < .001$.
Note. From "Effect of Classroom Environment on Shy Behavior, Aggressive Behavior, and Concentration Problems" by L. Werthamer-Larsson, S. G. Kellam, and L. Wheeler, 1991, *American Journal of Community Psychology, 19,* p. 595. Copyright 1991 by Plenum Publishing Corp. Reprinted by permission.

the highest percent to the lowest of male children receiving nominations for aggressive behavior. For females, the schools correspond to the ordering for male aggressive behavior.

As in Woodlawn, we found considerable variation in peer-rated aggressive behavior across schools for both genders. In fact, there was

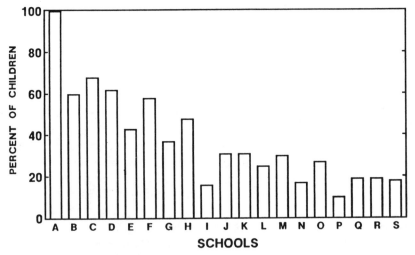

FIGURE 8.1. Prevalence of male aggressive behavior measured by classmates' nominations in 19 schools (one third or more of classmates).

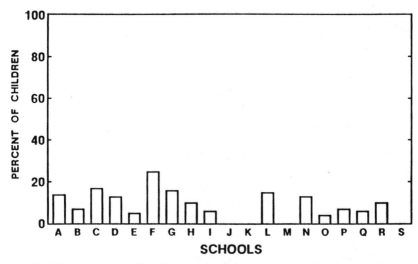

FIGURE 8.2. Prevalence of female aggressive behavior measured by classmates' nominations in 19 schools (one third or more of classmates).

a wider range of aggressive behavior as rated by peers across schools than of that rated by teachers. As Figure 8.1 indicates, in School A 100 percent of the children were nominated by a third or more of their classmates as aggressive. In School P less than 10 percent of the children were rated as aggressive by a third or more of their classmates.

Within schools, there was even more variation across classrooms in peer nominations for aggression. For example, in School B the prevalence of peer-rated aggressive behavior was about 60 percent, placing it among the top five schools in terms of prevalence of aggression. However, the variation across classrooms within the school in peer nominations for aggression was striking. In one classroom almost 85 percent of the children received nominations from classmates for aggression; in another classroom only about 33 percent of the children received aggressive behavior nominations.

Developmental and prevention research require understanding the influence of this variation in classroom environments over time on developmental course and on children's responses to preventive interventions. Classmate/peer groups with high rates of peer rejection or peer aggression may respond differently to preventive intervention than those with low rates, for example. Similarly, classmate/peer groups with high likability and low shy behavior levels may respond more positively to intervention than those exhibiting greater social isolation and less social warmth.

This variation occurred by the end of the first quarter of the school year in spite of random assignment of children within schools to classrooms. Presumably the variation reflects teacher, parent, and school behavior management effectiveness. It is important to underline the fact that random assignment did not equalize the child's behavior or learning across classrooms. Classroom, peer group, and family factors must continue to be included in analyses of impact. Richard Royall is particularly informative on the role of random assignment in clinical trials and much of his analysis appears appropriate to preventive trial design as well (Royall, 1976, 1991). His central point is that randomization may be an important device in experimental design, but it does not guarantee that selection bias is prevented or that relevant differences do not remain between experimental and control groups.

Baseline as a Developmental Model

As a first step in the assessment of impact of the two trials, baseline modeling was very important in revealing the evolving relationships among teacher ratings of shy and aggressive behaviors, concentration problems, achievement test scores (all social adaptational status measures), and self-reports of depression (a psychological well-being measure) (Kellam et al., 1991). These baseline modeling analyses were first derived from the first of two cohorts of first grade children in the Baltimore preventive trials, covering 1200 children who entered 19 public elementary schools in the eastern half of the city. This was at the time of the first report card, roughly 8 weeks into the school year.

Using multiple regression and log linear methods, we looked cross-sectionally at aggressive and shy behaviors and concentration first, then added school achievement test scores to these three, and finally added child self-reports of depressive symptoms to the model. To assess the evolving relationships and directions, we used a cross-lagged regression model in which pairs of variables were isolated to study the longitudinal relationships among the five variables from fall to spring. Only data from the 473 control children were analyzed for the longitudinal studies because the data from the other children were confounded over the course of first grade by the two preventive intervention trials. Analyses were done separately by gender (234 males, 239 females).

Baseline models derived from these methods show that maladaptation to classroom social task demands involving shy and aggressive behavior, concentration problems, and poor achievement are highly interrelated and are related to depressive symptoms as well, but in very specific ways with important gender differences (Kellam et al., 1991). The central role of concentration problems emerged in these baseline analyses. From fall to spring in first grade, concentration problems led to shy and aggressive behavior and poor achievement in both genders and to depressive symptoms among females. A summary of these cross-lagged relationships appears in Table 8.2.

Importantly, concentration problems almost never occurred by themselves; they were strongly associated with aggressive behavior, but equally strongly associated with shy behavior. A summary of the patterns of co-occurrence for each gender is contained in Figures 8.3 and 8.4. Based on these results, we hypothesize that concentration problems are a common latent condition underlying both social maladaptation and psychological well-being. Rather than a categorical attentional disorder, concentration/attention problems may be evidence of general developmental psychopathology with potential for expression in many forms including maladaptive shy and/or aggressive behavior, depressed affect, and poor learning.

Among females, but not males, there was evidence for reciprocal relationships between components of social adaptational status and between social adaptational status and psychological well-being (see Figure 8.4). For example, depressive symptoms led to poor achievement in both males and females, whereas poor achievement led to depressive symptoms in females but not males, at least over the first grade year. Similarly, for females, concentration problems in the fall preceded aggressive behavior in the spring, and aggressive behavior in the fall also predicted concentration problems later. The presence or absence of these reciprocal relationships may reflect an important aspect of gender differences that may be part of the explanation of later gender differences in prevalence of aggression and depression.

The reciprocal relationships that characterize first grade girls rather than boys suggest that girls show greater concern with the judgments of natural raters than boys. These results support recent findings showing that first grade girls are more responsive to parents' evaluation of their academic achievement, whereas first grade boys rely more on self-evaluations (Entwisle, Alexander, Pallas, & Cadigan, 1987; Roberts, 1991).

These results on reciprocities provide important epidemiological data on the developmental paths leading to problem outcomes and suggest further, more finely targeted, preventive trials. A plausible reciprocal effects hypothesis is that depression leads to poor achievement, which in turn leads to more depression, and so on with increasing effects. The prevention research question we are currently exploring in the periodic follow-up analyses of impact is whether this

TABLE 8.2. Summary of Cross-Lagged Regression Analyses: Fall to Spring

Predictor variable	Male			Female		
	b	*SE*	t	b	*SE*	t
Aggressive behavior						
Constant	0.60	0.07	6.99[c]	0.35	0.06	5.64[c]
Aggressive behavior	0.63	0.04	17.92[c]	0.73	0.03	21.24[c]
Concentration	0.07	0.03	2.66[c]	0.04	0.02	2.14[a]
	$R^2 = 0.52$			$R^2 = 0.58$		
Shy behavior						
Constant	0.57	0.10	5.93[c]	0.70	0.10	7.31[c]
Shy behavior	0.61	0.04	16.44[c]	0.60	0.04	16.46[c]
Concentration	0.11	0.03	4.31[c]	0.09	0.03	3.29[c]
	$R^2 = 0.53$			$R^2 = 0.48$		
Concentration						
Constant	0.32	0.10	3.11[c]	0.29	0.09	3.16[b]
Concentration	0.86	0.03	27.76[c]	0.73	0.03	25.14[c]
Aggressive behavior	0.01	0.04	0.29	0.18	0.05	3.56[c]
	$R^2 = 0.69$			$R^2 = 0.65$		
Constant	0.31	0.12	2.66[a]	0.49	0.10	4.77[c]
Concentration	0.86	0.03	26.72[c]	0.76	0.03	26.40[c]
Shy behavior	0.01	0.05	0.27	−0.02	0.04	−0.52
	$R^2 = 0.69$			$R^2 = 0.66$		
Constant	1.33	0.42	3.20[b]	1.08	0.37	2.91[b]
Concentration	0.82	0.03	24.35[b]	0.74	0.03	22.16[c]
Achievement	0.00	0.00	−2.48[b]	−0.00	0.00	−1.73
	$R^2 = 0.70$			$R^2 = 0.65$		
Constant	0.29	0.10	2.89[b]	0.39	0.09	4.33[c]
Concentration	0.85	0.03	28.77[c]	0.75	0.11	27.26[c]
Depression	0.13	0.12	1.13	0.22	0.03	2.00[a]
	$R^2 = 0.69$			$R^2 = 0.66$		
Achievement						
Constant	193.14	14.34	13.47[c]	227.33	13.02	17.46[c]
Achievement	0.56	0.05	12.43[c]	0.46	0.04	10.85[c]
Concentration	−11.29	1.16	−9.74[c]	−11.62	1.14	−10.21[c]
	$R^2 = 0.54$			$R^2 = 0.51$		
Constant	117.60	11.90	9.89[c]	151.49	10.75	14.09[c]
Achievement	0.77	0.04	18.02[c]	0.67	0.04	17.33[c]
Depression	−15.67	4.09	−3.84[c]	−17.06	4.03	−4.23[c]
	$R^2 = 0.46$			$R^2 = 0.43$		
Depression						
Constant	0.19	0.04	5.09[c]	0.10	0.04	2.76[b]
Depression	0.40	0.04	9.49[c]	0.42	0.05	8.97[c]
Concentration	0.00	0.01	0.36	0.04	0.01	−3.18[b]
	$R^2 = 0.21$			$R^2 = 0.23$		
Constant	0.21	0.12	1.72	0.53	0.12	4.51[c]
Depression	0.38	0.04	9.08[c]	0.42	0.05	9.14[c]
Achievement	0.00	0.00	−0.02	−0.00	0.00	−3.11[b]
	$R^2 = 0.19$			$R^2 = 0.24$		

[a] $p < .05$.
[b] $p < .01$.
[c] $p < .001$.

180

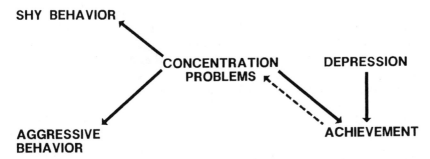

FIGURE 8.3. Course of classroom social adaptational status and depression from fall to spring of first grade, males (Cohort I 1985–1986).

reciprocity can be interrupted by improving achievement; and if so, whether the risk of more serious depressive disorder is reduced. Analyses of impact of the two preventive interventions are beginning to throw some light on this issue.

The results illustrate an important concept, baseline as a developmental model. Baseline measurement permits us to recognize the interrelationships among target antecedents and their evolving roles in development. We propose that in preventive trials the concept of baseline is best viewed as a developmental model that evolves over time, rather than as a cross-sectional model to be measured at a single point in time. Baseline consists of the developmental model over time without intervention, while the experimental group is the developmental model with the intervention.

Such trials allow testing of the developmental functions of target antecedents by informing us whether changing the antecedents re-

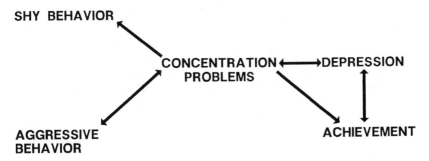

FIGURE 8.4. Course of classroom social adaptational status and depression from fall to spring of first grade, females (Cohort I 1985–1986).

duces the risk of the problem condition. Hence, developmental and etiological theory evolves at the same time that effective prevention methods do. Analyses of intervention impact need to take these inter-relationships of the target and other parts of the antecedent model into account. Simply treating the other conditions as covariates is insufficient. Assessment of variation in responses to intervention is a central part of the analytic work, the part that leads to strengthening the next stages of theory and trials.

The Early Impact of the Mastery Learning and Good Behavior Game Interventions

The two preventive trials in the Baltimore City Public Schools have been directed at the early behavioral responses of children to teachers' task demands in the classroom environment (as outlined in the previous section), which were demonstrated to be predictors for later depression, drug use, and delinquency. The first intervention was directed at learning problems and consisted of a strengthened reading curriculum for the entire class (Dolan et al., 1991). It was based on the literature on Mastery Learning (Block & Burns, 1976; Bloom, 1964).

A critical aspect of the Mastery Learning training program was the development of a group-paced approach to mastery, such that students did not proceed to the next learning unit until the majority (80% achieving 80–85% of objectives) of students fulfilled the learning objectives of the previous unit. Another primary goal of training was to develop a flexible corrective process targeted toward particular learners and particular learning problems or difficulties.

The second intervention, also directed at the entire class, was aimed at aggressive and shy-aggressive behavior and consisted of a behavior management method called the Good Behavior Game (Barrish, Saunders, & Wolfe, 1969; Dolan et al., 1991; Medland & Stacknik, 1972). The Good Behavior Game is a team-based behavior management strategy that promoted good behavior by rewarding teams that did not exceed maladaptive behavior standards. The strategy makes each child's behavior a matter of concern to all children in that team because the team reward is dependent on each child's behavior.

The Johns Hopkins Prevention Research Center has established very close collaboration with the Baltimore City Public Schools in all aspects of this prevention work. The interventions, measures, and all other procedures are jointly designed and are implemented after careful review by school officials, parents, teachers, and community organization leaders. Such a partnership is vital for this type of population and community-based research (Jason, 1982; Kellam &

Branch, 1971; Kellam et al., 1972; Kellam & Hunter, 1990; Rebok et al., 1991). From within the overall area of eastern Baltimore City, five quite varied urban areas were selected (see Table 8.3). In each urban area, three or four matched schools were chosen for a total of 19. Two population-based cohorts of 1,197 and 1,117 first grade children were studied.

One or two of the set of schools in each urban area was randomly assigned as a control school, another as a Mastery Learning school, and the third (or fourth) as a Good Behavior Game school. Within each intervention school, children were randomly assigned to an intervention classroom or a control classroom, with teachers also randomly chosen. The interventions were implemented over 2 years for each cohort after the intensive baseline assessments. Classrooms of children were kept together over the 2 years of the intervention.

The design for a preventive trial of this type must provide for some control over leakage or spillover effects that might happen if all or part of the intervention strategies were adopted in the comparison classrooms. These problems were addressed in the research design by having both internal control classrooms within the intervention schools and external control classrooms in the matched schools not receiving any special intervention. This also controlled for school level effects, a critical consideration in this type of research.

The results reported here focus on impact at the end of the first grade year. To be included in the analyses, all students had to remain in the same design condition for the entire year. Students who transferred into the school system or who left the system during the first grade year were not included in these analyses. For the Good Behavior Game condition, a total of 501 students met these criteria. The sample comprised 182 students from 8 classrooms for the Good Behavior Game intervention; the sample for the internal control condition comprised 107 students from 6 classrooms; and the sample for the external control condition comprised 212 students from 12 classrooms. For Mastery Learning, a total of 575 students remained in the same design condition for 1 year. The sample for the Mastery Learning condition comprised 207 students from 9 classrooms; the sample for the internal control condition comprised 156 students from 7 classrooms.

Teacher-rated concentration problems and aggressive and shy behavior, self-reported depressive symptoms, and standardized student achievement data from the California Achievement Test were all assessed for the Good Behavior Game, Mastery Learning, internal control, and external control conditions. Assessments were conducted in the fall of first grade at first report card time and in the following spring near the end of first grade.

TABLE 8.3. Characteristics of Five East Baltimore Areas from Which the Study Population Was Derived

Urban area	Ethnicity	Housing	Family structure	Income
1	Polish, Slavic, German, Italian, & Greek neighborhoods	Well-maintained small rowhouses passed from one generation to the next	Married couple with extended family members in close proximity	Low-middle
2	Predominantly black	Large public housing projects	Multigenerational with the grandmother as the primary parental figure	Very low to low
3	Totally black	Fairly well-maintained rowhouses; gradual decline of home ownership	Multigenerational with the grandmother as the primary parental figure	Middle; gradual decline
4	Integrated	Detached frame houses mostly owner-occupied	Married couples	Middle
5	White	Small detached or semi-detached homes mostly owner occupied	Married couples	Moderate

As hypothesized, short-term proximal or direct effects of both the Good Behavior Game and Mastery Learning interventions on their target antecedents were found in our initial analyses of impact (Dolan et al., 1991). For both males and females, the Good Behavior Game had a significant impact on aggressive and shy behavior as rated by teachers. Peer nominations of aggressive behavior by their classmates were also significantly reduced. It is notable that in both peer and teacher ratings of aggressive behavior, the more severely aggressive children responded the most to the Good Behavior Game. Of three peer-rated items for shy behavior only one showed significant impact ("has few friends"), and that was in the case of females only. We hypothesize that changes in aggressive behavior resulting from the Good Behavior Game intervention were due to group pressure to respond to team contingencies and classroom rewards for altering behavior, whereas changes in shy behavior may have resulted from an increase in very structured opportunities for nonthreatening interactions with others.

Cautions should be noted in the Good Behavior Game reports. Although teacher ratings are considered an important measure of social adaptational status, they are confounded by the fact that the teacher was an intervention agent and was knowledgeable about specific outcome targets. Therefore, the internal validity of the teacher ratings is at issue. Furthermore, teachers within the intervention school were aware that they were in a contrast condition and might want to improve the ratings within their classroom, assuming they liked the interventions. Peer ratings are also not without potential bias. The teams of classmates within the Good Behavior Game classrooms were reinforced for better behavior by their teacher. Hence the children may have reported better behavior among their peers than existed in reality. Alternatively, they and the teachers could have rated children more harshly because the cost of maladaptation had increased as a result of the Good Behavior Game. There was some evidence of this skewing in the results from the earlier Woodlawn prevention trials (Kellam et al., 1975).

Independent observers who were time-sampling classroom behavior were an important adjunct measure to gain control of this problem; and these revealed an increase in on-task behavior in the Good Behavior Game classrooms compared to the controls. Analyses of aggressive and shy behaviors assessed by the independent observers are now underway.

For the Mastery Learning intervention, we found significant short-term impact on reading achievement at the end of the spring of first grade for both males and females in covariance analyses controlling for baseline achievement. Importantly, the nature of the intervention impact differed by gender. Female high achievers benefited more from the Mastery Learning intervention than female low achievers, whereas male low achievers benefited more than male high achievers.

Depressed children were significantly lower in achievement in the fall of first grade. With Mastery Learning, their achievement levels in the spring were similar to those of the nondepressed children in Mastery Learning and significantly better than those of depressed children in either of the control conditions. We hypothesize that under Mastery Learning, the curriculum as used by the teachers maintained or increased depressed children's involvement in the teaching-learning process, and that the intervention clarified criteria for mastery and offered the children an experience of mastery.

Crossover Effects and Proximal/Distal Effects: The Core of Building Theory Through Preventive Trials

The essential element in this discourse on prevention trials and theory building lies in the possibility of (1) through dual trials changing the antecedent target condition of one trial by changing the target of the first trial (crossover effect); and (2) through each trial by changing an earlier antecedent along a developmental path and thereby shifting a distal target to a more healthy outcome later (proximal/distal effect).

Crossover Effects

The rationale for the dual trials in Baltimore rested on the correlation of aggressive behavior with poor achievement. To determine the etiological or developmental course leading to either of these, one intervention was aimed at aggressive behavior, the other at achievement test scores. The specificity was quite good in the case of each intervention in that only the specific proximal target was affected by the specific intervention. When we looked at the potential crossover effects, we were searching for the answer to our question of direction of development. If improved aggressive behavior resulting from the Good Behavior Game or other sources was associated with improved achievement, then we could hypothesize that aggressive behavior could actually lead to poor achievement and that such interventions as the Good Behavior Game could prevent poor achievement and, hypothetically, its distal consequences.

In the opposite way, if improvement in poor achievement was associated with improved aggressive behavior, then we would have hypothetical evidence that there was developmentally important linkage in that direction as well. With only two points of assessment analyzed thus far, we have a limited capacity to test whether it is the improved achievement that is driving the aggressive behavior, vice versa, or neither. However, if no crossover effect is found, then the hypothesis is supported that the proximal targets, aggressive behavior and poor achievement, derive from other sources than each other.

The results analyzed to date provide no evidence of any crossover effects of the two preventive interventions. Improvement in aggressive and shy behaviors occurred in the Good Behavior Game classrooms and in other contexts, but no improvement in achievement was associated with this behavioral improvement at least through the end of the first grade year. Similarly, the direct effects of Mastery Learning on improving reading achievement, its proximal target, produced no crossover reductions in aggressive behavior or shy behavior in the spring, as rated by teachers or peers.

Concentration problems may well be the shared underlying source of the correlation between aggressive and shy behavior and poor achievement. This hypothesis is suggested by the developmental baseline model results we described earlier (Kellam et al., 1991).

Proximal/Distal Effects

The purpose of the Mastery Learning intervention was to determine if by improving achievement, the risk of depressive symptoms and possibly depressive disorder could be improved. Similarly, the purpose of the Good Behavior Game was to test whether by improving aggressive and shy behaviors, the risk of the longer term outcomes of delinquency and heavy drug use could be reduced. The results provide powerful tools in understanding the relationship of the antecedents to the distal outcomes.

The antecedent becomes the proximal target of the intervention and the analyses must include the change in the proximal target to test the hypothesis. This theoretical function requires that new logical structure be applied to the analytic strategy. The randomized field trials we began with in Baltimore were no longer randomized field trials after the proximal targets were affected. Some children responded to each trial more or less than others, that is, they had differential nonrandom responses to the interventions. Treating the proximal target as simply a covariate while assessing impact on the distal target ignores, and may actually hide, the role of the proximal target in the hypothesized model. Mastery Learning was hypothesized, for example, to change reading scores and not to affect later depression directly. It was raised reading scores (mastery of a core task) that was hypothesized to improve the risk of depression. Also, treating the level of severity of the proximal target at baseline as a covariate rather than a potentially interacting variable may hide variation in impact of the intervention on the proximal target. Analyses of impact, therefore, must include the variation in reading scores (proximal target) as well as the variation in earlier and later depression.

The ways that the intervention may affect the proximal and distal targets are just now being explored, but we are finding major effects in the very relationships between the proximal and distal targets, or in the continuity and discontinuity of distal targets such as depression over time. Effects are frequently seen on the variances rather than on the means; indeed the means often are very poorly reflective of impact. For example, the impact of changing achievement appears to be on the continuity of depression from fall to spring among both boys and girls. Improving achievement is strongly associated with a marked drop in the continuity of depression from fall to spring, with those in Mastery Learning appearing to have a somewhat greater tendency toward lower continuity of depression with improved achievement. Children who did not improve in achievement had very strong correlations between fall and spring depression and higher levels of depression in the spring.

Redundant, Additive, or Synergistic Effects

The absence of crossover effects at least through first grade suggested the need for both the Mastery Learning and Good Behavior Game interventions since improving their proximal targets seemed to require specific interventions. The next set of preventive trials in Baltimore will include administering their combination in intervention classrooms. The combined impact may be redundant, that is, the impact of each may not be as great when done together in the same classrooms as when done separately. The effects could be additive or they could together provide synergism. Any of these outcomes allows interpretation that could be useful in building theory.

Combining the Mastery Learning and Good Behavior Game interventions may produce synergistic effects, however, in that the Good Behavior Game, by increasing attention to task and decreasing noncompliant and shy behavior, may make the child more available for the Mastery Learning intervention. In addition, the increased academic productivity associated with the Mastery Learning intervention could be improved by improving aggressive, shy, and off-task behaviors through the Good Behavior Game. Because there were only moderate improvements in reading and in aggressive and shy behaviors in the first prevention trials, there is room for improvement in both domains.

Negative Iatrogenic Effects

The consequences of children not responding well in preventive interventions is an area of current analysis. We are assessing negative effects on children who may be singled out by their classmates in the Good Behavior Game for costing their team rewards. Additionally, we are observant of children who may not improve in reading as much as their classmates and who may be at some increased risk of depression. If a child is referred to us by a teacher, principal, or parent who has a concern about extreme behavior or mood, or if an assessor or intervenor identifies a child who appears to be in severe distress during or soon after the time of assessment or intervention, our crisis response team has a crisis backup procedure in place. However, this leaves us with an analytic problem by potentially confounding the longer-term outcomes of the trial. We are just now attempting to integrate such post- or extratrial interventions into analyses of impact.

Introducing Malleability, Plasticity, and Elasticity into Developmental and Etiological Theory Building

In the prevention research approach we have described, the study populations and their environments are epidemiologically defined and deliberately varied. This enables us to examine the results as they apply to specific populations and determine whether the impact of the trial differs for subpopulations or under varying ecological conditions. We examine whether the effects of intervention are greatest among the groups with highest risk or whether the effects are greater, equal, or less among the lower risk groups (Brown, in press). Similarly, analyses are under way on the influence of classroom, peer, and family environments on children's development.

Impact in developmental terms is a reflection of malleability. Instead of conjecturing that a developmental process is changeable under certain conditions, the preventive trial allows us to test the question. Analyses of the results of the two Baltimore preventive interventions demonstrated impact particularly for children in high-risk groups. We were surprised to find that the Good Behavior Game appeared to reduce the level of aggressive behavior for children who were highly aggressive in the fall of first grade. Finding malleability in this subpopulation suggested that the level of severity in the fall was not a reflection of immutability, even with what might be considered a fairly low intensity of intervention. Severity did not equal immutability.

The Mastery Learning intervention led to significant gains in reading achievement scores on the California Achievement Test, compared to internal or external control conditions. Importantly, the reading scores for a subgroup of children in the fall of first grade who reported symptoms of depression were significantly lower than those of the other children. It was those initially depressed, low-scoring children who gained in reading through the Mastery Learning intervention. Again, we found malleability where we might not have expected it.

We are continuing to follow annually the same children through the transition to middle school and beyond to assess the slopes of impact in the children as a whole and to model variation in the slopes of impact among subgroups of the children. This follow-up analysis will also allow us to examine lagged effects of interventions across time and to test for the possibility of so-called sleeper effects. The follow-up analyses of the Baltimore preventive trials contribute to theory building by providing data on the malleability of the models being tested.

Theory building in developmental psychopathology and in human development generally is dramatically enhanced by testing malleability and two closely related concepts, plasticity and elasticity. Assessing the slopes of outcome turns our attention to the enduring qualities of the malleability in the model. If the results of the Good Behavior Game are short lived, they will have been informative about the character of the model. Those aspects that change with intervention but revert back to their earlier condition can be termed *elastic*, while those that change and remain changed can be termed *plastic*. We first learned of this important distinction from the Leightons and their colleagues (1963), who quoted from the biologist Paul Weiss (1949).

Developmental epidemiologically-based preventive trials are field experiments that provide us with a powerful means of addressing questions about etiology, vulnerability, development, and contextual influences on various subgroups within defined populations, across different social fields and life stages. Their promise is not for an immediate fix, but for an enduring and developing foundation for prevention and control of mental health problems, our public mental health mission.

ACKNOWLEDGMENTS

We acknowledge the contributions of the City of Baltimore, its families and children, and the administration of the Baltimore City Public Schools. The

Prevention Program is a collaboration between the Baltimore City Public Schools and the Prevention Research Center of the Department of Mental Hygiene, Johns Hopkins University School of Hygiene and Public Health. This work of the Prevention Program would not have been possible, let alone successful, without the active participation and continued support of the leadership, faculty, and staff of the school district and their guidance in our research and service enterprise. The Board of School Commissioners gave their strong endorsement.

The faculty and staff of the Baltimore Public Schools have made crucial contributions, specifically Dr. Walter Amprey, superintendent of Baltimore City Public Schools, and Drs. Lillian Gonzales and Patsy Blacksheare, deputy superintendents; Dr. Richard Hunter and Ms. Alice Pinderhughes, former superintendents of the Baltimore City Schools; and Dr. Charlene Griffin, former assistant superintendent for school management. The assistance and support of the following have been vital to our program: Dr. Leonard Wheeler, assistant superintendent for elementary schools, has been a major coordinator; Dr. Charlene Cooper-Boston, associate superintendent for external affairs; Dr. Herman Howard, associate superintendent for vocational and special education; Dr. Carla Ford, supervisor, office of early childhood education; Mr. Craig Cutter, former staff director, department of education; Mr. Clifton Ball, former executive director; and Ms. Jessie Douglas, former director of elementary schools. The leadership of Ms. Elva Edwards and her staff effort in community base-building and crisis backup are gratefully acknowledged. We acknowledge the scientific contributions of Drs. C. Hendricks Brown, James C. Anthony, Nick Ialongo, Lisa Werthamer-Larsson, Lawrence J. Dolan, Lawrence S. Mayer, and Gail Edelsohn. We also thank Ms. Maria Corrada-Bravo for her contribution to data analyses; Ms. Alice Brogden for manuscript control and production; and Ms. Fionnuala Regan for editorial preparation. The studies on which this chapter is based have been supported by the following grants, with supplements from the National Institute on Drug Abuse (NIDA): National Institute of Mental Health (NIMH), Grant Number P50 MH38725, Epidemiologic Prevention Center for Early Risk Behavior; NIMH Grant Number 1R01 MH42968, Periodic Outcome of Two Preventive Trials; and NIMH Grant Number 1R01 MH40859, Statistical Methods for Mental Health Preventive Trials; State of Illinois Department of Mental Health grants 17-224 and 17-322; NIMH Grant Number MH-15760; and Research Scientist Development Award Grant 1K01-MH47596; the Maurice Falk Medical Fund; and for the follow-up, NIDA Grant DA-00787.

REFERENCES

Anthony, J. C. (1990). Prevention research in the context of epidemiology, with a discussion of public health models. In P. Muehrer (Ed.), *Conceptual research models for preventing mental disorders* (DHHS Publication No. ADM 90-1713, pp. 1–32). Washington, DC: U.S. Government Printing Office.

Anthony, J .C., Folstein, M., Romanoski, A. J., Von Korff, M. R., Nestadt, G. R., Chahal, R., Merchant, A., Brown, C. H., Shapiro, S., Kramer, M., & Gruenberg, E. M. (1985). Comparison of the lay diagnostic interview schedule and a standardized psychiatric diagnosis. *Archives of General Psychiatry, 42,* 667–675.

American Psychiatric Association (1987). *Diagnostic and statistical manual of mental disorders* (3rd ed., rev.). Washington, DC: American Psychiatric Association.

Asarnow, J. R., & Carlson, G. A. (1985). Depression self-rating scale: Utility with child psychiatric inpatients. *Journal of Consulting and Clinical Psychology, 53,* 491–499.

Baltes, P. B. (1987). Theoretical propositions of life-span developmental psychology: On the dynamics between growth and decline. *Developmental Psychology, 23,* 611–626.

Baltes, P. B., Reese, H. W., & Lipsitt, L. P. (1980). Life-span developmental psychology. *Annual Review of Psychology, 31,* 65–110.

Bank, L., Dishion, T. J., Skinner, M., & Patterson, G. R. (1990). Method variance in structural equation modeling: Living with "GLOP." In G. R. Patterson (Ed.), *Depression and aggression in family interaction* (pp. 248–279). Englewood Cliffs, NJ: Erlbaum.

Barrish, H. H., Saunders, M., & Wolfe, M. D. (1969). Good Behavior Game. Effects of individual contingencies for group consequences and disruptive behavior in a classroom. *Journal of Applied Behavior Analysis, 2,* 119–124.

Block, J., Block, J. H., & Keyes, S. (1988). Longitudinally fore-telling drug usage in adolescence: Early childhood personality and environmental precursors. *Child Development, 59,* 336–355.

Block, J., & Burns, R. (1976). Mastery learning. In L. Shulman (Ed.), *Review of Research in Education* (Vol. 4, pp. 3–49). Itasca, IL: Peacock.

Bloom, B. S. (1964). *Stability and change in human characteristics.* New York: Wiley.

Brim, O. G., Jr., & Kagan, J. (1980). Perspectives on continuity. In O. G. Brim, Jr., & J. Kagan (Eds.), *Constancy and change: A view of the issues* (pp. 26–74). Cambridge: Harvard University Press.

Brown, C. H. (in press). Statistical methods for preventive trials in mental health. *Statistics in Medicine.*

Dolan, L. J., Kellam, S. G., Brown, C. H., Werthamer-Larsson, L., Rebok, G. W., Mayer, L. S., Laudolff, J., Turkkan, J. S., Ford, C., & Wheeler, L. (1991). *Short-term impact of two classroom-based preventive interventions on aggressive and shy behaviors and poor achievement.* Manuscript submitted for publication.

Edelsohn, G., Ialongo, N., Werthamer-Larsson, L., Crockett, L., & Kellam, S. (1992). Self-reported depressive symptoms in first-grade children: Developmentally transient phenomena? *Journal of the American Academy of Child and Adolescent Psychiatry, 31,* 282–290.

Ensminger, M. E. (1990). Sexual activity and problem behaviors among black urban adolescents. *Child Development, 61,* 2032–2046.

Ensminger, M. E., Kellam, S. G., & Rubin, B. R. (1983). School and family origins of delinquency: Comparisons by sex. In K. T. Van Dusen & S. A. Mednick (Eds.), *Prospective studies of crime and delinquency* (pp. 73–97). Boston: Kluwer-Nijhoff.

Entwisle, D. R., Alexander, K. L., Pallas, A. M., & Cadigan, D. (1987). The emergent academic self-image of first graders: Its response to social structure. *Child Development, 58,* 1190–1206.

Farrington, D. P., Gallagher, B., Morley, L., St. Ledger, R. J., & West, D. J. (1988). Are there successful men from criminogenic backgrounds? *Psychiatry, 51,* 116–130.

Farrington, D. P., & Gunn, J. (Eds.). (1985). *Aggression and dangerousness.* New York: Wiley.

Gordon, R. S. (1983). An operational classification of disease prevention. *Public Health Reports, 98,* 107–109.

Hans, S. L., Marcus, J., Henson, L., Auerbach, J. G., & Mirsky, A. F. (1991). *Interpersonal behavior of children at risk for schizophrenia.* Manuscript submitted for publication.

Jason, L. A. (1982). Community-based approaches in preventing adolescent problems. *School Psychology Review, 11,* 417–424.

Kazdin, A. E., Rodgers, A., & Colbus, D. (1986). The Hopelessness Scale for Children: Psychometric characteristics and concurrent validity. *Journal of Consulting and Clinical Psychology, 54,* 242–245.

Kellam, S. G. (1990). Developmental epidemiologic framework for family research on depression and aggression. In G. R. Patterson (Ed.), *Depression and aggression in family interaction* (pp. 11–48). Englewood Cliffs, NJ: Erlbaum.

Kellam, S. G. (1991). A developmental epidemiological research program for the prevention of mental distress and disorder, heavy drug use, and violent behavior. In W. LL Parry-Jones & N. Queloz (Eds.), *Mental health and deviants in inner cities* (pp. 101–108). Geneva: World Health Organization.

Kellam, S. G., Adams, R. G., Brown, C. H., & Ensminger, M. E. (1982). The long-term evolution of family structure of teenage and older mothers. *Journal of Marriage and the Family, 44,* 539–554.

Kellam, S. G., & Branch, J. D. (1971). An approach to community mental health: Analysis of basic problems. *Seminars in Psychiatry, 3,* 207–25.

Kellam, S. G., Branch, J. D., Agrawal, K. C., & Ensminger, M. E. (1975). *Mental health and going to school: The Woodlawn program of assessment, early intervention, and evaluation.* Chicago: University of Chicago Press.

Kellam, S. G., Branch, J. D., Agrawal, K. C., & Grabill, M. E. (1972). Woodlawn Mental Health Center: An evolving strategy for planning in community mental health. In S. E. Golann & E. Eisdorfer (Eds.),

Handbook of community mental health (pp. 711–727). New York: Appleton-Century-Crofts.

Kellam, S. G., Brown, C. H., Rubin, B. R., & Ensminger, M. E. (1983). Paths leading to teenage psychiatric symptoms and substance use: Developmental epidemiological studies in Woodlawn. In S. B. Guze, F. J. Earls, & J. E. Barrett (Eds.), *Childhood psychopathology and development* (pp. 17–51). New York: Raven Press.

Kellam, S. G., & Ensminger, M. E. (1980). Theory and method in child psychiatric epidemiology. In F. Earls (Ed.), *Studies of children* (pp. 145–180). New York: Prodist.

Kellam, S. G., Ensminger, M. E., & Turner, R. J. (1977). Family structure and the mental health of children. *Archives of General Psychiatry, 34,* 1012–1022.

Kellam, S. G., & Hunter, R. C. (1990). Prevention begins in first grade. *Principal, 70,* 17–19.

Kellam, S. G., & Werthamer-Larsson, L. (1986). Developmental epidemiology: A basis for prevention. In M. Kessler & S. E. Goldston (Eds.), *A decade of progress in primary prevention* (pp. 154–180). Hanover, NH: University Press of New England.

Kellam, S. G., Werthamer-Larsson, L., Dolan, L., Brown, C. H., Mayer, L., Rebok, G. W., Anthony, J. C., Laudolff, J., Edelsohn, G., & Wheeler, L. (1991). Developmental epidemiologically based preventive trials: Baseline modeling of early target behaviors and depressive symptoms. *American Journal of Community Psychology, 19,* 563–584.

Kovacs, M. (1983). *The children's depression inventory: A self-rated depression scale for school-age youngsters.* Unpublished Manuscript, University of Pittsburgh: Pittsburgh, PA.

Leighton, D. C., Harding, J. S., Macklin, D. B., Macmillan, A. M., & Leighton, A. H. (1963). *The character of danger: Vol. 3. Psychiatric symptoms in selected communities.* New York: Basic Books.

McCord, J. (1988). Parental behavior in the cycle of aggression. *Psychiatry, 51,* 14–23.

Medland, M. B., & Stacknik, T. J. (1972). Good Behavior Game: A replication and systematic analysis. *Journal of Applied Behavior Analysis, 5,* 45–51.

Neugarten, B. (1969). Continuities and discontinuities of psychological issues into adult life. *Human Development, 12,* 121–130.

Pekarik, E., Prinz, R., Leibert, C., Weintraub, S., & Neale, J. (1976). The Pupil Evaluation Inventory: A sociometric technique for assessing children's social behavior. *Journal of Abnormal Child Psychology, 4,* 83–97.

Rebok, G. W., Kellam, S. G., Dolan, L. J., Werthamer-Larsson, L., Edwards, E. J., Mayer, L. S., & Brown, C. H. (1991). Early risk behaviors: Process issues and problem areas in prevention research. *Community Psychologist, 24,* 18–21.

Reynolds, C. R. & Richmond, B. O. (1985). Revised Children's Manifest Anxiety Scale (RCMAS) Manual. Los Angeles: Western Psychological Services.

Roberts, T. (1991). Gender and the influence of evaluations on self-assessments in achievement settings. *Psychological Bulletin, 109*, 297–308.

Robins, L. N. (1978). Sturdy childhood predictors of adult antisocial behavior: Replications from longitudinal studies. *Psychological Medicine, 8*, 611–622.

Royall, R. M. (1976). Current advances in sampling theory: Implications for human observational studies. *American Journal of Epidemiology, 104*, 463–474.

Royall, R. M. (1991). Ethics and statistics in randomized clinical trials. *Statistical Science, 6*, 52–58.

Rutter, M. (1989). Pathways from childhood to adult life. *Journal of Child Psychology and Psychiatry, 30*, 23–51.

Schwartzman, A. E., Ledingham, J. E., & Serbin, L. A. (1985). Identification of children at-risk for adult schizophrenia: A longitudinal study. *International Review of Applied Psychology, 34*, 363–380.

Shedler, J., & Block, J. (1990). Adolescent drug use and psychological health: A longitudinal inquiry. *American Psychologist, 45*, 612–630.

Tomas, J. M., Vlahov, D., & Anthony, J. C. (1990). Association between intravenous drug use and early misbehavior. *Drug and Alcohol Dependence, 25*, 79–89.

Tremblay, R. E., Masse, B., Perron, D., LeBlanc, M., Schwartzman, A. E., & Ledingham, J. E. (1992). Early disruptive behavior, poor school achievement, delinquent behavior, and delinquent personality: Longitudinal analyses. *Journal of Consulting and Clinical Psychology, 60*, 64–72.

Uttal, D. H., & Perlmutter, M. (1989). Toward a broader conceptualization of development: The role of gains and losses across the life span. *Developmental Review, 9*, 101–132.

Weiss, P. (1949). The biological basis of adaptation. In J. Romano (Ed.), *Adaptation* (pp. 7–14). Ithaca, NY: Cornell University Press.

Werthamer-Larsson, L., Kellam, S. G., & Wheeler, L. (1991). Effect of classroom environment on shy behavior, aggressive behavior, and concentration problems. *American Journal of Community Psychology, 19*, 585–602.

CHAPTER 9

◆ ——— ◆

The Cambridge-Somerville Study:
A Pioneering Longitudinal Experimental Study of Delinquency Prevention

JOAN MCCORD

Claims linking family inadequacies with criminal behavior are far from new. In the 17th century, for example, William Gouge (1627) described the duties of family members toward one another by writing that "children well nurtured and by correction kept in filiall awe, will so carry themselves, as their parents may rest somewhat secure" (p. 311). In the 19th century, convinced that "all sources of crime . . . may be traced to one original cause, namely, the neglect of parents as to a proper care of their children," Jevons urged that parents, rather than their children, be punished for their children's delinquency (1834/1970, p. 153). In 1848, the New York City chief of police described the delinquents he encountered as "the offspring of always careless, generally intemperate, and oftentimes immoral and dishonest parents" (Matsell, 1850, p. 14).

By the first quarter of the 20th century, such observations had become common enough to encourage a movement aimed at preventing crime through use of child guidance clinics. As part of this movement, teams of workers consisting of a psychologist, a psychiatrist, and a social worker joined forces to combat problems believed to be at the root of crime. In 1917, Judge Frederick Cabot invited William Healy, M.D., director of the Juvenile Psychopathic Institute in Chicago, to become head of the Judge Baker Foundation (Mennel, 1973).

Healy (1917) believed that delinquents lacked close emotional ties. Delinquents, he wrote, "never had any one near to them, particularly in family life, who supplied opportunities for sympathetic confidences" (p. 327).

As director of the Judge Baker Foundation (later known as the Judge Baker Guidance Centre), Healy and his codirector, Augusta Bronner, worked closely with Judge Cabot. The Judge Baker Foundation reviewed juvenile court cases, making recommendations to the court regarding placement and treatment. Careful case reviews not only served as bases for their recommendations but also enabled Healy and Bronner (1926) to identify common features in the backgrounds of delinquents. Among the discoveries they reported was the fact that less than 10% of 2000 young recidivists had come from "reasonably good conditions for the upbringing of a child" (p. 129). When they compared delinquents with their nondelinquent siblings, they gained additional support for the view that lack of warm interaction in the family was at least partially responsible for crime. Healy and Bronner (1936) discovered that the nondelinquents received more affection. Naturally, recommendations made by the Judge Baker Foundation reflected the perspectives of its directors.

Meanwhile, Sheldon Glueck, who had taken a seminar with Richard Clark Cabot (a cousin of Judge Cabot) in 1925, began to study the impact of the juvenile justice system on later criminal careers (Glueck & Glueck, 1945). As part of this assessment, Sheldon and Eleanor T. Glueck retraced delinquents 5 years after official control by the Boston court ended. Disconcertingly, Glueck and Glueck (1934) reported that of the 905 delinquents who could have become recidivists, 798 (88.2%) had done so. Rates of recidivism were only slightly lower among the subset of cases in which the Judge Baker recommendations had been followed. These results produced calls for stronger interventions and greater attention to the broader life setting of delinquents. Healy had suggested attacking the problem of delinquency as it could "be seen developing in school life" (1934, p. 94). This was the climate into which the Cambridge-Somerville Youth Study was born.

In 1934 Dr. Cabot retired from Harvard, where he had served as professor of clinical medicine and of social ethics. His medical work included texts on diagnosis. He had made a mark in the field by showing how to differentiate typhoid fever from malaria, and his etiological study of heart disease was widely recognized as an important medical contribution. Cabot introduced social services to Massachusetts General Hospital and became president of the National Conference on Social Work in 1931. He wrote about social work, the relationship between psychotherapy and religion, and the meaning of right and wrong. His scientific writing and teaching had been broadly critical, and it was reported that the Massachusetts Medical Society considered expelling him for publicly criticizing general practitioners by claiming that most diagnoses were wrong (Deardorff, 1958).

Richard C. Cabot reviewed the Gluecks' study of recidivism for the journal *Survey* and was convinced of the need for more information about the development of criminal behavior. He concluded his review with an expression of admiration that shaped the future of his work: "What piece of social work . . . is able to declare (with good grounds for its belief) that it has not failed in 88 percent of its endeavors? I honor the Judge Baker Foundation and the Boston Juvenile Court for having welcomed this piece of investigation. They have trusted in the spirit of science though their hopes of success may perish at the hands of that spirit" (1934, p. 40).

Cabot hypothesized that even rebellious youths from ghastly families "may conceivably be steered away from a delinquent career and toward useful citizenship if a devoted individual outside his own family gives him consistent emotional support, friendship, and timely guidance" (Allport, 1951, p. vi). The Cambridge-Somerville Youth Study would test this hypothesis.

METHOD

The Cambridge-Somerville Youth Study grafted scientific methods onto a social action program. The Youth Study was designed both to learn about the development of delinquent youngsters and to test Cabot's belief about how a child could be steered away from delinquency. Cabot selected as the sites for his study an area of eastern Massachusetts in which poverty was widespread and crimes were common. Within these areas, boys whose ages were less than 12 became potential targets for intervention.

To avoid stigmatizing participants, boys without difficulties as well as those who seemed headed for trouble were included in the program. Between 1935 and 1939 the Youth Study staff used information collected from schools, neighborhoods, courts, physicians, and families to match pairs of boys similar in age, intelligence, physiques, family environments and backgrounds, social environments, and delinquency-prone histories. In the absence of intervention, both boys in a pair would be expected to have similar lives. The selection committee flipped a coin to decide which member of the pair would receive treatment and which would be placed in the control group.[1]

Each boy in the treatment group was assigned to a social worker who tried to build a close personal relationship with the boy and assist both the boy and his family in a variety of ways. Counselors were not allowed to have contact with criminal justice agencies or with boys in the control group, though, naturally, no attempt was made to prevent their receiving assistance from other sources.

Supported by the Ella Lyman Cabot Foundation, the program started with 325 matched pairs of boys. This number was reduced as the United States entered World War II, counselors joined the armed forces, and gas rationing made it more difficult to travel. When a boy was dropped from the treatment program, his "matched mate" was dropped from the control group. In 1942, when 253 boys remained in the treatment program and an equal number remained in the control group, the research staff compared the groups (Powers & Witmer, 1951).

No reliable differences were discovered in comparisons of age, IQ, or whether referral to the Youth Study had been as difficult or not difficult. The two groups had almost identical delinquency prediction scores, as these were assigned by the selection committee summarizing the boys' family histories and home environments. No reliable differences appeared in comparisons regarding the boys' physical health as rated by the doctor after a medical examination, or in mental health, social adjustment, acceptance of authority, or social aggressiveness as reflected by teachers' descriptions of the boys. Nor were reliable differences found in ratings regarding adequacy of the home, disruption of the home, delinquency in the home, adequacy of discipline, standard of living, occupational status of the father, "social status level" of the elementary school attended by the boy (a measure based on the occupational levels of fathers whose children attended the school), or quality of the neighborhood in which the boys resided (Powers & Witmer, 1951).

The average age of the boys at the start of treatment was 10.5. Social workers, psychologists, tutors, a shop instructor, consulting psychiatrists, and medical doctors formed the treatment staff. Boys were seen in their homes, on the streets, and in the headquarters of the project.

1. An exception to random assignment was made for eight cases who were matched after the treatment began. In addition, brothers were assigned to that group to which the first of siblings was randomly assigned. This involved 21 boys in the treatment group and 19 in the control group.

To the innovative design in which matched groups provided a basis for random assignment to a treatment or control group, Cabot added the requirement of keeping excellent records. Following any encounter of the staff with a boy in the study or his family, the staff member dictated a report about what had transpired. Throughout the years of the project, counselors reviewed case records at staff meetings. (See Powers & Witmer, 1951, for further details.)

Case workers offered the boys as well as their parents counseling for personal problems; they referred cases to specialists when that seemed advisable. When the program terminated in 1945, boys in the treatment group had been visited, on the average, two times a month for 5½ years. Over half the boys had been tutored in academic subjects; over 100 received medical or psychiatric attention; almost half had been sent to summer camps; and most of the boys had participated with their counselors in such activities as swimming, visits to local athletic competitions, and woodwork in the project's shop. Boys in the treatment group were encouraged to join the Y.M.C.A. and other community youth programs. The boys and their parents called upon the social workers for help with a variety of problems including illness and unemployment.

Boys assigned to the control group were excluded from activities provided to the treatment group. Members of the control group did receive help, of course. Families, churches, and community organizations provided assistance. The difference between treatment and control groups was not whether boys received help, but rather whether boys received the integrated, friendly guidance provided by the Cambridge-Somerville Youth Study.

RESULTS

The men were born between 1925 and 1934 (mean = 1928; SD = 1.7). The most recent follow-up began when the men were an average of 47 years old. The Youth Study had been designed to prevent antisocial behavior, so measures of criminal behavior were particularly appropriate to its evaluation. Court records had the advantage of objectivity and were independent of self-reporting biases. Although court records yield incomplete records of criminal activities and are likely to reflect cultural, racial, and social class biases, the treatment and control groups would be equally affected by these influences.

In order to evaluate the impact of treatment, names and pseudonyms of the 506 men were checked through the Massachusetts Department of Probation centralized records in 1975–76. If treatment and control group men had migrated differentially from Massachusetts, the evaluations might have produced biased results. To check this possibility, we searched for the men themselves. By the end of 1979, 248 men from the treatment group and 246 men from the control group had been found. Equal proportions in each group, 76%, were living in Massachusetts.

As we discovered the men, we expanded record searches to the states where men were known to have lived. To obtain additional objective information about the men, files of the Massachusetts Department of Mental Health, the Division of Alcoholism, state alcoholic clinics, and the Department of Vital Statistics were searched. Records of these agencies yielded information showing which of the men had died and which had been treated for mental illness or alcoholism.

To use a single objective measure for evaluating whether the Cambridge-Somerville Youth Study had affected the lives of its clients, each of the 506 men was classified as having or not having an objectively defined "undesirable" outcome. If and only if a man had been convicted for a crime indexed by the F.B.I., had died prior to age 35, or had received a medical diagnosis as alcoholic, schizophrenic, or manic-depressive was a man's outcome counted as undesirable. All other men were classified as having no undesirable outcome. Each pair was then placed in one of four categories: (1) neither the man from the treatment group nor the man from the control group had an undesirable outcome; (2) both men had undesirable outcomes; (3) only the man from the control group had an undesirable outcome; or (4) only the man from the treatment group had an undesirable outcome.

Discrepancies within pairs would be interpreted as evidence for effects of the treatment program. Pairs in which only the man from the control group had an undesirable outcome would be considered pairs in which the treatment program had been helpful.

Unfortunately, the objective measure for evaluating outcome indicated that the program had an adverse effect (See Table 9.1).

If some of the families resented intervention, failures might be due to their refusals to accept assistance or to that resentment. It therefore seemed reasonable to look at differences in effects of treatment based on whether the treatment group boys had been recipients of the intended program. To make the comparison, families were divided into those who presented problems of cooperation and those who did not. Counselors dictated reports about each of their interactions with the boys or the families, so that most of the case records included several hundred pages. Cases were considered to have shown

TABLE 9.1. Effects of Treatment

Outcome	Number
Neither an undesirable outcome	109 pairs
Both an undesirable outcome	42 pairs
Only control group man an undesirable outcome	*39 pairs
Only treatment group man an undesirable outcome	*63 pairs
Total	253

$^*z = .0226$, two-tailed test.

problems of cooperation if the counselor reported such difficulties or if the case record was exceptionally short (fewer than 25 pages), indicating little interaction. The results, shown in Figure 9.1, indicate that only the cooperative families were affected by the treatment program.

Among the pairs in which the treatment family was uncooperative, the control and treatment boys were equally likely to turn out badly. Among the pairs in which the treatment family was cooperative, however, there were 27 pairs in which the treatment boys turned out better but 52 pairs in which the treatment boys turned out worse. These findings strongly suggest that the treatment itself had been harmful.

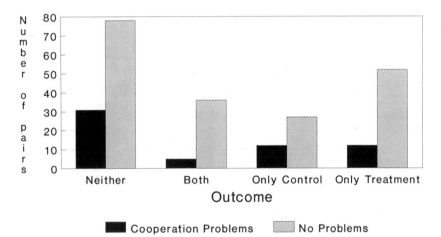

FIGURE 9.1. Case–control comparison: Bad outcomes (convicted for index crime, treated for psychoses or alcoholism, or died before age 35).

The general impact of treatment appeared to have been damaging. Nevertheless, some subgroups of those who received treatment might have been helped. Beneficial effects might have resulted from starting treatment when the child was particularly young, from providing more frequent help, or from treatment being available over an especially long period of time. None of these possibilities received support. Nor was there evidence to show that some particular variation of treatment had been effective. Moreover, when comparisons were restricted to those with whom a counselor had particularly good rapport or those whom the staff believed it had helped most, the objective evidence failed to show that the program had been beneficial. (See McCord, 1981, 1990a, for details.)

DISCUSSION

Why did the treatment have harmful effects? Part of the reason, it seems to me, has been the compensatory model on which treatment was based. Cabot—and many others—have assumed that an appropriate treatment would undo deficits in backgrounds of people at high risk for developing problems. This can be a critical error. A child rejected by parents may not be best served by someone else who tries to take the role of parent. Such a strategy might result in an exaggerated sense of loss; it might produce expectations for or dependence on assistance.

We know that supervision or "monitoring" is an efficient predictor of socialized behavior. But absence of supervision is likely to have resulted in a set of expectations, adaptations, and (perhaps) skills. So a child who has not been supervised may become *more* antisocial if he is placed under close supervision.

Children who are not good in school may not be best served by tutoring them. Self-identity or peer labeling may make such tutoring reinforce perceptions of inadequacy. Timing could be critical in determining whether a particular intervention would be beneficial or harmful.

In a strange sort of way, we may have come close to assuming that there is a single mold that would be appropriate for all. So we assume that children who are not loved should be given love; children who are doing badly in school should be taught to do better.

Certainly there are alternatives to academic success for satisfactory lives. The same might be said regarding social success.

Despite failure of the treatment program, the records of the Cambridge-Somerville Youth Study provided a rich field for mining information about the homes of 253 boys. These records were coded in 1957, prior to collection of the follow-up data. They therefore were not contaminated by retrospective biases. (See McCord & McCord, 1960, for a complete description of the coding.)

Analyses based on these records have shown that the criminogenic impact of paternal absence depends largely on the nature of the family interaction (McCord, 1990b), that differences between families with and without alcoholic fathers are permeating in terms of variables related to child rearing (McCord, 1988), and that home environments during early adolescence are strong predictors of both juvenile delinquency and of adult criminal behavior (McCord, 1991a).

It has been possible to learn, also, that some patterns of family interaction seem to promote alcoholism (McCord, 1988), while others contribute to competence (McCord, 1991b). It is doubtful that these relationships could have been discovered had not evidence been collected by direct observation and over a relatively long period of time. The opportunity for observation was generated by the treatment provided (Cabot, 1940).

On the one hand, the Cambridge-Somerville Youth Study could be considered a failure because it harmed some of the boys given treatment through its auspices. On the other hand, the study should be considered a success. It was a success because:

1. It showed the importance of using random assignment to treatment and control groups in order to assess the validity of cherished beliefs about helping others. Despite good intentions, iatrogenic effects occurred.
2. It showed that providing supportive friendly guidance was not a sufficient antidote for criminogenic conditions.
3. It showed that careful records collected in the process of providing treatment can yield scientifically valuable information about developmental issues.
4. It demonstrated that intervention can have long-term effects.

On a theoretical level, results of the Cambridge-Somerville Youth Study have two implications. First, they provide grounds for doubting that deficit approaches to reducing crime can be effective. And second, they provide grounds for doubting the adequacy of control theory as an explanation for crime.

Control theory explains crime as the result of failure to develop attachments to family, school, and norms. The Cambridge-Somerville Youth Study succeeded in developing conventional ties—but nevertheless failed to prevent deviant behavior.

ACKNOWLEDGMENTS

This study was partially supported by U.S. Public Health Service Research Grant MH26779, National Institute of Mental Health (Center for Studies of Crime and Delinquency). The author expresses appreciation to the Department of Probation of the Commonwealth of Massachusetts, to the Division of Criminal Justice Services of the State of New York, to the Maine State Bureau of Identification, and to the states of California, Florida, Michigan, New Jersey, Pennsylvania, Virginia, and Washington for supplemental data about the men. The author thanks Richard Parente, Robert Staib, Ellen Myers, and Ann Cronin for their work in tracing the men and their records and Joan Immel, Tom Smedile, Harriet Sayre, Mary Duell, Elise Goldman, Abby Brodkin, and Laura Otten for their careful coding. The author is responsible for the statistical analyses and for the conclusions drawn from this research.

REFERENCES

Allport, G. (1951). Foreword. In E. Powers & H. Witmer, *An experiment in the prevention of delinquency: The Cambridge-Somerville Youth Study*. New York: Columbia University Press.

Cabot, P. S. deQ. (1940). A long-term study of children: The Cambridge-Somerville Youth Study. *Child Development, 11*, 143–151.

Cabot, R. C. (1934). 1000 delinquent boys: First findings of the Harvard Law School's survey of crime. *Survey, 70*(2), 38–40.

Deardorff, N. R. (1958). Richard Clarke Cabot. In R. L. Schuyler & E. T. James (Eds.), *Dictionary of American biography* (Supplement 2, pp. 83–85). New York: Scribner's.

Glueck, S., & Glueck, E. T. (1934). *One thousand juvenile delinquents*. Cambridge: Harvard University Press.

Glueck, S., & Glueck, E. T. (1945). *After-conduct of discharged offenders*. London: Macmillan.

Gouge, W. (1627). *The works of William Gouge: Vol. 1 Domesticall duties*. London: John Beal.

Healy, W. (1917). *Mental conflicts and misconduct*. Boston: Little Brown.

Healy, W. (1934). Comments. *Survey, 70*(3), 94.

Healy, W., & Bronner, A. F. (1926). *Delinquents and criminals: Their making and unmaking*. New York: Macmillan.

Healy, W., & Bronner, A. F. (1936). *New light on delinquency and its treatment*. New Haven: Yale University Press.

Jevons, T. (1834/1970). Remarks on criminal law; with a plan for an improved system and observations on the prevention of crime. London. Reprinted in W. B. Sanders (Ed.), *Juvenile offenders for a thousand years* (pp. 152–154). Chapel Hill: University of North Carolina Press.

Matsell, G. W. (1850). Report of the chief of police concerning destitution and crime among children in the city. In T. L. Harris (Ed.), *Juvenile depravity and crime in our city. A sermon* (pp. 14–15). New York: Norton.

McCord, J. (1981). Consideration of some effects of a counseling program. In S. E. Martin, L. B. Sechrest, & R. Redner (Eds.), *New directions in the rehabilitation of criminal offenders* (pp. 394–405). Washington, DC: National Academy of Sciences.

McCord, J. (1988). Identifying developmental paradigms leading to alcoholism. *Journal of Studies on Alcohol, 49*(4), 357–362.

McCord, J. (1990a). Crime in moral and social contexts. *Criminology, 28*(1), 1–26.

McCord, J. (1990b). Long-term perspectives on parental absence. In L. N. Robins & M. Rutter (Eds.), *Straight and devious pathways from childhood to adulthood* (pp. 116–134). Cambridge: Cambridge University Press.

McCord, J. (1991a). Family relationships, juvenile delinquency, and adult criminality. *Criminology, 29*(3), 397–417.

McCord, J. (1991b). Competence in long-term perspective. *Psychiatry, 54*(3), 227–237.

McCord, W., & McCord, J. (1960). *Origins of alcoholism.* Stanford, CA.: Stanford University Press.

Mennel, R. M. (1973). *Thorns and thistles: Juvenile delinquents in the United States 1825–1940.* Hanover, NH: University Press of New England.

Powers, E., & Witmer, H. (1951). *An experiment in the prevention of delinquency: The Cambridge-Somerville Youth Study.* New York: Columbia University Press.

◆ —— ◆

PART IV

PREVENTION EXPERIMENTS DURING ADOLESCENCE

CHAPTER 10

The Interplay of Theory and Practice in Delinquency Prevention:
From Behavior Modification to Activity Settings

CLIFFORD R. O'DONNELL

This chapter describes the mutual influence of theory and practice in the delinquency prevention work conducted with my colleagues over the 20 years from 1970 to 1990. Conceptually, this work began as an application of behavior modification and has developed into a generic theory of community intervention based on activity settings. This chapter begins with discussion of the theory of behavior modification that prevailed in 1970. A specific project that was based on this prevailing theory, the Buddy System, is then described. The results of this project were unexpected and puzzling. Efforts to understand these results led to a reexamination of prevailing theory.

This reexamination changed the theory used to guide our delinquency prevention projects. The reexamination began with a review of the physical and social factors of environments and proceeded to a focus on the importance of social networks. Eventually, it benefited a new program called the Youth Development Project and contributed to theoretical change in community intervention. This process is described below. The chapter concludes with a discussion of the current theoretical development based on activity settings and the implications for future projects in delinquency prevention.

PREVAILING THEORY AND THE BUDDY SYSTEM

Behavior Modification and the Triadic Model

Historically, the theory of behavior modification is based on the early work of Thorndike (1898, 1913) and Skinner (1938). Thorndike developed the first stimulus-response theory, described in his dissertation, using hungry cats in a puzzle box. In the typical experiment, the cat would learn to move the latch to obtain the food outside of the box. Over trials, the cat would take less time to move the latch. Thorndike stated that the food served as a "satisfying state of affairs" and strengthened the response. This finding was the basis for his famous law of effect.

The law of effect was developed into the principles of operant conditioning by Skinner's experimental work, mostly with pigeons. These principles were based on how a variety of events affected the probability of a response. These events included such principles as reinforcement, which increased the probability of a response, schedules of reinforcement, which affected the rate of response; extinction, to eliminate a response; secondary reinforcement, by which a new stimulus became reinforcing through association with an already reinforcing stimulus; and shaping, in which a behavior occurred through the reinforcement of successive approximations to the behavior.

Attempts to use the principles of operant conditioning to improve human behavior began with the work of Fuller (1949) with an institutionalized patient. Particularly influential was the work of Ayllon and Azrin (1964, 1965, 1968) with mental patients. Their work led to the widespread use of token economies in which secondary reinforcers (tokens or points) were used to reinforce improvements in behavior. Another influential publication was the edited book by Ullmann and Krasner (1965) which compiled many of the early case studies in a field that was now being called behavior modification. By 1968, this field had its own journal, the *Journal of Applied Behavior Analysis*.

Applications of behavior modification to child behavior began with the use of extinction for tantrums (Williams, 1959). Important work with autistic and schizophrenic children was conducted by Ferster, Lovaas, and their colleagues (Ferster, 1968; Ferster & DeMyer, 1961; Ferster & Simons, 1966; Lovaas, 1966, 1967, 1968; Lovaas, Berberich, Perloff, & Schaeffer, 1966; Lovaas, Freitag, Gold, & Kassorla, 1965; Lovaas, Freitag, Kinder, Rubenstein, Schaeffer, & Simmons, 1966; Lovaas, Freitas, Nelson, & Whalen, 1967; Lovaas, Schaeffer, & Simmons, 1965). In addition, Wahler showed how parents and nonprofessionals could use these techniques to change the behavior of their children (Wahler, 1969; Wahler & Erickson, 1969; Wahler, Winkel, Peterson, & Morrison, 1965). Bijou and Baer (1967) edited a book on behavior modification in child development and Patterson and Gullion (1968) followed with one for parents and teachers.

Other researchers were evaluating the use of behavior modification with delinquents (Burchard & Tyler, 1965). Phillips (1968) incorporated the token economy into a home for "predelinquent" boys called Achievement Place. Thorne, Tharp, and Wetzel (1967) showed how the techniques could be used by probation officers. This work with delinquents offered much promise in a field where so many other approaches had failed.

Overall, the extension of the principles of behavior modification to new populations and to behaviors that typically did not respond to treatment was important and exciting. Applications were often innovative. Rarely, however, did these applications contribute to the development of theory until the classic work of Tharp and Wetzel (1969).

In their book, *Behavior Modification in the Natural Environment*, they introduced the triadic model. Conceptually, the triadic model is a chain consisting of a consultant (perhaps with supervisors), a mediator, and a target. The *consultant* is a person with intervention expertise, the *mediator* is a person who has regular contact with the target in everyday life, and the *target* is the person whose behavior is the focus of change. The consultant could be a psychologist, social worker, parent, teacher, or anyone with the required knowledge. Likewise, the mediator could be a parent, teacher, older sibling, friend, or anyone who has regular contact with the target.

This model serves as a system for the application of behavior modification theory to the behavior of the target. The mediator is trained by the consultant to follow the target's desirable behavior with a reinforcing event and to withhold the event following undesirable behavior. In turn, the behavior of the mediator is influenced by the reinforcement from the consultant and the changes in the target's behavior. Similarly, the consultant's behavior is influenced by the effectiveness of the mediator and the reinforcement from a supervisor. In this model, the task of the consultant is to select the mediator and the behaviors to be used as reinforcers. Each individual in the chain modifies the next individual's behavior.

The triadic model was an elegant addition to the behavior modification literature. It incorporated the basic principles and the increasing use of nonprofessionals into a system for the use of contingencies and relationships in the everyday lives of people. It served as the model for the Buddy System.

The Buddy System

In psychology, attempts to change the antisocial behavior of children date back to the work of Witmer (1906–1907). As we have seen, by 1970 these attempts were increasingly based on the principles of behavior modification. With the introduction of the triadic model, it was now possible to apply these principles on a larger scale. A small number of consultants could supervise a larger number of nonprofessionals who could intervene with a still larger number of youths.

The Buddy System used this model. It operated from 1970 through 1973 with Model Cities funds administered by the Department of Housing and Urban Development and with demonstration grants from the Office of Juvenile Delinquency and Youth Development in the U.S. Department of Health, Education, and Welfare to the First Circuit Family Court in Hawaii.

Four graduate students, supervised by faculty members, served as consultants. These students were referred to as "behavior analysts." Mediators were indigenous nonprofessionals, referred to as "buddies," who were recruited through advertisements in newspapers. The target population was youth referred for behavior management problems such as truancy, fighting, classroom disruption, and poor academic achievement.

Buddies lived in the same communities as the youngsters, included males and females, were from 17 to 65 years of age, had an educational range from fourth grade to a master's degree, and represented diverse ethnicities and occupations. They were paid up to $144 per month for making contact each week with each of their assigned youngsters, submitting data, completing assignments with their youngsters, and attending training sessions.

Youths were from 11 to 17 years of age ($x = 14$) and had a variety of ethnic backgrounds, including Hawaiian, Filipino, Japanese, Chinese, and Caucasian. Most were in the seventh and eighth grades. Each was referred for a specific behavior problem by the public schools, police, parents, neighbors, Family Court, and various social welfare agencies.

Specific behaviors of both the youths and the buddies were targeted and programed for reinforcement. The role behaviors of the buddies and the consultants were specified and organized for this purpose. Buddies were trained in the following mediator behaviors:

(a) meet weekly with each of their target youths and participate in social and recreational activities with them; (b) establish a warm, positive, and trusting relationship with their youngsters; (c) identify problem areas and specify them in behavioral terms; (d) count the frequency of occurrence of the targeted behaviors and submit weekly behavioral data to the behavior analyst; (e) draw up and carry out intervention programs aimed at ameliorating the youngsters' target behaviors; and (f) serve as an advocate for the youngsters in their dealings with persons in their environment. (Fo & O'Donnell, 1974, p. 165)

Consultants consisted of the graduate-student behavior analysts and their supervisors. The behaviors specified for the behavior analysts were to:

(a) maintain responsibility for the day-to-day details of managing the behaviors of the buddies; (b) provide the buddies with intensive, ongoing training in behavioral principles and techniques; (c) provide the buddies with continuous consultation and supervision in case management both by telephone and in the field; (d) design intervention plans for ameliorating behavior problems of the target youths; (e) collect and graph weekly behavioral data submitted by the buddies; (f) trouble shoot difficulties as they arise in the buddy-youngster relationship and in the intervention program; and (g) monitor the behaviors of the buddies and supervise the administration of the point system. (Fo & O'Donnell, 1974, p. 165)

Tasks were also specified for the supervisors. They were to

(a) maintain overall administrative responsibility for the training, research, and evaluation of the project; (b) conduct ongoing program planning and development; (c) provide the behavior analysts with expertise and training in behavioral technology; (d) provide ongoing consultation and supervision to the behavior analysts in designing and implementing intervention programs for the target youths; (e) monitor the record keeping functions of the behavior analysts to ensure decision-making consistent with the data; (f) collect and analyze the data for research and evaluative purposes; (g) oversee the behaviors of the behavior analysts and provide necessary feedback to maximize their success in working with the buddies; and (h) monitor the operations of the project at every organizational level so as to ensure efficient and effective functioning consistent with the goals of the program. (Fo & O'Donnell, 1974; p. 165)

These role behaviors were specified to allow each role to influence the next one in the triadic chain as part of the system designed to improve the behaviors for which the youths were referred.

To assess whether this system improved the referred behaviors, an experiment was designed. Youths ($n = 42$) were randomly assigned to one of four conditions, three experimental and one control, and compared across three time periods. In all three experimental conditions, buddies were trained to establish a warm and positive relationship with each of their youngsters. In one experimental condition, this relationship was not contingent on any improvement in the referral behavior; in the second it was contingent; in the third of these conditions, the $10 per month that every buddy had to spend on each youth was also contingent on the youth showing improvement. Youth in the control condition were referred, but not invited to participate.

The results were convincing. Youths in the contingency conditions improved, while those in the noncontingency and control conditions did not. In the third time period, when youth in the noncontingency condition were switched to contingency, they also improved. Additional statistical analysis showed that, with one exception, all of the youths in the contingency conditions showed the improvement, while only three youths in the other conditions did so (Fo & O'Donnell, 1974).

The Buddy System was developed as a delinquency prevention program. During the 3 years of its operation, 553 juveniles were referred. Of these, 335 (206 boys and 129 girls) were accepted. Because of the excess of referrals over openings, the remaining 218 (151 boys and 67 girls) were randomly assigned to the control condition. The implicit assumption was that youngsters who showed improvement in the problem behaviors for which they were referred would be less likely to commit delinquent offenses.

This assumption was evaluated by comparing the arrest records of all of those who participated in the Buddy System with the records of the control youths, first in a preliminary study (Fo & O'Donnell, 1975) and later using the complete sample (O'Donnell, Lydgate, & Fo, 1979). The comparison using the complete sample was made for a 3-year period beginning with their referral. Separate comparisons were made for those who were arrested for a major offense in the year prior to their referral ($n = 73$) and for those who were not arrested ($n = 480$). The major offenses excluded juvenile status offenses, technical violations, traffic violations, and minor vice offenses.

The percentage of all 553 youngsters arrested over the 3 years was 25.7. This overall rate varied between 10.8% and 81% depending on gender, recent offense history, and participation in the Buddy System. As would be expected, those who had been arrested in the year prior to their referral had a higher arrest rate (63%) than did those who had not been arrested (20%), and males (30.3%) had a higher rate than females (17.3%).

The most important results were the comparisons of those who participated in the Buddy System with those who did not. The arrest rate was lower for those who participated in the Buddy System (56%) than for those who did not (78.3%), but only if they had an arrest in the year prior to their referral. If they had not been arrested, the arrest rate for participants (22.5%) was higher than that for controls (16.4%). This finding meant that the Buddy System was helpful for the 13.2% of the youths with a prior arrest, but harmful for the remaining 86.8%! Moreover, additional analyses revealed that the harmful effect occurred among those youth who participated in the Buddy System for more than 1 year ($n = 67$) and was not likely to be due to a sampling bias.

This result was, of course, unexpected. How could participation produce such a result? Interpretation focused on the possibility that some of those without a prior arrest formed friendships with those already arrested. The program provided opportunities for such contacts among participants through group gatherings several times each year. In addition, some buddies met with all three of their assigned youths at the same time and thereby provided additional opportunities for these contacts.

The prevailing theory of behavior modification, however, suggested that the improvement in targeted behaviors did not generalize to the delinquent behaviors and settings. Interest then turned to the topic of generalization in other studies. The expectation was that these other studies could provide information that would increase the likelihood of generalization.

THE REEXAMINATION OF PREVAILING THEORY

A review of these studies focused on the application of behavior modification in community settings (O'Donnell, 1977). Included were studies on aftercare programs for those released from hospitals, correctional programs, family intervention programs, and general community programs for litter control, energy conservation, and employment.

Results of these studies were highly consistent. Most found improvement in behavior while the participants were in the program. However, the results of studies with follow-up data were virtually unanimous in showing that the improved behaviors were not maintained after the participants left the program. In short, there was no generalization to nonprogram settings.

Since this finding occurred across all types of programs and areas reviewed, it was suggested that "perhaps we have been asking the wrong question. Is it reasonable to expect that the effect of any intervention will generalize to a postintervention setting and improved behavior will be maintained? . . . Indeed, perhaps the primary evaluation of whether behavior has been maintained should depend on the assessment of postintervention environments" (O'Donnell, 1977, p. 96).

Prevailing theory stated that the question was one of the generalization of learned behavior. Once the behaviors had been learned in the program, the task was to generalize the behavior to other settings. The greater the similarity between settings, the greater the possibility of generalization. What was now being suggested was that the question was not generalization, but performance. Given that the person was capable of the behavior, its occurrence would depend on many characteristics of the setting other than similarity to the setting in which the behavior was learned. The emphasis shifted from the conditions of learning to the context of performance. So began the reexamination of prevailing theory.

The implication of this change in the question was that special programs would be needed only if they were necessary for the learning of new behavior. Influencing the occurrence of these behaviors, however, would require understanding of the settings of everyday life. The difficulty was that while much was known about the construction of program settings, little was known about the functioning of everyday settings. Therefore, the review closed with a presentation of research areas that could lead to an increase in our knowledge of these settings.

One of these research areas was the relationship between behavior and its physical context. Growth of interest and productivity in the field of environmental psychology in the 1970s led to the suggestion that the field could contribute to, and perhaps even be integrated with, the field of behavior modification (Willems, 1974). Therefore, the literature of environmental psychology was reviewed for the purpose of both understanding everyday settings and developing applications to address psychological problems, including crime and delinquency (O'Donnell, 1980).

This review showed that the physical environment "influences the frequency and nature of participation in activities with others, that our attachments and responsibilities to others are based in the social interaction inherent in this participation, and that these relationships contribute to the prevention and alleviation of many psychological problems" (O'Donnell, 1980, p. 280). It was found that the physical environment affects our social interactions through the physical design of the environment. For example, social contact can be facilitated or inhibited by the proximity among people created by variables such as the partitioning of space, seating arrangements, and access to group activities.

Proximity provides the opportunity for social interaction and participation in the activities of the setting. However, the degree of interaction and participation that occurs over time depends on the manning level of the setting (Barker, 1960, 1968). "The degree of manning depends on the number of people available to fulfill the roles of a setting. Settings with relatively few people for the number of roles are said to be undermanned. In these settings demands to participate are greater and standards for participation lower. As a result, those with marginal abilities are more likely to be sought out and accepted. In overmanned settings, of course, the reverse is true. Therefore, the concept of manning helps to explain the degree of participation and interaction. Participation is encouraged in undermanned settings and withdrawal is encouraged in overmanned settings" (O'Donnell, 1980, p. 284).

There was also evidence that psychological problems were affected by participation and social interaction. Those with less social contact were found to have higher rates of unemployment, illness, hospitalization, and death. Participation and social interaction over time leads, of course, to relationships and to the development of a social network. This social network can serve to alter or maintain behavior, including psychological problems.

This review contributed to the reexamination of prevailing theory by suggesting that the key variables of environmental design were proximity and manning level, and that these variables affected social interaction and the development of networks, which influenced the occurrence of problem behavior. It was now apparent that prevailing theory would have to be changed to include nonbehavioral concepts if the settings of everyday life were to be understood.

The question remained: Why didn't behavior that had been acquired in one (program) setting not occur in other (nonprogram) settings? One answer suggested so far was that the proximity among people and the manning level of the setting could influence social interaction and participation within the setting. O'Donnell and Tharp (1982) suggested an additional possibility: perhaps the setting actually prevented the occurrence of the behavior.

They presented examples based on the work of Tharp, Gallimore, and their colleagues at Kamehameha Schools, a school for Native Hawaiian children. The Hawaiian children were raised in a culture that strongly supports peer-initiated cooperative activities. These children showed initiative and responsibility within the cooperative structure at home. The classroom, however, emphasized individual performance and teacher-initiated activities. Therefore, the children performed less competently at school than they did at home until the classroom setting was restructured to emphasize cooperative, peer-related activities. This strategy was successful in improving both academic performance and social behavior. The classroom setting now allowed the desired behaviors to occur (O'Donnell & Tharp, 1982). This finding supported the learning-performance distinction that although a behavior may have been learned, the *occurrence* of the learned behavior is a function of the variables within the setting.

Overall, this reexamination provided concepts that could be evaluated in new delinquency-prevention projects and used to change prevailing theory. One of these concepts was the social network. Studies of the importance of social networks in delinquency prevention, with an example of a new project that benefited from these studies, is presented in the next section. This presentation is followed by a section on the development of theoretical changes.

SOCIAL NETWORKS AND THE YOUTH DEVELOPMENT PROJECT

Interpretation of the results of the Buddy System centered on the possibility that some youths who had been arrested for a major offense in the previous year had formed friendships with youths who had not been arrested and thereby increased the subsequent arrest rates of these youths. A review of diversion and neighborhood delinquency programs lent considerable support to this interpretation (O'Donnell, Manos, & Chesney-Lind, 1987). An overview of these programs is presented below, followed by a discussion of a delinquency-prevention program that is designed to assess the effect of peer networks on delinquency.

Studies of diversion and neighborhood delinquency-prevention programs have included youths who have been arrested, convicted, or placed on probation, and youths in programs that take them to visit adult prisons, provide social services, or offer alternatives to gang membership. Most of these studies show that these programs do not reduce delinquency, and sometimes may even increase it. For example, self-report data comparing youths engaging in similar delinquent activity show that those who are arrested or convicted are more likely to continue delinquent behavior than are those whose offenses are not detected or those who are not convicted (Ageton & Elliott, 1974; Farrington, 1977; Gold & Williams, 1969).

Another study compared youths on probation who were contacted by their probation officers with those who were never contacted (McEachern, Taylor, Newman, & Ashford, 1968). Those who were not contacted had fewer and less serious subsequent offenses than those who received probation services. Even more surprising, those who were not contacted had a worse prior record.

Historically, many programs have looked for a "magic bullet" to prevent delinquency. A recent example of such a panacea is the prison visit. The original prison visit study was conducted at Rahway State Prison in New Jersey and presented in the film *Scared Straight*. In this program, youths were taken to the adult prison, shown the problems of prison life, and intimidated; often they became upset and cried. The purpose was to "scare them straight." Initial results appeared promising, but later evaluations indicated higher arrest rates among those who participated in the program (Finckenauer, 1979) and a lack of support for program effectiveness (Lewis, 1983; Subcommittee on Human Resources of the Committee on Education and Labor, 1979).

In Hawaii, a similar program was developed. Instead of "Scared Straight," it was called "Stay Straight." The idea was to befriend rather than to scare. In the program, youths visited the old Oahu Prison where a select group of prisoners described prison life and related their lives and experiences to those of the youths. The program centered on an intense emotional experience too, but relied on empathy instead of intimidation. But again, results showed higher arrest rates for some of the youths who participated in the program. Specifically, the higher arrest rates occurred for those who participated in organized groups as members of other delinquency prevention programs (Buckner & Chesney-Lind, 1983).

Of the studies that provided social services to youths, including the remarkable 30-year follow-up to the Cambridge-Somerville study (McCord, 1978), several showed that the few differences among groups favored the controls (e.g., Berleman, Seaberg, & Steinburn, 1972).

What all these studies have in common is that the youths came into contact with each other in order to participate in the program. Contact could occur among arrested youths, those appearing in court, those receiving probation services, those visiting prisons, and certainly among those participating in social service programs. The results suggest, among other possible alternatives, that this contact may lead to friendships that are carried on outside of the program and continue after the program is completed. These social networks may well diminish any effectiveness of the programs.

Studies of juvenile gangs support this conclusion. For example, in the Group Guidance Project (Klein, 1971) activities such as athletic events, dances, and academic tutoring were offered to four gangs with a total membership of about 800. Despite satisfaction with the program, an analysis of age-adjusted offense frequencies revealed an *increase* in delinquency among the gang members. Additional analyses showed that this increase occurred because the program activities attracted the fringe members of the gangs and increased their contact with core gang members.

To his credit, Klein altered his strategy and began the Ladino Hills Project (Klein, 1971). This program was designed to reduce contact among gang members and thereby reduce gang membership. Employment opportunities were developed. Direct observation by means of regular driving patrols revealed that employed youth were less likely to be on the street. As a result of this project, gang cohesiveness and the total number of offenses decreased because of reduction in the size of the gang.

These findings illustrate the potential importance of the contribution of social networks to delinquency. Networks form as a result of participation in the activities in specific settings. Therefore, we need to look not only at the networks, but also at the activities and settings that facilitate their formation. For example, youngsters living in the same neighborhood, of similar age, and attending the same school are likely to have contact with each other in the course of everyday life. When they also are facing similar problems at home or school, some will be at higher risk for delinquency. If they also come from multi-problem families, they may receive less adult supervision and have more free time for peer contact. Several studies have linked peer-controlled activities to a higher likelihood of delinquency (Schwendinger & Schwendinger, 1982; Wilson, 1980).

One implication of these findings for current programs is to give serious consideration to providing services individually, instead of in groups, to discourage contact among participants. This change may increase program effectiveness by removing the possible negative influence of a program-based social network. Another implication is that current programs should develop a means to assess the social networks of their participants and the impact of these networks on program effectiveness. Since friendships formed within a program may continue after the program, it is especially important to assess the impact of networks on program effects over time and in nonprogram settings.

The implication for future program development and research is to consider shifting the emphasis from individual to network change.

By promoting the development of prosocial networks, delinquency may be reduced.

An example of such a program is the Youth Development Project in Hawaii (Manos, 1988). It is a school-based, social skills training and student-team learning program. Entire classes (K–12) are taught social skills and participate in student-team learning assignments in the classroom. Cooperation among the students is required to complete the assignment and receive the individual and group credit. These student teams provide the opportunity to alter contact among students and potentially to affect their friendship patterns.

Current research on the project includes a social network assessment in which each student lists the friends with whom he or she has regular contact. Analyses of changes in student networks from sixth through twelfth grade are planned. These changes can then be compared to changes in school performance and delinquency. Preliminary data collected so far indicate that students who are rated by teachers to be at high risk for behavior problems are more likely to have regular contact with other high-risk students and to maintain that contact. If these preliminary data are substantiated, they suggest that intervention may be required to alter the networks of high-risk students. Failure to do so may result in problem behavior being maintained through continued contact with other high-risk peers.

If intervention is warranted, membership in the student teams could be arranged to discourage contact among high-risk students and to promote contact with prosocial peers. Additional possibilities include an assessment of the activities and settings outside of school where the contact occurs among high-risk students. It may then be possible to alter these activities or settings in ways that will lower the likelihood of delinquent behavior. Overall, the Youth Development Project is a good example of a current program with a greater emphasis on social networks and with the potential for network intervention and the prevention of delinquency.

THEORETICAL DEVELOPMENT

The reexamination of prevailing theory showed that behavior was strongly influenced by the setting in which it occurred; that participation in settings led to the formation of a social network; and that this network influenced the settings and activities in which people became involved. The question now became: How could these concepts be synthesized with prevailing theory? Efforts to do so have been presented in two publications (O'Donnell, 1984; O'Donnell & Tharp, 1990).

The first publication examined behavioral community psychology and the natural environment (O'Donnell, 1984). In this presentation, settings were described as either micro or macro. Microsettings were those in which one could have personal contact with the majority of people. Macrosettings were larger and consisted of a combination of microsettings. The purpose of this division was to illustrate how individual behavior was influenced within a (micro)setting and how microsettings interact as part of a macrosetting.

Microsettings were defined as consisting of "typically organized activities which take place in a specified physical environment. They provide their participants with roles which specify the behaviors expected for the activities, and with access to the available resources. These roles and the use of the resources influence participation in the setting and affect the behavioral development and social networks of the participants" (O'Donnell, 1984, p. 503). Behavior within a microsetting is influenced through the *roles and resources* provided in the setting.

A *role* refers to a pattern of behavior, "typically arranged to perform some function in the activities of a setting. These roles help to define the behaviors expected of people" (O'Donnell, 1984, p. 503). This definition specified why certain behaviors were expected of each person in the setting: because the behaviors composed a role that was needed to perform some function in the setting. This definition also implicitly showed how a particular behavior could occur in one setting and not in another: because the role of the person may be different in the two settings. The behavior might be expected in one role, but not in the other. This, of course, was the case in the classroom with Hawaiian children discussed above. Peer-initiated, cooperative behavior was a part of the role for Hawaiian children at home, but not at school. When the roles at school were restructured, the behavior was allowed to occur.

Two other concepts affect the occurrence of role behavior. The first is manning level, borrowed from Barker (1960, 1968), and used to predict the degree of participation, obligation, and responsibility to others in a setting. An overmanned setting, in which there are more people available for a given role than are needed, may prevent a desired behavior by discouraging participation and commitment to others. The other concept is the relative skill level of people in similar roles. Acceptable competency is relative to that which is available. When some are more proficient in some behavior, others may be discouraged from engaging in the behavior. Therefore, "roles in which relatively few people in the setting are highly competent may be considered 'underskilled,' while those in which many are competent would be considered 'overskilled.' The effects noted in studies of manning levels may also occur among those in under-and-overskilled roles" (O'Donnell, 1984, pp. 504–505).

Resources in a setting influence behavior through social interaction. People are the most important resource in a setting. People can be sources of support, information, skills, and so forth. Behavioral development of people occurs through social interaction. Stress can be reduced when the stressful situation is a shared experience. Cognitive development also occurs when people interact to resolve conflict within a setting.

Macrosettings were used to discuss the involvement of people in several microsettings. Such involvement provides people with different roles, opportunities for behavior development, and a more extensive social network. An interesting effect of these studies is that when participation is limited in one microsetting, people are more likely to become involved in another. For example, when the participation of adolescents in school is limited by overmanning, they are more involved in peer activities outside of school. This involvement can increase their commitment to their peers and affect their behavioral development for better or worse, depending on the activities of their peers (O'Donnell, 1984).

A potentially harmful effect can occur when a person's participation is limited in many microsettings and leads to relative social isolation. Social isolation has been associated with a litany of social ills, including higher rates of psychological problems, illness, prescription-drug use, suicide, child abuse, and death (O'Donnell, 1984).

The second publication changed the concept of a microsetting, added other concepts, and enriched the synthesis with prevailing theory (O'Donnell & Tharp, 1990). The neo-Vygotskian concept of an activity setting was used instead of a microsetting. Activity settings were defined as "events in which collaborative interaction, intersubjectivity, and assisted performance occur; they incorporate cognitive and motoric action within the objective features of the setting (Tharp & Gallimore, 1988). . . . The activity setting is not dependent on the experience of any given person, but is the social process common to the participants from which cognition develops. The activity setting is the unit in which the development of cognitive processes and structures of meaning occur" (O'Donnell & Tharp, 1990, p. 253), and is therefore the unit by which community and cultural life are propagated.

The advantage of the concept of the activity setting is that it unifies setting, action, and experience into a common phenomenon. The internal process of cognition and the external features of the setting become one through the social interaction inherent in the activities. For these reasons, it was proposed as the basic unit of analysis for community psychology.

The components of the activity setting were expanded over those of the microsetting. These components include time, funds, and symbols as well as the physical environment, positions, and people. The most important of these additions was symbols, because "symbols, including language, reflect the meaning of the activity setting. The understanding, explanation, and meaning of the activity are a part of why activity settings exist and continue" (O'Donnell & Tharp, 1990, p. 254).

The heart of the activity setting is human interaction. Interaction is the foundational process by which skills are acquired, cognitions develop, relationships are formed, activities are carried out, and goals are achieved. The most important form of interaction is reciprocal participation in which each person both assists and is assisted during the activity. Reciprocal participation facilitates learning from those who are more competent in some aspect of the activity and creates a pattern of interdependency among members of the activity setting.

In addition, the reciprocal relationship between behavior in settings and social networks is explicit:

> Settings are sites for activity in which human action is supported by the available resources. In the course of this activity, participants acquire and develop specific behaviors and initiate and maintain social contact with other participants. Both their behavioral repertoires and their social networks are affected. The reciprocal nature of the relationship between behavioral repertoires and social networks is rooted in the common seed of activity.
>
> The repertoire contributes to successful participation in the activity, participation establishes relationships with others, and these relationships and skills provide access to new settings. Participation in the activities of new settings offers the opportunity for the continued development of both networks and repertoires. They are the product of activity and through their reciprocal relationship, they germinate new activities. . . . Behavior and relationships form a cycle linked by activities in which who you know leads to who you are to who you know, until who you are is who you know. (O'Donnell & Tharp, 1990, pp. 256-257)

This reciprocal relationship is an outcome of participation in an activity setting. In well-functioning activity settings there is another important outcome: intersubjectivity. Intersubjectivity is the harmony among emotions, cognitions, values, goals, and shared experiences that develops among people working together in activity settings. These people develop common bonds, come to think and experience the world in similar ways, and become more interdependent. Intersubjectivity is developed in activity settings as people confront and overcome common problems, experience similar events and emotions, and use common language and symbols to give meaning to their activities. Productivity increases with intersubjectivity. "In joint productive activity settings, intersubjectivities are created. Who you are—the intramental, cognitive, value-laden selfhood—arises in the social plane, and is made individual through the processes of communication and shared activity. To a major extent, each of us psychologically becomes those people with whom we work, share, and grow. Through the processes of intersubjectivity, culture and cognition create each other (Cole, 1985) and community and individual create each other" (O'Donnell & Tharp, 1990, p. 258).

The presentation of the theory concluded with the implications for intervention—implications that also apply to delinquency prevention. The goal of intervention is always to affect interaction, for behavioral and cognitive development occurs through interaction. To affect interaction is to intervene in an activity setting because that is where all interaction takes place. Intervention can be direct through one or more of the six components of an activity setting or indirect through a related activity setting.

Direct intervention requires an assessment of the *process, means,* and *conditions* of assistance within the setting. An assessment of the *process* of assistance involves an identification of those who need assistance, those who could provide it, and those whose behavior could be harmed by assistance.

The next task is to select and implement one or more *means* of assistance. Six were suggested: modeling, feedback, contingency management, instructing, questioning, and cognitive structuring. Studies have supported the effectiveness of each (Tharp & Gallimore, 1988; Tharp & Note, 1989).

The *conditions* of assistance refer to the factors that influence whether assistance is likely to occur:

> The conditions of assistance are determined by the components of the activity setting: (1) physical resources, (2) funds, (3) time, (4) symbols, (5) people, (6) positions, and the activity itself. To increase the likelihood of a pattern of reciprocal participation, it is necessary to use one or more of the components as a lever of intervention. A change in the component will directly affect the activity because the components are integral to the activity. The change in the activity can create the

conditions for a pattern of reciprocal participation. To assess whether assistance is likely to occur, it is necessary to assess the components. (O'Donnell & Tharp, 1990, p. 262)

Assessment of time, funds, and the physical features of the environment is straightforward. Symbols can be assessed through the examination of language and other signs used in the setting; people and positions through skill levels, manning levels, and the behaviors used to compose each role. Intervention can then proceed by using one or more of these components to affect interaction, develop reciprocal participation, and increase intersubjectivity.

CONCLUSIONS

This intellectual odyssey began in 1970 with the start of the Buddy System Project. The results of the Buddy System Project prompted a seemingly simple question that eventually led to the publication of "Community Intervention Guided by Theoretical Development" (O'Donnell & Tharp, 1990). What has been learned during these 20 years has changed the nature of the question, of the prevailing theory, and of the intervention projects that need to be developed.

The question, prompted by the results of the Buddy System Project, was: Why does the behavior of an individual occur in one setting and not in another? Or in the terms of the theory prevailing at the time: Why does the behavior not generalize from the program setting to other settings? Neither the question nor the answer were as simple as they seemed.

The work of many researchers over these 20 years has shown that the occurrence of a behavior is a function of the characteristics of the setting, only one of which is whether the individual is capable of the behavior. That the individual is capable of the behavior, that it is desirable for the behavior to occur, and that the individual wishes to engage in the behavior, does not mean that the behavior necessarily will occur. The behavior of an individual is part of the interaction with others in a setting and cannot be accurately assessed in isolation from the ongoing activities.

These activities, and therefore individual behaviors, are influenced by the components of the setting and their related variables, such as the relative levels of skill and manning levels. Over time, the behavioral capabilities of individuals interacting in an activity setting will be changed to correspond more closely with such characteristics of the setting as the behaviors used to compose the roles, the functions of each role in the ongoing activities, the availability of assistance, the relationships that form, and the degree of reciprocal participation and intersubjectivity that are developed.

This understanding of the important functions of activity settings shows that the focus of delinquency-prevention projects should be on the settings and networks of participants rather than be limited to individual behavior change. Peer settings based on delinquent activities have the same components and characteristics as other activity settings. The behavior of the individuals within the setting also is influenced by the components of the setting and their related variables. Over time, the behavioral capabilities of these individuals also will be changed to correspond more closely with the characteristics of the setting. Intersubjectivity can be developed in settings based on delinquent activities as easily as in any other type of activity setting.

For these reasons, the long-term effectiveness of delinquency-prevention projects are a function of their effect on settings and networks. The effectiveness of projects with a sole focus on individual behavior change is likely to be reduced if the participants maintain networks with delinquent peers and their settings. Worse yet, as we have seen, projects may increase delinquency by facilitating relationships with participants who are involved in delinquent activities. An understanding of the functioning of activity settings shows how these harmful social-network effects occur and emphasizes the importance of promoting relationships with prosocial peers.

Research and theoretical developments over the past 20 years also shows that the prevailing theory of behavior modification was not wrong, but it was limited in the scope of its effective application. What was needed was a theoretical context in which it could be placed. The current theory incorporates behavior modification and integrates it with the important theoretical contributions of Barker (1960, 1968), Bronfenbrenner (1979), and Vygotsky (1978, 1981). It provides the activity setting as the context for individual behavior. By changing the basic unit of analysis from the individual to the activity setting, the current theory shows how the individual and the setting create each other.

From this perspective, to study either the individual or the setting independently is to distort the phenomena. Activity settings literally cannot exist without individuals and individual behavior occurs in an activity setting. This point is important in a comparison of the Buddy System and the Youth Development Project. In the Buddy System, individual behavior change (e.g., reduced truancy) was promoted outside of the activity settings where the behavior was expected to occur (school classrooms). Since the improved behavior was not a function of the activity setting where it occurred, the improvement was unlikely to continue after the youths left the program. In addition, other settings of importance, such as peer activity settings, were influenced only inadvertently (both positively and negatively) through network changes.

In contrast, the Youth Development Project, although not developed from the current theory, directly alters the classroom activity setting through the structuring of student-team learning and the introduction of social skills training. The combination of both may facilitate prosocial networks and reduce delinquency. It is also possible that the project may have to expand to include intervention in peer settings to affect delinquency, but if so the theory can help to guide that intervention. Whichever turns out to be the case, the Youth Development Project represents a step in the right direction, for it intervenes in the everyday classroom settings of the participants instead of in a separately designed program setting.

In general, the current theory offers many alternative forms of direct intervention. Any of the six means of assistance may be implemented through any of the six components of an activity setting or through various combinations. All forms affect interaction because they are inherent in the process and thereby influence the nature of the setting and the individuals within it. The theory is the key link in a complex chain of events that began with a simple question and, hopefully, will proceed to more effective delinquency prevention.

REFERENCES

Ageton, S. S., & Elliott, D. S. (1974). The effects of legal processing on delinquent orientations. *Social Problems, 22,* 87–100.

Ayllon, T., & Azrin, N. (1964). Reinforcement and instructions with mental patients. *Journal of the Experimental Analysis of Behavior, 7,* 327–331.

Ayllon, T., & Azrin, N. (1965). The measurement and reinforcement of behavior of psychotics. *Journal of the Experimental Analysis of Behavior, 8,* 357–383.

Ayllon, T., & Azrin, N. (1968). *The token economy: A motivational system for therapy and rehabilitation.* New York: Appleton-Century-Crofts.

Barker, R. G. (1960). Ecology and motivation. In M. R. Jones (Ed.), *Nebraska symposium on motivation* (pp. 1–49). Lincoln: University of Nebraska Press.

Barker, R. G. (1968). *Ecological psychology.* Stanford, CA: Stanford University Press.

Berleman, W. C., Seaberg, J. R., & Steinburn, T. W. (1972). The delinquency prevention experiment of the Seattle Atlantic Street Center: A final evaluation. *Social Service Review, 46,* 323–346.

Bijou, S. W., & Baer, D. M. (1967). *Child development: Readings in experimental analysis.* New York: Meredith.

Bronfenbrenner, U. B. (1979). *The ecology of human development.* Cambridge: Harvard University Press.

Buckner, J. C., & Chesney-Lind, M. (1983). Dramatic cures for juvenile crime: An evaluation of a prisoner-run delinquency prevention program. *Criminal Justice and Behavior, 10,* 227–247.

Burchard, J., & Tyler, V. (1965). The modification of delinquent behavior through operant conditioning. *Behaviour Research and Therapy, 2,* 245–250.

Cole, M. (1985). The zone of proximal development: Where culture and cognition create each other. In J. V. Wertsch (Ed.), *Culture, communication, and cognition: Vygotskian perspectives* (pp. 146–161). Cambridge: Cambridge University Press.

Farrington, D. P. (1977). The effects of public labelling. *British Journal of Criminology, 17,* 112–125.

Ferster, C. B. (1968). Operant reinforcement of infantile autism. In S. Lesse (Ed.), *An evaluation of the results of the psychotherapies* (pp. 221–236). Springfield, IL: Thomas.

Ferster, C. B., & DeMyer, M. K. (1961). The development of performance in autistic children in an automatically controlled environment. *Journal of Chronic Disease, 13,* 312–345.

Ferster, C. B., & Simons, J. (1966). Behavior therapy with children. *Psychological Record, 16,* 65–71.

Finckenauer, J. O. (1979). Scared crooked. *Psychology Today, 13,* 6–11.

Fo, W. S. O., & O'Donnell, C. R. (1974). The buddy system: Relationship and contingency conditions in a community intervention program for youth with nonprofessionals as behavior change agents. *Journal of Consulting and Clinical Psychology, 42,* 163–169.

Fo, W. S. O., & O'Donnell, C. R. (1975). The buddy system: Effect of community intervention on delinquent offences. *Behavior Therapy, 6,* 522–524.

Fuller, P. R. (1949). Operant conditioning of a vegetative human organism. *American Journal of Psychology, 62,* 587–590.

Gold, M., & Williams, J. R. (1969). National study of the aftermath of apprehension. *Prospectus, 3,* 3–12.

Klein, M. W. (1971). *Street gangs and street workers.* Englewood Cliffs, NJ: Prentice-Hall.

Lewis, R. V. (1983). Scared straight—California style: Evaluation of the San Quentin Squires Program. *Criminal Justice and Behavior, 10,* 209–226.

Lovaas, O. I. (1966). Program for establishment of speech in schizophrenic and autistic children. In J. Wing (Ed.), *Childhood autism* (pp. 115–144). London: Pergamon Press.

Lovaas, O. I. (1967). A behavior therapy approach to the treatment of childhood schizophrenia. In J. P. Hill (Ed.), *Minnesota symposia on child psychology* (Vol. 1, pp. 131–154). Minneapolis: University of Minnesota Press.

Lovaas, O. I. (1968). Some studies on the treatment of childhood schizophrenia. In J. M. Shlien (Ed.), *Research in psychotherapy* (pp. 102–121). Washington, DC: American Psychological Association.

Lovaas, O. I., Berberich, J. P., Perloff, B. F., & Shaeffer, B. (1966). Acquisition of imitative speech in schizophrenic children. *Science, 151,* 705–707.

Lovaas, O. I., Freitag, G., Gold, V. J., & Kassorla, I. C. (1965). Experimental studies in childhood schizophrenia: Analysis of self-destructive behavior. *Journal of Experimental Child Psychology, 2,* 67–84.

Lovaas, O. I., Freitag, G., Kinder, M. I., Rubenstein, B. D., Schaeffer, B., & Simmons, J. Q. (1966). Establishment of social reinforcers in two schizophrenic children on the basis of food. *Journal of Experimental Child Psychology, 4,* 109–125.

Lovaas, O. I., Freitas, L., Nelson, K., & Whalen, K. (1967). The establishment of imitation and its use for the development of complex behavior in schizophrenic children. *Behaviour Research and Therapy, 5,* 171–181.

Lovaas, O. I., Schaeffer, B., & Simmons, J. Q. (1965). Building social behavior in autistic children using electric shock. *Journal of Experimental Studies in Personality, 1,* 99–109.

Manos, M. J. (1988). *Youth development project: Preventive intervention in delinquency. Three year evaluation report: 1984–1987,* (Report No. 338). Honolulu: University of Hawaii-Manoa, Center for Youth Research.

McCord, J. (1978). A thirty-year follow-up of treatment effects. *American Psychologist, 33,* 284–289.

McEachern, A. W., Taylor, E. M., Newman, J. R., & Ashford, A. E. (1968). The juvenile probation system: Stimulation for research and decision making. *American Behavioral Scientist, 11,* 1–45.

O'Donnell, C. R. (1977). Behavior modification in community settings. In M. Hersen, R. M. Eisler, & P. M. Miller (Eds.), *Progress in behavior modification* (Vol. 4, pp. 69–117). New York: Academic Press.

O'Donnell, C. R. (1980). Environmental design and the prevention of psychological problems. In M. P. Feldman & J. F. Orford (Eds.), *The social psychology of psychological problems* (pp. 279–309). New York: Wiley.

O'Donnell, C. R. (1984). Behavioral community psychology and the natural environment. In C. M. Franks (Ed.), *New developments in behavior therapy: From research to clinical application* (pp. 495–523). New York: Hawthorn Press.

O'Donnell, C. R., Lydgate, T., & Fo, W.S.O. (1979). The buddy system: Review and follow-up. *Child and Family Behavior Therapy, 1,* 161–169.

O'Donnell, C. R., Manos, M. J., & Chesney-Lind, M. (1987). Diversion and neighborhood delinquency programs in open settings: A social network interpretation. In E. K. Morris & C. J. Braukmann (Eds.), *Behavioral approaches to crime and delinquency* (pp. 251–269). New York: Plenum Press.

O'Donnell, C. R., & Tharp, R. G. (1982). Community intervention and the use of multi-disciplinary knowledge. In A. S. Bellack, M. Hersen, & A. E. Kazdin (Eds.), *International handbook of behavior modification and therapy* (pp. 291–318). New York: Plenum Press.

O'Donnell, C. R., & Tharp, R. G. (1990). Community intervention guided by theoretical development. In A. S. Bellack, M. Hersen, & A. E. Kazdin (Eds.), *International handbook of behavior modification and therapy* (2nd ed., pp. 251–266). New York: Plenum Press.

Patterson, G. R., & Gullion, M. E. (1968). *Living with children: New methods for parents and teachers.* Champagne, IL: Research Press.

Phillips, E. L. (1968). Achievement Place: Token reinforcement procedures in a home-style rehabilitation setting for "pre-delinquent" boys. *Journal of Applied Behavior Analysis, 1,* 213–223.

Schwendinger, H., & Schwendinger, J. (1982). The paradigmatic crisis in delinquency theory. *Crime and Social Justice, 17,* 70–78.

Skinner, B. F. (1938). *The behavior of organisms: An experimental analysis.* New York: Appleton-Century-Crofts.

Subcommittee on Human Resources of the Committee on Education and Labor. (1979). *Oversight on "Scared Straight."* Washington, DC: U.S. Government Printing Office.

Tharp, R. G., & Gallimore, R. (1988). *Rousing minds to life: Teaching and learning in social context.* New York: Cambridge University Press.

Tharp, R. G., & Note, M. (1989). The triadic model of consultation: New developments. In F. West (Ed.), *School consultation: Interdisciplinary perspectives on theory, research, training, and practice* (pp. 35–51). Austin: University of Texas at Austin, Research and Training Project on School Consultation.

Tharp, R. G., & Wetzel, B. J. (1969). *Behavior modification in the natural environment.* New York: Academic Press.

Thorndike, E. L. (1898). Animal intelligence: An experimental study of the associative processes in animals. *Psychological Review, 2*(Suppl. 8), 1–109.

Thorndike, E. L. (1913). *The psychology of learning.* New York: Teachers College.

Thorne, G. L., Tharp, R. G., & Wetzel, R. J. (1967). Behavior modification techniques: New tools for probation officers. *Federal Probation, 31,* 21–27.

Ullmann, L. P., & Krasner, L. (Eds.). (1965). *Case studies in behavior modification.* New York: Holt, Rinehart and Winston.

Vygotsky, L. S. (1978). *Mind in society: The development of higher psychological processes.* (M. Cole, V. John-Steiner, S. Scribner, & E. Souberman, Trans. and Eds.). Cambridge: Harvard University Press.

Vygotsky, L. S. (1981). The genesis of higher mental functions. In J. V.

Wertsch (Ed.), *The concept of activity in Soviet psychology* (pp. 144–188). Armank, NY: Sharpe.

Wahler, R. G. (1969). Oppositional children: A quest for parental reinforcement control. *Journal of Applied Behavior Analysis, 2,* 159–170.

Wahler, R. G., & Erickson, M. (1969). Child behavior therapy: A community program in Appalachia. *Behaviour Research and Therapy, 7,* 71–78.

Wahler, R. G., Winkel, G. H., Peterson, R. F., & Morrison, D. C. (1965). Mothers as behavior therapists for their own children. *Behaviour Research and Therapy, 3,* 113–124.

Willems, E. P. (1974). Behavioral technology and behavioral ecology. *Journal of Applied Behavior Analysis, 7,* 151–165.

Williams, C. D. (1959). The elimination of tantrum behavior by extinction procedures. *Journal of Abnormal and Social Psychology, 59,* 269–270.

Wilson, H. (1980). Parental supervision: A neglected aspect of delinquency. *British Journal of Criminology, 20,* 203–235.

Witmer, L. (1906–1907). Clinical psychology. *Psychological Clinic, 1,* 1–9.

◆ ──────── ◆

CHAPTER 11

The St. Louis Experiment:
Effective Treatment of Antisocial Youths in Prosocial Peer Groups

RONALD A. FELDMAN

A detailed review of the available research literature by the author and his colleagues (Feldman, Caplinger, & Wodarski, 1983) has clearly demonstrated that treatment programs for antisocial youths must be significantly restructured if they are to achieve maximum success. Put briefly, it is essential to offer treatment in nonstigmatizing environments and in contexts that are comprised of large numbers of prosocial peers. The treatment setting ought to be as similar as possible to the antisocial youth's natural environment and, if feasible, an integral part of it. Such conditions are likely to promote easier transferability of behavior gains and to maximize the likelihood that they will be stabilized and sustained within the youth's natural environment. Throughout, the subjects should receive maximum exposure to prosocial peers and minimum exposure to antisocial peers. To the extent possible, the requisite interventions also should enable antisocial youngsters to perform conventional social roles and to assume maximum responsibility for their own behavior and its consequences.

The potential therapeutic role of prosocial peers is clearly suggested by two studies. Friday and Hage (1976), for example, found that peers are likely to play an especially prominent role in shaping a youth's behavior when the youth's relationship with his or her parents is weak. They identified five major patterns of role relationships that can influence a youth's behavior: (1) kin, (2) community or neighborhood, (3) school, (4) work, and (5) peers not otherwise defined by the four others. When there was little intimacy in the first four contexts, Friday and Hage found peer group relationships to be especially potent. Thus, as youths spent more time with peers they became isolated from other socializing agents and tended to develop criminal tendencies. Indeed, the investigators discovered a particularly strong negative correlation ($-.81$) between interaction in the family and interaction with friends. Hence, with reference to delinquent activity, a weak familial relationship seems to contribute toward heightened reliance upon one's peers.

Even more instructive in this regard is a major study of peer influence reported by Linden and Hackler (1973). Based upon interviews with 200 working-class boys who ranged in age from 13 to 15, they obtained data regarding self-reported delinquency, closeness of ties to parents, closeness of ties to delinquent peers, and closeness of ties to conventional (that is, nondelinquent) peers. The greatest proportion of delinquency was found among subjects with weak ties to conventional associates but with moderate or strong ties to deviant peers; 58.3% of this group was delinquent. Nearly 43% of boys with weak or nonexistent ties to adults or peers (be they conventional or delinquent) considered themselves delinquent. Boys who had ties to conventional peers and adults but not to deviant peers were the least delinquent (15.2%). The researchers' data are especially illuminating when one considers boys who had weak or nonexistent ties to their parents. In such instances, ties with conventional peers largely offset the disposition toward delinquency. Among subjects who reported moderate or strong ties to deviant peers and only weak or nonexistent ties to conventional ones, more than half were delinquent. However, if moderate or strong ties with deviant peers were countervailed by concurrent moderate or strong ties with conventional peers, the incidence of delinquency dropped to 26.3%.

Likewise, 42.9% of Linden and Hackler's subjects reported delinquent behavior when they had weak or nonexistent ties with deviant peers and weak or nonexistent ties with conventional ones. This figure dropped to 25% for boys who had weak or nonexistent ties to deviant peers and moderate or strong ties to conventional peers. Hence, it is evident that the adverse influence of deviant peers can be largely neutralized by providing youths with opportunities for meaningful social relationships with conventional peers. Indeed, this formulation is consistent with the vast majority of theoretical formulations concerning the development of antisocial and delinquent behavior including, in particular, theories of differential association (Akers, 1973; Sutherland & Cressey, 1978).

This analysis leads to the supposition that antisocial youths ought to be treated primarily—perhaps exclusively—in prosocial environments. To minimize dysfunctional role models and deviant peer reinforcement systems, it is posited that antisocial youths should be treated among youngsters who display positive social behavior themselves and who reward and reinforce it when it is displayed by others. Further, by situating treatment programs in settings such as community centers and neighborhood houses, it should prove possible not only to reduce peer-based obstacles to effective treatment but also to minimize the undue labeling and stigma that attend intervention in more traditional treatment settings. The forces that encourage positive behavior change ought to be at their maximum when only one antisocial youth is placed in an activity group that consists entirely of youths who are regarded as prosocial, that is, who exhibit acceptable and stable patterns of prosocial behavior in a variety of contexts.

Given the fact that few, if any, intervention programs have thus far been devised upon the basis of such premises, what has militated against their establishment? Perhaps the most important factor in this regard is concern about the prosocial youths who would take part. Parents may fear that their prosocial children will adopt deviant behaviors as a result of their exposure to antisocial or delinquent peers. Indeed, such fears are not likely to be vitiated in the absence of rigorous empirical evidence to the contrary. And, the latter cannot accrue in the absence of a carefully designed experimental study.

RESEARCH DESIGN

While the basic theoretical premises of the above-described intervention approach are few and relatively simple, they raise a series of questions that, in turn, pose complex challenges for research design and implementation. Thus, for instance, how can one ascertain whether the behavior gains, if any, of antisocial youths in mixed, or integrated, groups surpass those of antisocial youths who are treated in the conventional manner, that is, solely among antisocial peers? Similarly, how can one ascertain whether the prosocial youths who take part in mixed groups fare any worse, if at all, than comparable prosocial youths who participate in groups that are comprised solely of prosocial peers? In small-group research of this kind, how can one avert a "placebo" effect or, at least, measure the extent to which it obtains? How can one determine whether this particular form of group treatment fares better or worse than alternative types of group treatment, or even than no treatment at all? How can one ascertain whether the treatments being measured were, in fact, actually implemented by the putative intervention agents? And how can one accurately determine whether the resultant behavior patterns actually differ from those that obtained prior to the implementation of treatment? These questions and others were addressed, at least in part, by the research design described below.

Known locally as the Group Integration Project and nationally as the St. Louis Experiment (Center for Studies of Crime and Delinquency, 1974), the research program was established at a suburban community center, namely, the Jewish Community Centers Association (JCCA) of St. Louis, Missouri. A total of 701 subjects took part in the research. In simplest terms, only two categories of subjects participated in the research: nonreferred youths and referred youths. The former were boys between 7 and 15 years old who were regularly enrolled members at the JCAA. The latter were boys of the same age who were referred to the program by the professional staff of juvenile courts, special schools, mental health facilities, and residential treatment centers. A referral checklist was devised in order to facilitate referrals to the program. The checklist required a referral agent to estimate the number of times during the preceding 7 days that a referred youth engaged in a variety of criterion behaviors deemed to hurt, disrupt, or annoy others. These included antisocial motor behaviors, physical contacts, verbalizations, object interference, and distracting others. For a boy to qualify for an enrollment interview, the referral agent had to report that the youth had engaged in at least 21 antisocial behaviors per week. However, referral agents were never told about this quantitative enrollment criterion. When a referred youth scored above the criterion, he and his parents were invited to an intake interview. A similar checklist was then completed by the parents. To gain admission to the St. Louis Experiment, the youth's parents had to confirm independently that he engaged in 21 or more antisocial acts per week. The product–moment correlation for scores on the referral agent and parent checklists was .51 ($p < .001$).

The mean age of the referred subjects was 11.2 years. Sixty-five percent were white, 34% were black, and 1% were classified as "other." As inferred from data regarding their mother's religion, 66.3% of the referred boys were Protestant, 23.4% were Catholic, 5.6% were Jewish, and 4.8% were "other." Using Census Bureau occupational categories (Reiss, Duncan, Hatt, & North, 1961), 12.5% of the referred boys' fathers were classified as professional, 13.0% as managerial, 32.3% as skilled, 33.2% as unskilled, 3.8% as unemployed, and 5.3% as "other."

The research employed a $3 \times 3 \times 2$ factorial design succinctly summarized in Table 11.1. Three major sets of variables were studied: mode of group composition (referred groups vs. nonreferred groups vs. mixed, or integrated, groups), group treatment method (social learning method vs. traditional group work vs. minimal treatment), and extent of group leader's prior experience (experienced vs. inexperienced). All groups were stratified by age. The referred groups ($n = 25$) consisted of 237 referred youths. The nonreferred groups ($n = 13$) consisted of 174 nonreferred youths. The mixed groups ($n = 22$) consisted of 264 nonreferred youths plus one or two referred youths ($n = 26$) in each group who had been assigned to them on a random basis. All told, this design yielded four discrete samples of subjects: referred youths in unmixed groups, referred youths in mixed groups, nonreferred youths in mixed groups, and nonreferred youths in unmixed groups.

The group treatment methods employed during the St. Louis Experiment are fully described elsewhere (Feldman & Wodarski, 1975). In brief, the social learning method primarily entailed the use of group-level behavior modification. The traditional group work method, in contrast, entailed the application of interventions that were based upon social psychological and social group work principles. No systematic training or interventions were entailed on the part of minimal-treatment group leaders. Instead, they were encouraged to interact with group members in a purely natural and spontaneous fashion. Only after the conclusion of an 8-week baseline period were the respective treatment methods assigned and taught to the group leaders. At various intervals throughout the research, trained nonparticipant observers completed a checklist that indicated which type of intervention method was actually being implemented by each group leader. This permitted a rudimentary assessment of the extent to which the independent variable, or particular type of group intervention method, had been, in fact, administered.

The experienced group leaders were students at a graduate school of social work; the inexperienced leaders were untrained undergraduate students. Assignment of virtually all group leaders and treatment methods was made on a random basis. Utilizing the above-described research design, two cohorts of subjects participated in a wide range of recreational and leisure activities in small groups that met approximately once per week during the school year.

Throughout the research, the subjects' behavior was examined by means of a variety of measures. The most important are proportionate behavioral profiles. Most research on antisocial youths has focused exclusively on their deviant behavior and therefore has neglected to

TABLE 11.1. Research Design Implemented for the St. Louis Experiment by Leader Training, Treatment Method, and Mode of Group Composition: Total n = 701 Subjects and 60 Groups

Group composition	Experienced leaders			Inexperienced leaders			Total
	Behavioral method	Traditional method	Minimal method	Behavioral method	Traditional method	Minimal method	
Referred	Ss = 61 Gs = 6 (5)	Ss = 41 Gs = 4	SS = 37 Gs = 4	Ss = 34 Gs = 4	Ss = 25 Gs = 3	Ss = 39 Gs = 4	SS = 237 Gs = 25
Mixed	Ss = 55 Gs = 4	Ss = 50 Gs = 4 (5)	Ss = 44 Gs = 3 (4)	Ss = 30 Gs = 4 (4)	Ss = 61 Gs = 4 (4)	Ss = 50 Gs = 3 (4)	Ss = 290 Gs = 22 (26)
Nonreferred	Ss = 38 Gs = 3	Ss = 22 Gs = 2	Ss = 14 Gs = 1	Ss = 40 Gs = 3	Ss = 30 Gs = 2	Ss = 30 Gs = 2	Ss = 174 Gs = 13
Total	Ss = 154 Gs = 13	Ss = 113 Gs = 10	Ss = 95 Gs = 9	Ss = 104 Gs = 10	Ss = 116 Gs = 9	Ss = 119 Gs = 9	Ss = 701 Gs = 60

Note. Ss = Number of subjects per cell; Gs = Number of groups per cell; ( ) = Number of referred subjects assigned to each group category.

238

simultaneously examine their constructive behavior. To avert this bias three types of behavior were studied concurrently. *Prosocial behavior* was defined operationally as any action by a group member that was directed toward completion of a peer group's tasks or activities. *Antisocial behavior* was defined as any action that disrupts, hurts, or annoys other members, or that otherwise prevents them from participating in the group's tasks or activities. *Nonsocial behavior* was defined as any action that is not directed toward completion of a group's tasks or activities but that does not interfere with another youth's participation in the group's tasks or activities. By analyzing these respective behaviors it was possible to calculate each subject's proportionate behavioral profile at any particular juncture of the research program. Hence, delinquent behavior was not treated merely as a dichotomous attribute, or as something that one either is or is not.

At pretest and posttest, behavioral checklists were completed by the referral agents, parents, group leaders, and the youths themselves. The checklists requested the respondents to estimate the frequency with which a given youth exhibited various types of prosocial, nonsocial, and antisocial behavior during a 7-day period. In addition, throughout the entire project trained nonparticipant observers employed a 10-second summated partition sampling system that classified each subject's actual behavior into similar prosocial, nonsocial, or antisocial categories. All observations for each subject were tabulated after each group meeting. As a result, it was possible to tabulate the proportion of each subject's behavior that was either prosocial, nonsocial, or antisocial during a given group meeting. An arc sine transformation was performed for all of the proportionate behavioral scores in order to meet the customary requirements for the statistical analysis of percentage and proportionate data (Winer, 1971, p. 400). Furthermore, to facilitate the identification of longitudinal trends, the data for all sessions were collapsed into four successive periods of approximately 8 weeks each: baseline, T1, T2, and T3. The nonparticipant observers were evaluated every 2 weeks by comparing their ratings of different videotapes of group interaction with those of an "expert judge." They were permitted to work only if their reliability was consistently at a level of .90 or above. Across all sessions, the mean reliability ratio for observers was 92.2.

The nonparticipant observers and group leaders also provided data that enabled the determination of each subject's extent of normative, functional, and interpersonal integration into his respective peer group. An individual's *normative integration* into a group refers to the extent to which he adheres to basic norms that are shared by his groupmates. *Functional integration* refers to the extent to which he contributes effectively to the attainment of key group goals such as goal attainment, pattern maintenance, and external relations. *Interpersonal integration* refers to the extent to which he likes others in the group and, in turn, is liked by them. The theoretical rationales and mathematical procedures for calculating subjects' scores on each of these dimensions are described elsewhere (cf. Feldman, 1973; Feldman et al., 1983). Pretest and posttest responses to the Manifest Aggression subscale of the Jesness Inventory (Jesness, Derisi, McCormick, & Wedge, 1972) also were acquired from the subjects.

In addition to conventional univariate analyses, multivariate analyses of the data were performed by means of composite measures that distinguished between the referred and nonreferred samples. Typically, these combined information from each of the five basic self-report instruments that were employed during the research (mean manifest aggression scores, absolute frequencies of antisocial behavior, and proportionate mean incidences of antisocial, nonsocial, and prosocial behavior). Differences between the two samples were ascertained by means of standardized discriminant analyses (Kaplan & Litrownik, 1977). By averaging the discriminant scores for all cases within a particular group, it was possible to obtain group centroids, or means, for the multiple measures that defined a discriminant function. The group centroids constituted a graphic mechanism for depicting complex multivariate findings in a relatively succinct fashion.

Analyses of covariance were employed for the assessment of pretest-posttest changes among the subjects in order to avert some of the analytical problems that are associated with classical experimental designs. Pretest data were employed as the concomitant variable in the analysis of covariance, thereby partialing out that portion of variance in the subjects' scores that can be predicted from pretest scores (Huck & McLean, 1975; Roscoe, 1969). Unlike simple analyses of gain scores, covariance analyses result in the reduction of error variance. Furthermore, they help to reduce errors in interpretation that might be due to regressions to the mean. This is accomplished by subtracting from the raw measures of change (or postscores) a function of the subjects' initial level of performance. Nevertheless, it is essential to correct for measurement errors in analyses of covariance that are attributable to the unreliability of subjects' prescores (Cronbach & Furby, 1970). Therefore, the assessments reported here employ a method for reliability-corrected covariance analyses wherein the subjects' "true" prescores are estimated and then utilized to determine pretest-posttest "gains" (Porter, 1967).

Endpoint analyses, dropout analyses, and survivor analyses were employed in order to determine longitudinal variations in the subjects' scores. Endpoint analyses were performed by examining each subject's behavioral profile for the last time period (that is, T1, T2, or T3) during which he participated in the program. Analyses of endpoint data were performed by means of a multivariate analysis of covariance in which the subjects' observed baseline behaviors served as the concomitant variate. These analyses could be performed either for dropouts (that is, youths who quit the program after the baseline period but before the commencement of T3) or for survivors (that is, youths who remained in the program for the full year, or throughout T3). Finally, whenever indicated, a posteriori tests for individual comparisons were conducted by means of Hotelling's T-square statistic (Bock, 1975).

In brief, then, the St. Louis Experiment was characterized by a large variety of methodological features. These include: a factorial design; randomized assignment of group leaders, subjects, and treatment methods; comparison groups; a no-intervention baseline period; nonparticipant observers who were checked for reliability on a biweekly basis; a multiple time-series research design; measures that accounted for subjects' prosocial and nonsocial behavior as well as their antisocial behavior and, also, that viewed the latter from the perspective of each subject's proportionate behavioral profile; multiple independent judges, including referral agents, group leaders, parents, trained nonparticipant observers, and the participating youths themselves; independent measures regarding the extent to which the independent variables, or modes of intervention, actually were implemented; a blind intake criterion applied by two sets of independent judges; a standard measure of manifest aggression; arc sin transformations of proportionate data; reliability-corrected analyses of covariance that adjusted for differences in the subjects' pretest behavioral profiles; multiple discriminant analyses; and, endpoint, dropout, and survivor analyses. Clearly, the research design sought to guard against numerous threats that could compromise the integrity with which valid and reliable inferences can be drawn from experimental data. The major pretest and posttest measures are summarized succinctly in Table 11.2. While the research design hardly approaches perfection, it does enable certain conclusions to be drawn from the data with somewhat greater assurance than typically has been the case for field studies of antisocial youths.

SELECTED FINDINGS

The above-described data permit the examination of numerous interrelationships among a multitude of variables. Only a few of the

TABLE 11.2. Schedule for Administration of Research Instruments, by Respondents and Time Period

Time period	Respondents				
	Referral agents	Parents	Group leaders	Children	Observers
Intake	1	1			
Baseline*			1,3,4,5,6	1,2	3,4,5,6,7,8
T1					7,8
T2					7,8
T3	1	1	1,3,4,5,6	1,2	3,4,5,6,7,8
Follow-up**	1	1			

Research instruments: 1, behavioral inventory; 2, Jesness inventory, manifest aggression subscale; 3, normative integration index, individual and group; 4, interpersonal integration index, individual and group; 5, functional integration index, individual and group; 6, social power index, individual and group; 7, behavioral ratings; 8, report of treatment method.
*Approximately 8 weeks after first group session; thereafter, approximately 8 weeks transpired between successive treatment periods.
**Approximately 1 year following termination of treatment.

central findings are reported here insofar as a fully detailed report is available elsewhere (Feldman et al., 1983). The subjects' pretest behavior will be examined first and then the experimental outcomes will be reviewed as reported by a variety of different sources, namely, nonparticipant observers, group leaders, the youths, their parents, and referral agents.

Pretest Behavior of the Subjects

Using the behavioral checklist, the parents of the referred youths estimated at intake that their sons engaged in 26.5 antisocial acts per week, or about 4 per day. On a proportionate basis, about 35% of their sons' behavior was regarded as antisocial. The referral agents reported even higher incidences of antisocial behavior on the part of referred youths, to wit, 62.7 antisocial acts per week. This represented 59% of their total behavior. Self-reports from the referred and nonreferred youths indicated considerably less pretest variation between the two samples. Nevertheless, the referred youths reported significantly higher pretest scores on manifest aggression than did the nonreferred youths ($p < .001$). Moreover, the two samples differed significantly at pretest on the basis of the multivariate composite measure of self-reported behavior ($\chi^2 (5) = 31.05$, $p < .001$).

The group leaders and the nonparticipant observers also reported that the referred youths had significantly lower pretest scores than

nonreferred youths with respect to social power and normative, functional, and interpersonal integration ($p < .001$). Hence, even from the
outset of the intervention program, nonreferred boys may have been
better able than the referred boys to resist undue peer pressures
toward antisocial behavior. Mixed, or integrated, groups were characterized by relatively high norm consensus and this may have been
one of the key factors that contributed to prosocial behavior change
on the part of the referred youths in such groups.

Behavior Changes from the Perspective of Nonparticipant Observers

Initial analyses of data from the St. Louis Experiment focused upon
behavior changes in accord with variations in leader experience,
treatment method, and peer group composition. The effects of each
variable are reviewed separately.

Leader Experience

The endpoint data that were reported by the nonparticipant observers
revealed significant posttest behavioral differences. Boys who were
treated by experienced leaders benefited considerably more from the
program than did boys who were treated by inexperienced leaders.
The former exhibited marked reductions in proportionate antisocial
($M = -3.1\%$, $p < .001$) and nonsocial ($M = -1.9\%$, $p < .001$) behavior. By the end of treatment, 96.7% of these boys' observed behavior
was prosocial. This represents a substantial upturn in prosocial behavior ($M = +5.0\%$, $p < .001$) from their mean pretreatment incidence.
In contrast, at the end of treatment merely 2.4% of their behavior was
antisocial.

About 6.9% of the behavior of boys with inexperienced group
leaders was antisocial at end point. This is nearly three times the
incidence for boys with experienced leaders. Equally important,
83.2% of the latter boys manifested prosocial gains during the program while only 54.7% of the former did so. Moreover, longitudinal
analyses demonstrated that the experienced group leaders were able to
bring about marked declines in the subjects' antisocial behavior quite
rapidly (that is, during T1) and to sustain them over time. In comparison, boys who were treated by inexperienced group leaders exhibited
negative behavioral outcomes, especially if they quit the program at
an early point. Nevertheless, above and beyond the youths' baseline
behavior, only 9.6% of the variance in treatment outcomes was explained by the differential effectiveness of experienced and inexpe-

rienced leaders. Hence, additional factors must account for the observed changes in the youths' behavior.

Treatment Method

In contrast with the findings for leader experience, the particular method of group treatment exerted little or no impact on the subjects' behavior change. The behavioral method promoted significantly better outcomes than traditional group work ($p < .001$) but it fared no better than the minimal method ($p < .79$). In part, this may be due to the fact that the traditional group work method was difficult to implement. Reports by the nonparticipant observers indicated that it was, in fact, appropriately implemented far less often than were the other two methods. Consistent with this finding, an assessment of interaction effects suggested that experienced leaders achieved relatively positive outcomes regardless of which treatment method they applied while inexperienced leaders had relatively negative outcomes, especially when they tried to implement traditional group work.

Group Composition

Although the observational data suggested a rather weak relationship between group composition and treatment outcomes, most of the trends were in the expected direction. For example, while the observed antisocial behavior of referred boys in unmixed groups did not decline over time ($M = +0.3\%$, $p < .70$), such antisocial behavior fell significantly among referred boys in mixed groups ($M = -2.2\%$, $p < .01$). At end point, 5.7% of the observed behavior for the former boys was antisocial and barely half of them (50.9%) had achieved any discernible decline in antisocial behavior. In contrast, only 3.2% of the behavior of the latter boys was antisocial and 91.3% of them had achieved a decline in antisocial behavior. In fact, by end point the behavioral patterns of the referred boys in mixed groups differed very little from those of the nonreferred members of their groups ($p < .26$). Moreover, no significant differences were found between the endpoint behavioral profiles of the nonreferred boys in mixed groups and the nonreferred boys in unmixed groups. Hence, it appears that the behavior of the former boys was not affected adversely by sustained interaction with one or two putatively antisocial youths.

The data also permitted examination of the behavior patterns of subjects who discontinued from the program prior to the end of T3. These findings reinforce the trends noted above. When placed in mixed groups, for instance, referred youths benefited from treatment regardless of whether they continued for the full duration of the program or quit at an early point. Antisocial behavior constituted only 2.5% of the endpoint behavioral profile of referred boys in mixed groups who discontinued early while it constituted 10.4% for referred boys in unmixed groups who quit early. The former boys, therefore, tended to discontinue from treatment primarily after they had established relatively stable patterns of prosocial behavior. Hence, in their case early discontinuance ought not be regarded as an instance of treatment failure.

The treatment potential of mixed groups is demonstrated even more by the fact that referred boys in such groups achieved notable gains in prosocial behavior ($M = +2.7\%$, $p < .02$) even when they were led by inexperienced leaders. They also displayed significant declines in antisocial ($M = -1.7\%$, $p < .05$) and nonsocial ($M = -1.0\%$, $p < .01$) behavior. Although they did not benefit as much as referred boys in mixed groups that were led by experienced leaders, they nonetheless improved markedly. Hence, the therapeutic features of mixed groups may compensate in large part for the deficits of inexperienced leaders. The validity of this supposition is strengthened by the finding that referred youths fared very poorly when treated in unmixed groups that were led by inexperienced leaders. At end point, 9.1% of the behavior of these youths was antisocial; this represents a significant increase from baseline ($M = +3.6\%$, $p < .01$). Hence, the combination of experienced leaders and mixed peer groups surpasses the separate treatment contributions of either variable alone.

Behavior Changes from the Perspective of Youths and Group Leaders

Whereas the nonparticipant observers gathered time-sampling data on a continuous basis, the youths and group leaders provided self-report data at only two junctures, namely, at the end of the 8-week baseline period and at the conclusion of treatment.

Leader Experience

The self-report data from the youths themselves revealed trends that were similar to those reported by the nonparticipant observers. Youths with experienced leaders reported relatively positive outcomes, while youths with inexperienced leaders reported relatively negative outcomes. However, the differences between the two samples fell short of statistical significance. Comparable data reported by the group leaders indicated that boys with experienced leaders benefited far more than did boys with inexperienced leaders. Thus, for example, 28.3% of the former boys' posttest behavioral profile was antisocial, representing a significant decline ($M = -4.5\%$, $p < .001$). In contrast, 35.7% of the latter boys' behavior was antisocial, reflecting a slight increment in such behavior ($M = +2.9\%$, $p < .13$). Furthermore, experienced leaders reported improvements among 60.1% of the boys in their groups while inexperienced leaders reported gains among only 45.0% ($\chi^2(1) = 6.54$, $p < .01$). In concert with the data from the nonparticipant observers, these findings lend further credence to the conclusion that leader experience is a key determinant of favorable treatment outcomes on the part of antisocial youths.

Treatment Method

As with the nonparticipant observers, the self-report data from group leaders and the youths themselves did not indicate that one type of group treatment method was particularly more effective than the others.

Group Composition

Significantly better outcomes were reported by the referred boys in mixed groups than by the referred boys in unmixed groups (T-square = 14.1, $p < .01$). Again, therefore, the data suggest the efficacy of treating antisocial youths among peers who have no identifiable behavioral problems. Further, an examination of self-report data concerning the behavior of nonreferred youths in mixed groups indicates the absence of deleterious treatment outcomes on their part. In their own judgment, their behavioral outcomes did not differ significantly from the ones reported by nonreferred boys in unmixed groups ($p < .20$). In fact, at posttest the former boys reported 35% fewer antisocial acts than the latter. Moreover, pretest-posttest comparisons revealed no significant changes in proportionate incidences of antisocial, nonsocial, or prosocial behavior on the part of either category of subjects.

Similarly, the group leaders reported relatively positive outcomes for referred boys in mixed groups and negative outcomes for referred boys in unmixed groups. However, the differences did not attain statistical significance. Like the youths, the group leaders also reported no adverse behavioral outcomes on the part of nonreferred boys in mixed groups vis-à-vis nonreferred boys in unmixed groups. In fact, the leaders' reports indicated a sharp decline in proportionate antisocial behavior among the former subjects ($M = -6.9\%$, $p < .001$) but virtually no change on the part of the latter.

Behavior Changes from the Perspective of Referral Agents and Parents

The posttest data from referral agents and parents were limited. Due to their extensive caseloads and high rates of job turnover, the referral agents provided complete pretest-posttest data for only 74 youths. The parents provided complete pretest-posttest data for only 140 youths. Both groups of respondents reported significant pretest-posttest declines in the antisocial behavior of the referred youths. Moreover, they expressed a high degree of consensus about the youths' behavioral gains ($r = .73$, $p < .001$). Nevertheless, unlike other respondents, they did not report differential treatment gains in accord with the main variables under consideration, that is, leader experience, mode of group treatment, and type of group composition.

THE DYNAMIC NATURE OF GROUP COMPOSITION

Throughout the St. Louis Experiment, some youths discontinued from the program. While many left after achieving stable behavioral gains others left with decidedly antisocial behavior profiles. These early departures raised an important conceptual and operational question, namely, does the nature of the variable denoted as "group composition" change over time in accord with the behavioral profiles of the subjects who remain in the group? If, for example, three or four of the most antisocial members of a referred group quit the program early, would not the group become a relatively more prosocial vehicle for fostering behavior gains among its remaining members?

To examine this question, the respective behavior profile of each treatment group in the program was examined for the particular time period (that is, baseline, T1, or T2) that immediately preceded the specific time period being studied (that is, T1, T2, or T3). The initial peer behavior that had been reported in the preceding time period was regarded as a relatively precise indicator of the actual behavior profiles of the group's members at that particular moment in time, and therefore of its "group composition." Each youth's behavior in the group either had or had not been modified in the preceding time period by interventions attempted by the group leader and by the behavior of his groupmates. His resulting behavior in the treatment group then contributed to further behavior changes on the part of each of his peers in the group.

Hence, unlike the conceptualization that had been reflected in the original research design for the St. Louis Experiment, none of the putative treatment groups could be considered as purely antisocial or purely prosocial throughout the course of treatment. Rather, each group varied in the degree to which it was prosocial or antisocial and, moreover, each group's status in this regard varied from one phase of the program to the other. Consequently, group composition was reconceptualized as a dynamic phenomenon that influences members' behavior over time rather than as a static one. While this formulation further complicates the difficulties of performing empirical research concerning group composition, it also yields a more veridical picture of a group's characteristics at each point in time throughout the course of treatment. This approach is far superior to the original one in which group composition was defined simply and statically in terms of the pretreatment designations of group members as being either prosocial or antisocial.

The utility of this perspective is demonstrated in Table 11.3 where it is seen that antecedent changes in the behavior of peers, as measured by trained nonparticipant observers, account for 70% of the variance of behavior changes in youths in referred groups, 50% of the variance in mixed groups, and 29% of the variance in nonreferred groups. Hence, for all three modes of group composition, prior behavioral changes among one's peers is the single best predictor of treatment outcomes. Moreover, the power of this predictor varies directly with the concentration of referred antisocial youths in the group. This is as it ought to be since the need for behavioral change is likely to be least among the members of nonreferred groups, slightly higher in mixed groups, and at a maximum in referred groups.

This more complex and dynamic perspective regarding the study of behavior change in small groups enables one to view each peer group primarily in terms of the changing behavior profiles of their members. Accordingly, it recognizes that the composition of a peer group can vary over time. A group can become more or less prosocial as treatment progresses and as various members leave it. Cross-lag analyses indicate further that the initial direction of influence in group treatment flows from the leader to the group. Modifications in peer group behavior that are initiated by the leader then promote desirable changes on the part of individual members. Experienced leaders generated particularly favorable outcomes precisely because they were effective at fostering antecedent changes within the group itself. In groups that were treated by experienced leaders, nearly 59% of the variance in individual members' outcomes was predicted by the antecedent behavioral changes of their peers. This represents 89% of the total explained variance. Consonant with the basis tenets of social group work, the data clearly indicate that effective group leaders

TABLE 11.3. Variance Explained in Predicting Change in Antisocial Behavior Among Youths by Mode of Group Composition

Variable category	Referred groups (n = 175)		Mixed groups (n = 167)		Nonreferred groups (n = 110)	
	Proportion of variance added to R^2	% Explained variance	Proportion of variance added to R^2	% Explained variance	Proportion of variance added to R^2	% Explained variance
Initial youth behavior	.0508	6	.0610	9	.1429	29
Initial peer behavior	.0086	1	.0069	1	.0153	3
Peer change in behavior	.7004	84	.4979	72	.2867	57
Leader behavior	.0575	7	.0461	7	.0265	5
Program activity	.0162	2	.0577	8	.0234	5
Leader experience	.0004	0	.0068	1	.0000	0
Treatment method	.0033	0	.0108	2	.0040	1
Total	.8362	100	.6872	100	.4988	100

modified the peer group and it in turn altered the behavior of individual group members.

IMPLICATIONS FOR RESEARCH, THEORY, AND PROGRAM DESIGN

Only a portion of the research findings derived from the St. Louis Experiment have been reported here. Nevertheless, even these have significant implications for future research, theory, and programs that seek to reduce antisocial behavior on the part of youths. With regard to future research, for example, it is evident that rigorous and comprehensive field experiments must be designed in order to identify and evaluate the complexities of behavior change. Indeed, it is probable that the methodological rigor of the St. Louis Experiment was in itself a major factor that enabled favorable treatment outcomes to be delineated.

Time sampling studies that include a nonintervention baseline period are needed in future research so as to enable longitudinal treatment processes and outcomes to be clearly identified. Multiple indicators provided by a variety of independent judges can significantly strengthen the ability to draw tenable conclusions from a data base. Similarly, endpoint data that contrast a program's differential effects upon dropouts and survivors can greatly illuminate the dynamics of behavior change. Further, by examining the extent to which the independent (that is, treatment) variables actually are implemented, the researcher can better determine the extent to which observed behavior changes, or the lack thereof, are attributable to the particular modes of treatment under study. And the presence of minimal-treatment or no-treatment comparison groups further enables one to ascertain whether the outcomes attributable to a given group treatment are stronger than those that might obtain merely from expectational effects.

The findings of the St. Louis Experiment also have import for extant theoretical formulations about the etiology of antisocial behavior and prosocial behavior. The data are supportive of current theories of peer group influence and differential association. Even more, they shed light upon the ways in which treatment groups become integrated; individual members become more or less integrated into their respective peer groups; and youths' normative integration, functional integration, interpersonal integration, and social power affect their susceptibility toward peer group pressures that conduce toward behavior change. During the past 2 decades field experiments concerning the social psychological dynamics of intervention groups have been few; yet, the above data point clearly to the need to renew and revitalize field research concerning such phenomena.

ACKNOWLEDGMENT

This study was supported by means of Research Grant MH-18813 from the Center for Studies of Crime and Delinquency, National Institute of Mental Health. It draws largely from previous work published by the author and his colleagues (cf., in particular, Feldman & Caplinger, 1983, and Feldman, Caplinger, & Wodarski, 1983).

REFERENCES

Akers, R. L. (1973). *Deviant behavior: A social learning approach.* Belmont, CA: Wadsworth.

Bock, R. D. (1975). *Multivariate statistical methods in behavioral research.* New York: McGraw-Hill.

Center for Studies of Crime and Delinquency, National Institute of Mental Health. (1974). *The St. Louis experiment: Treating antisocial children in the open community* (Research Report No. 3). Rockville, MD: U.S. Department of Health, Education, and Welfare, Alcohol, Drug Abuse and Mental Health Administration.

Cronbach, L. J., & Furby, L. (1970). How should we measure "change," or should we? *Psychological Bulletin, 74,* 68–80.

Feldman, R. A. (1973). Power distribution, integration and conformity in small groups. *American Journal of Sociology, 79*(3), 639–664.

Feldman, R. A., & Caplinger, T. E. (1977). Social work experience and client behavioral change: A multivariate analysis of process and outcome. *Journal of Social Service Research, 1*(1), 5–34.

Feldman, R. A., & Caplinger, T. E. (1983). The St. Louis experiment: Treatment of antisocial youths in prosocial peer groups. In James R. Kluegel (Ed.), *Evaluating Juvenile Justice* (pp. 121–148). Beverly Hills, CA: Sage.

Feldman, R. A., Caplinger, T. E., & Wodarski, J. S. (1983). *The St. Louis conundrum: The effective treatment of antisocial youths.* Englewood Cliffs, NJ: Prentice Hall.

Feldman, R. A., & Wodarski, J. S. (1975). *Contemporary approaches to group treatment.* San Francisco, CA: Jossey-Bass.

Feldman, R. A., Wodarski, J. S., Goodman, M., & Flax, N. (1973). Prosocial and antisocial boys together. *Social Work, 18*(5), 26–36.

Friday, P. C., & Hage, J. (1976). Youth crime in postindustrial societies: An integrated perspective. *Criminology, 14,* 347–368.

Huck, S. W., & McLean, R. A. (1975). Using a repeated measures ANOVA to analyze the data from a pretest/posttest design: A potentially confusing task. *Psychological Bulletin, 82,* 511–518.

Jesness, C. F., Derisi, W. J., McCormick, P., & Wedge, R. F. (1972). *The youth center research project.* Sacramento: CA: California Youth Authority.

Kaplan, R. M., & Litrownik, A. D. (1977). Some statistical methods for the assessment of multiple outcome criteria in behavioral research. *Behavior Therapy, 8,* 383–392.

Linden, E., & Hackler, J. C. (1973). Affective ties and delinquency. *Pacific Sociological Review, 16,* 27–46.

Porter, A. C. (1967). *The effects of using fallible variables in the analysis of covariance.* Unpublished doctoral dissertation, University of Wisconsin.

Reiss, A. J., Jr., Duncan, O. D., Hatt, P., & North, G. (1961). *Occupations and social status.* New York: Free Press.

Roscoe, J. T. (1969). *Fundamental research statistics for the behavioral sciences.* New York: Holt, Rinehart, and Winston.

Sutherland, E. H., & Cressey, D. R. (1978). *Principles of criminology* (10th ed.). Philadelphia: Lippincott.

Winer, B. J. (1971). *Statistical principles in experimental design.* New York: McGraw-Hill.

CHAPTER 12

An Experimental Test of the Coercion Model:
Linking Theory, Measurement, and Intervention

THOMAS J. DISHION
GERALD R. PATTERSON
KATHRYN A. KAVANAGH

INTRODUCTION

Theoretical Overview

At times, innovations in child-rearing models appear to be no more than new ways to pitch old messages. Many assume that the scientific study of child-rearing practices would relieve us from the arbitrary cycle of rhetoric. Improved understanding of parent–child socialization mechanisms should enhance control over childhood outcomes. An empirical knowledge base of optimal child-rearing practices could be systematically promoted within larger social units, such as in communities (Biglan, Glasgow, & Singer, 1990). The case will be made in this chapter that the coercion model (Patterson, 1982) provides a basis for better understanding the parent–child processes associated with serious child antisocial behavior, and that this understanding can be applied to enhance early adolescents adaption within the family and school.

The coercion model (Patterson, 1982) emerged from a program of research focused on child antisocial behavior. During the late 1960s and 1970s, this activity involved developing a treatment technology (Patterson, 1985), accompanied by the use of naturalistic observations in the homes of antisocial children to evaluate treatment outcome (Reid, 1978). The combination of observation in natural settings and the simultaneous development of interventions to alter problem behaviors led to the identification of parenting skills as the key to successful treatment outcomes. Random assignment designs using the parent training intervention with postobservation measures have shown that such procedures provide significant reductions in child antisocial behavior (Patterson, Chamberlain, & Reid, 1982; Walter & Gilmore, 1973). Similar effects have been produced by other investigators as well (e.g., Webster-Stratton, 1984).

These initial successes led us to believe that existing models of antisocial behavior and delinquency had underemphasized the role of parenting practices in child socialization. Researchers at the Oregon Social Learning Center began longitudinal studies to develop a model of child antisocial behavior in children and adolescents related to parenting practices. We have worked from a social interactional perspective, studying the moment-by-moment interchanges between parents and the child. The social interactional framework specifies that global traits (i.e., "antisocial" or "prosocial") are attributed to people, based on their patterns of social exchange. These personality traits can be seen as a "cloak" (see Figure 12.1) "covering" the primary patterns of interpersonal exchange that facilitate interpretation and action by participants. However, it is the orderliness of the interpersonal processes and their relation to shifts in behavioral rates that are of primary interest to investigators with an interactional focus.

The early studies of parent–child interaction patterns associated with antisocial behavior were individually oriented clinical studies. Functional analyses were conducted at dyadic levels to assess the relation between antecedents and consequences to children's aggressive acts. The intervention task was to change the controlling stimuli and consequences to reduce the problem behavior. Although clinically powerful, the behavior analytic strategy fell short of an etiological theory, in respect to providing a more general explanation of child antisocial behavior across samples that would guide preventive interventions.

Coercion theory poses that a child's interpersonal style is learned within the family, and under more extreme conditions carries over to a child's interactions with others outside the family, including peers and teachers. Coercion is seen as a probable pattern of interactions involving both negative and positive reinforcement arrangements. Repeated over thousands of trials, these interactions train the child to

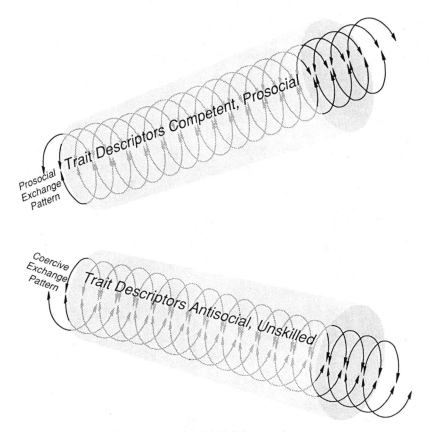

FIGURE 12.1. Trait descriptors as the "cloak" for social interaction patterns.

use aversive interpersonal behavior to gain control over disruptive, chaotic, or aversive circumstances. These parent–child patterns are overlearned, not consciously driven. In the absence of counterveiling forces, the child may progress from the display of trivial aversive behaviors and engage in behaviors that potentially inflict harm to people or property. The major regulator in coercive interactions is the parent's skill and effectiveness in setting limits. Because parents are frequently unaware of their automatic action-reaction patterns, parent report is an unreliable measure. Thus direct observations are necessary to measure parent–child interactions.

The development of an operational model of childhood and adolescent problem behavior requires two formidable steps. First, it is necessary to develop a means of measuring the key theoretical constructs in such a way as to assure validity and reliability when these measures are applied to large samples. As we will argue in a latter section of this chapter, measurement models are inextricably linked to theory development. The measurement aspect of model development in the behavioral sciences is frequently underestimated, and serves as the Achilles heel to hypothesis testing (Meehl, 1978). Second, once the measurement strategy is established, it is helpful if the constructs in the model show predictive validity across a number of samples, that is, the model is generalizable across age, sex, and for normal and at-risk samples. This statement represents the ideal in scientific parsimony, that one model would apply across settings, cultures, and population definitions. This assumption is accepted as an empirical starting point, with the expectation that variations in models will emerge. Progress through the first two stages of model development provides a readiness for experimental field studies. A brief review of research conducted on the coercion model for the first two stages will be provided before discussion of the experimental study. For a more detailed review, see Forgatch (1991).

Model Development

All measures in social sciences are biased in one sense or another. An indicator for a parent practice concept could be perfectly reliable but extremely biased. For example, a series of laboratory studies showed that mothers of problem children were biased in overclassifying relatively trivial events as deviant (Holleran, Littman, Freund, & Schmaling, 1982). Fiske (1986, 1987) identified the problem of understanding method variance as one of the key difficulties impeding the development of the social sciences. Research on parenting has been especially plagued by measurement strategies that depend heavily on parent's retrospective global reports with questions that pull for socially desirable responses.

The problem of differentiating method variance from true-score variance was clarified in the classic statement of Campbell and Fiske (1959). Defining two kinds of parent practices would require several different kinds of data (e.g., interview and observation) for each concept (i.e., construct). If the correlations among indicators *within* a construct were greater than those *between* construct but within methods, then the constructs are differentiated. Patterson and Bank (1987) reported on a successful attempt to differentiate the measurement of parental discipline from monitoring using a multimethod and multitrait approach. It was clear from these studies that parental reports of discipline practices correlated little with behavior observations and observer impression ratings nor with measures of child antisocial behavior. Parental reports of their monitoring practices did not perform much better. The conclusion that more objective estimates of parenting behavior are needed is supported by classic longitudinal studies showing the predictive validity of home visitor impressions of parenting to adolescent antisocial behavior (Loeber & Dishion, 1983; McCord, McCord, & Howard, 1963).

Correlational research provided the initial basis for developing a more general model of children's antisocial behavior. The first step was to develop a model that applied to two independent cohorts of 100 boys in the Oregon Youth Study (OYS). Patterson, Reid, and Dishion (in press) tested a correlational model (shown in Figure 12.2) that posed inept parent discipline practices as the proximal correlate of boys' antisocial behavior. Parent discipline was defined by home observations scores of parent nattering, explosive discipline, observer impressions of evenhandedness, and the mother's interview of discipline practices. The mother's interview contributed little to the definition of the construct, as Figure 12.2 indicates. The model, however, provided a statistically reliable fit to the data in the two independent OYS cohorts of 9- to 10-year-old boys.

A unique feature of this model is the bidirectional effect (statistically constrained to be equal) between parent discipline practices and

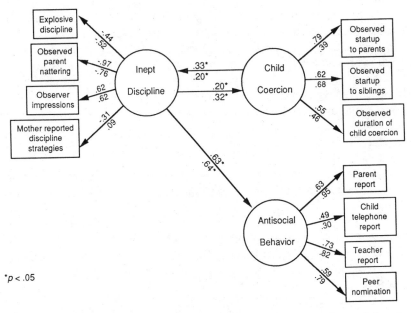

*p < .05

FIGURE 12.2. Basic training for antisocial behavior. Upper number refers to Cohort I and lower to Cohort II of the Oregon Youth Study.

child coercion. From a social interactional view, poor parent discipline practices increase the likelihood of child coercive responses, and high rates of child coercion impede parent's attempts to provide evenhanded, consistent, and effective discipline. It is in this sense that parental limit setting for behaviors such as lying, stealing, or fighting often fail in the quagmire of the child's arguments, excuses, and counteraccusations.

The data in the model are correlational, so the bidirectional path between these two constructs is by no means proven with this model. Previous research (Patterson, 1982), however, has established the importance of parental antecedents and consequences to moment-by-moment coercive behavior of the child. Experimental manipulations of specific controlling stimuli and consequences in the parent's behavior resulted in immediate reductions in the child's coercive response rate. Studies (Barkley, Karlsson, Strzeleck, & Murphy, 1984) show that administering medication to difficult children also reveals subsequent reductions in parental negative reactive behavior. From an academic point of view, the parent and child reciprocally influence one another. On the other hand, from the perspective of intervention, focusing on the parent's behavior in these transactions provides the only firm handle on adaptive behavior change in families with problem children.

The child's antisocial behavior decreases his or her adjustment in other social contexts. Failure in developing peer relations (Coie & Kupersmidt, 1983; Dishion, 1990; Dodge, 1983) and poor adjustment in school take on a life of their own, particularly as the child becomes increasingly active in creating and shaping his or her social niche (Scarr & McCartney, 1983). For example, academic failure, peer rejection, antisocial behavior, and poor parental monitoring all contribute statistically to account for variance in early adolescent involvement with antisocial peers (Dishion, Patterson, Stoolmiller, & Skinner, 1991).

The relation between poor discipline practices and child behavior has been replicated across several different samples. Forgatch (1991) compared the parent model for three different samples: two were at risk and one was a clinical sample referred for treatment. The model, which showed both parent monitoring and parent discipline practices to be directly related to child antisocial behavior, provided an acceptable fit to all three samples. The correlations between parent practices and child antisocial behavior were in the expected direction, that is, poor parenting practices covaried with high rates of antisocial behavior.

Although the coercion model of the contribution of parenting to child antisocial behavior appears robust in a variety of samples, it is clear that social and cultural contexts can impact the basic socialization process. A useful conceptualization of the impact of context on socialization is the ecological model provided by Bronfenbrenner (1989) where the social environment is conceptualized at various levels, ranging from basic momentary social exchanges to face-to-face interactions to larger contextual units. A number of studies (e.g., Caspi & Elder, 1988; Elder, Van Nguyen, & Caspi, 1985) have shown that the effects of contextual variables such as stress, unemployment, social status, and parent pathology on child adjustment are mediated through measures of parenting behavior. McLloyd (1990) integrates issues of ethnic status along with contextual effects on families in an effort to better understand the disruption of minority families residing in high-risk urban settings. Although there is higher pathology associated with high-risk urban context (Rutter, 1983), there is also variability that requires explanation. Not all parents living in a ghetto produce delinquent youth; however, youth with poor parent supervision seem to be at great risk (Wilson, 1980). These studies indicate that parenting practices in high-risk settings or in stressful circumstances may be especially important to child outcome.

Field Experimentation

The correlational analyses showed that a good fit for the general idea that parent practices and child maladjustment seem to covary. However, it is easy to invoke some third variable that might well account for the covariation, for example, the shared genetic endowment of parents and children. While any of the correlational models might have falsified the hypothesis that parent practices and child adjustment are related in some way, none of the studies demonstrate that one bears a causal relation to the other. An experimental study by Forgatch and Toobert (1979) showed that teaching mothers of preschool oppositional children better discipline practices resulted in greater compliance. These children were not particularly antisocial, and none of the data included showed that the improvements were associated with changes in discipline practices.

The data for a clinical sample of older children address both of these omissions (Forgatch, 1991). Her analyses of a sample of treated cases showed that those families that improved significantly on parent discipline or monitoring were characterized by significant reductions in child antisocial behavior (as measured by three indicators). But since there was no random assignment design or a comparison group that did not receive parent training, it is impossible to draw a firm conclusion about the causal status of parent practices.

The remainder of this chapter discusses our initial outcome results to an experimental manipulation of parenting practices on young (11- to 14-year-old) adolescent's antisocial behavior. The Adolescent Transitions Program (ATP) field experiment arose out of the research of the OYS and the relation to onset of substance use in early adolescence. Research by Dishion and Loeber (1985) indicated that family management (parent monitoring and discipline) and associations with deviant peers jointly contributed to boys' early substance use. The boys who were antisocial in respect to their peer and family environments and were patterned substance users were most at-risk. These analyses were later extended to early drug experimentation in middle childhood (Dishion, Reid, & Patterson, 1988). Other research documents the relation between parenting practices and substance use (e.g., Baumrind, 1985) and antisocial behavior (Block, Block, & Keyes, 1988; Kellam, Brown, Rubin, & Ensminger, 1983; McCord, 1979), and deviant peer environments (e.g., Elliott, Huizinga, & Ageton, 1985; Huba & Bentler, 1982) to adolescent substance use. Thus, these variables became the intervention targets for the ATP field experiment. Because antisocial behavior is highly correlated with substance abuse and problem behavior, the design and intervention procedures lend themselves to assessing two basic hypotheses: (1) a technology of parent training exists that is effective in improving parenting practices; and (2) improvement in parenting (i.e., discipline) is associated with less antisocial behavior. Data related to the impact of the interventions on the youngsters substance use progression are not available as of this writing.

METHODS

Sample and Design

One hundred and nineteen at-risk families participated in the ATP field experiment. The sample consisted of 58 boys and 61 girls between the ages of 10 and 14 (mean age 12). The children were enrolled in middle school (sixth grade through eighth grade), and the mean grade level for the sample was seventh grade. Ninety-five percent of the sample was European-American.

Families were self-referred and learned about the program through a number of sources, including newspaper advertisements, community flyers, school counselors, and other community professionals. Following parent inquiry, a telephone screening was conducted using a 10-question screening instrument, based on risk-factor research by Bry and colleagues (Bry, McKeon, & Pandina, 1982). Over the telephone, parents were interviewed on 10 dimensions of child risk: closeness to parents, emotional adjustment, academic engagement, involvement in positive activities, experience seeking, problem behaviors, the child's substance use, peer substance use, family substance-use history, and stressful life events. If the child was judged at risk on at least four dimensions, the family was randomly assigned to an intervention condition. Fifty percent of the families were excluded as not meeting these screening criteria.

At the time of admission, families were randomly assigned to one of the four intervention conditions: (1) Parent Focus only; (2) Teen Focus only; (3) Parent and Teen Focus; and (4) Self-Directed Change. A cluster sampling approach was used to achieve random assignment. This procedure provides a preestablished order of assignment of families to each of the four intervention conditions until all conditions are filled. Boys and girls received assignment separately to assure equal distribution of gender across conditions. The interventions were carried out over the course of 2 years, with four cohorts of approximately 30 families per cohort. Each intervention group consisted of approximately seven to eight families within each cohort.

In this study, there was not a pure "no-treatment" control group. At the onset of the research, we hypothesized that the Self-Directed Change condition would be an inactive intervention. Research by Webster-Stratton, Kolpacoff, and Hollinsworth (1988) indicated, however, that videotape curricula alone can be effective in producing short-term change in young children's problem behavior.

For the purpose of the hypotheses addressed in this study, the interventions targeting family management skills (Parent Focus only and Parent and Teen Focus) were collapsed into one group and compared to those conditions (Teen Focus only and Self-Directed Change) not providing direct family management training to parents. Consistent with the coercion theory, it was hypothesized that direct family management training would result in improvement in parents' discipline practices that would lead to improvements in children's antisocial behavior.

Table 12.1 provides the sample demographic characteristics broken down into Parent and No Parent Intervention. Table 12.1 reveals that the sample was primarily low income. Approximately one-fourth of the families had an annual income of less than $10,000 and more than half of the families were receiving some type of governmental financial assistance. On the other hand, the sample was moderately well educated. More than 50% of the mothers and 45% of the fathers had some college (see Table 12.1). The Parent and No-Parent Intervention

TABLE 12.1. Demographic Characteristics of the Adolescent Transitions Program Test Sample ($n = 119$)

	Parent training ($n = 56$)	No parent training ($n = 63$)
Family characteristics		
Single parent	51.8%	38.1%*
Two parent	48.2%	61.9%*
Average number of children in home	2.09	2.33
Target child—male	46.4%	50.8%
Target child—female	53.6%	49.2%
Average age of target child	12.19	12.27
Parents with some college education, degree, or graduate education		
Mothers	41.8%	46.7%
Fathers	16.0%	29.7%
Financial assistance		
Food stamps	39.3%*	23.6%*
Aid to Dependent Children (ADC)	28.6%	17.5%
Welfare (Not ADC)	3.6%	3.2%
Unemployment insurance	7.1%	4.8%
Other financial aid	28.6%	39.7%
Child Adjustment		
Conduct problems (T > 69 PCBCL Delinquency Scale)	30.4%	29.5%
Depressed	23.2%*	37.7%*
Nonstatus police contact	22.0%	19.0%

*Indicates significant (< .10) mean differences between groups.

groups were significantly different on the percentage of single parents, percentage receiving food stamps, and percentage of children in the depressed range. There were more families receiving food stamps and single parenting in the Parent Intervention compared to the No-Parent Intervention condition. However, there was more child depression in the latter compared to those families assigned to parent training.

The termination assessment occurred 3 months after baseline was completed by 107 of the 119 families (90% retention; 10% drop-out). Families who dropped out of ATP were represented in the following way across the four interventions: (A) Parent Focus (1); (B) Teen Focus (2); (C) Parent and Teen Focus (4); (D) Self-Directed Change (5). Inspection of these rates reveals a trend toward families dropping out of those conditions that either appeared ineffective (e.g., Self-Directed Change) or required considerable time commitment from both the parents and the teenager (Parent and Teen Focus). Drop-out rates in the Parent (8.9%) and No-Parent Intervention (11.1%) groups was approximately equal.

Intervention Overview

The ATP intervention phase lasted for 12 weeks. All families were first visited in their home by the therapists for their group. Families in Teen and/or Parent Focus interventions attended 90-minute weekly meetings. All weekly sessions were based on the Parent and Teen Focus Curricula. The Parent Focus intervention targeted the parent's family management practices and communication skills. The Teen Focus intervention targeted early adolescent self-regulation and pro-social behavior in the context of parent and peer environments.

Parent Focus

The Parent Focus curriculum (Kavanagh & Dishion, 1990) is based on four key family management skills determined, by 20 years of clinical and research investigations, to be critical for healthy child adjustment: monitoring, prosocial fostering, discipline, and problem solving. Social learning parent training is a step-wise, skill-based approach for developing effective parenting skills and strategies for maintaining change. Groups optimally consist of 8 families, therefore including a minimum of 8 to a maximum of 16 parents who attend each session. The content of the sessions was preestablished by the curriculum. Sessions usually began with some discussion of home practice for the previous week, followed by the therapist's introduction of a family management skill. Considerable time within each session was allocated to exercises, role play, and discussion focused on family management issues and skills. The groups were buttressed by four individual sessions for specific family issues related to the change processes addressed in the group meetings.

A key component of the Parent Focus intervention is the use of a parent consultant to assist two staff therapists and act as a bridge between parents and group leaders. The parent consultant has an adolescent child and he or she has already successfully completed the ATP. The role of the consultant is to model appropriate parenting skills and provide both in-session and between-session support to parents trying to implement these skills.

Teen Focus

The Teen Focus curriculum (Dishion, Moore, Prescott, & Kavanagh, 1990) attempts to enhance the teenager's regulation of his or her own prosocial and disruptive behavior in the context of parent and peer environments. Deficits in self-regulation (Miller & Brown, 1991) are central to a cognitive-behavioral perspective of addictive behaviors. Longitudinal studies indicate that early antisocial behavior is prognostic of subsequent problems in substance use (Kellam et al., 1983; McCord, 1979; Miller, 1990). Recent analyses on the Oregon Youth Study boys indicate that early antisocial behavior accounts independently for the degree of early adolescent substance use over and above exposure to deviant peers, poor parent monitoring, and depression (Dishion & Ray, 1991).

In an effort to enhance young adolescent's self-regulation, the behavior change process successful in parent training was applied to the teenagers. The following sets of skills were targeted: self-monitoring/tracking, prosocial goal setting, developing peer environments supportive of prosocial behavior, setting limits with friends, and problem solving and communication skills with parents and peers. Teenagers were responsible for defining their own behavior change goals. At least 75% selected, on their own initiative, some aspect of improved school performance. Other goals included abstinence from drug experimentation and improved family relations.

The approach to the weekly session was structured with the curriculum determining the focus of each meeting. The groups consisted of seven to eight teenagers, equally distributed between boys and girls. Sessions began by discussing home practice and events occurring in the previous week. Therapists then introduced a new skill or topic for the week, followed by role play and discussion. Groups ended with a home practice assignment for the coming week. Group incentives (e. g., pizza, art projects, etc.) were offered to the teenagers for meeting preestablished levels of attendance, home practice completion, and supportive behavior to other groups members during the sessions.

Peer counselors were also a critical aspect of the Teen Focus groups. These were represented by older high school adolescents who had made significant behavior change, in terms of reducing substance use and/or antisocial behavior. Out of four peer counselors, one had successfully completed an earlier version of ATP, and three others had successfully completed drug treatment programs. These youngsters were instrumental in modeling and endorsing prosocial goals including substance abstinence as well as avoidance of antisocial behavior. Peer counselors were also helpful in initiating role plays and other group activities, as well as modeling important interpersonal behaviors such as peer support for prosocial behavior.

Self-Directed Change

The Self-Directed Change intervention did not involve weekly group meetings or therapist contact. These families simply received the intervention materials that accompanied the Parent and Teen Focus interventions. These materials consisted of six newsletters and five brief videotapes. These materials covered the informational content of the group sessions and highlighted critical skills of the Parent and Teen Focus intervention programs. Materials were mailed on a biweekly basis and videotapes were made available to the parent and child for viewing.

Measurements

Following a screening and a consent to participate, the families completed an individual interview, participated in a videotaped family problem-solving task (3 hours), received six brief telephone interviews (2 hours), and school information was collected. Each family member was paid $10 per hour of assessment.

Observational data are critical to testing the social interactional basis of the coercion model. The videotaped problem-solving task provided the minimum of data needed to assess the parent–child interactions hypothesized to change under experimental intervention. Prior to the problem-solving task a revised version of the Issues Checklist was administered to parent(s) and child. The parent(s) and child independently identified conflictual issues in the family, accompanied by ratings of how "hot" (i.e., emotionally upsetting) the topics were. The "hottest" issue identified by the parent and child was selected for the parent and child problem, respectively. Following this, families participated in a 25-minute problem-solving session consisting of three parts: (1) 5 minutes of planning a family activity; (2) 10 minutes of discussion of a parent-identified problem; and (3) 10 minutes of discussion of a child-identified problem. Instructions for each phase of the problem-solving task were to make their best effort to: (1) plan an activity, something they could potentially do in the next week, and (2) solve the identified problem.

The observation scores described below were based on all 25 minutes of videotaped family interaction, collapsed across the 3 parts. The Family Process Code (Dishion, Gardner, Patterson, Reid, Thibodeaux, & Spyrou, 1983) was used to code these interactions.

Construct Development

The focus of this chapter is on the short-term impact of the Parent Focus intervention on parent discipline practices and child antisocial behavior (Patterson, 1986; Patterson, Reid, & Dishion, 1991). Two constructs are critical to this model: Mother Negative Discipline and Child Antisocial Behavior. The formulation of these constructs was based on previous research by Patterson and colleagues; a more detailed account of the two constructs as developed in the Oregon Youth Study is found in Capaldi and Patterson (1989).

Mother Negative Discipline

This construct measures poor or maladaptive discipline practices shown to be associated with child antisocial behavior in previous studies (e.g., Dishion, 1990; Patterson, 1986). Since roughly 50% of the families were single-parent, this score was based entirely on the mother's behavior with her child during the problem-solving session. Three observation scores from the family problem-solving task define Mother Negative Discipline: Nattering, Punishment Density, and Observer Impressions. The Observer Impression score reflects impressions that the mother was ineffective, unfair, inconsistent, and not even handed in her discipline practices.

The nattering score measures the mother's noncontingent aversiveness with the child, represented by the likelihood that the parent was coded as negative in the interaction with the child regardless of the child's behavior. Eight negative content codes were defined on a rational basis to describe this parent discipline tactic (e.g., Negative Verbal). In the Oregon Youth Study, the retest stability of the Mothers Nattering indicator was found to be .36 over a 2- to 3-month interval ($n = 29$).

The second mother-to-child interactional measure was the Punishment Density score. This score was used in lieu of the Explosive Discipline indicator (Patterson, 1986), as previous research indicated a normal distribution. This score reflects the density (i.e., relative frequency) of mother-to-child negative exchanges in respect to positive mother–child interactions. The rate-per-minute of all mother-to-child positive content codes was subtracted from the rate of negative codes. Mothers who scored high on the Punishment Density score were frequently and predominantly negative. The correlation between two observers on mother's Punishment Density was .75 ($n = 8$).

Considered together, the three scores describe a parenting style that is coercive, irritable, and frequently negative. Table 12.2 reveals

TABLE 12.2. Convergent and Predictive Validity for Indicators of Mother Negative Discipline

	Convergent validity			Predictive validity of baseline indicator scores	
				Arrests	Child report
All children					
Lab observer impressions	1.0	.35[a]**	.55**	.25*	.22*
Observer mother nattering	.41**	1.0	.34**	.07	−.10
Observer mother punishment density	.69**	.36**	1.0	.16	.25*
Boys, $n = 50$					
Lab observer impressions	1.0	.44**	.57**	.36*	.30
Observer mother nattering	.36*	1.0	.34**	.13	−.12
Observer mother punishment density	.58**	.41**	1.0	.23	.38**
Girls, $n = 61$					
Lab observer impressions	1.0	.25	.52**	.20	.17
Observer mother nattering	.45*	1.0	.35*	.04	−.09
Observer mother punishment density	.77**	.32*	1.0	.13	.16

[a]Correlations above the diagonal represent convergent validities at termination.
*$p < .05$.
**$p < .01$.

excellent convergent validity among these discipline indicators for baseline (below the diagonal in Table 12.2) and termination (above the diagonal in Table 12.2). The convergent validity stands when considering boys and girls separately as well. The observer impressions of the mother's negative discipline interactions showed statistically reliable predictive validity for the number of child arrests and the child's self-reported antisocial behavior. Comparing boys and girls, the predictive validity of negative discipline practices was greater for boys than for girls. There were no gender differences within this sample on the mean level of these parenting behaviors.

Child Antisocial

In previous research (Capaldi & Patterson, 1989) teacher, parent, and child reports were used to define child antisocial behavior. In this study, we relied on the parent and teacher reports of child antisocial behavior to provide more objective estimates of problem behavior by reporting agents other than the child. Two indicators comprised this construct: the parent telephone reports of antisocial behavior (10-item scale) and the teacher's ratings of antisocial behavior (19-item scale) on the Child Behavior Checklist (Achenbach & Edelbrock, 1986). These particular measures were used because they include a recall time frame of less than 3 months, which was the time lapse between baseline and termination assessments.

The convergent and predictive validity of the parent and teacher indicators of antisocial behavior are shown in Table 12.3. Parent and teacher reports at baseline show statistically reliable convergence across gender as well as for boys and girls considered separately. The convergence is somewhat less robust at termination. Across gender, the predictive validity to arrests and child self-report is weak, where only teacher ratings correlated reliably with the child's report of antisocial behavior. There predictive validities were not statistically reliable for boys. Teacher and parent reports of girls antisocial behavior correlated with the child's report of antisocial behavior and arrests, respectively. Inspection of the scatter plots for girls showed the magnitude of these predictive validities was accounted for by a few girls who tended to be more extreme on both sets of measures.

It is interesting that the only reliable gender difference in all indicators in the model are the teacher's rating of antisocial behavior. Girls showed half the level of antisocial behaviors compared to boys in the school setting, in contrast, girls showed the same level of negative behavior within their families.

TABLE 12.3. Convergent and Predictive Validity for Indicators of Child Behavior

| | Termination | | Predictive validity of baseline indicator scores | |
	Convergent validity		Arrests	Child report
All children				
Teacher ratings, antisocial	1.0	.24*	.02	.22*
Parent telephone, antisocial	.36**	1.0	.13	.19
Boys, $n = 50$				
Teacher ratings, antisocial	1.0	.28	−.06	.17
Parent telephone, antisocial	.33*	1.0	.10	.26
Girls, $n = 61$				
Teacher ratings, antisocial	1.0	.16	−.05	.36**
Parent telephone, antisocial	.34**	1.0	.27*	.11

*$p < .05$.
**$p < .01$.

Analysis Strategy

Structural equation modeling (SEM) was used to test the mediational model: parent training produced improvements in mother discipline practices that were associated with reductions in child antisocial behavior. A particular advantage of the SEM approach to evaluating models of longitudinal change is that the program provides the capability of modeling correlated error. It is assumed that errors in measuring each of the indicators at baseline and termination are correlated. Failure to specify these correlated errors in a multiple regression, for example, results in biased estimates of effect coefficients estimating the level of association between the independent and dependent constructs (Dwyer, 1983; Judd & Kenny, 1982). Random assignment to parent training was represented as a latent construct (Dwyer, 1983), measured without error, and scored dichotomously (1 = parent training; 0 = no parent training). In addition to the SEM analyses, the multivariate and univariate effects for all indicators within the construct were examined. A MANCOVA format for these analyses used baseline measures of the dependent variables as covariates.

INTERVENTION RESULTS

Mother Negative Discipline

The model in Figure 12.3 summarizes the SEM analysis of the short-term impact of the parent training on mother discipline practices. It was hypothesized that involvement in parent training would be negatively related to the mother's use of negative discipline, after controlling for the stability in her parenting from baseline to termination. In the model shown in Figure 12.3, the longitudinal correlated error was statistically significant for the Nattering and Punishment Density indicators.

Figure 12.3 shows the model was consistent with the observed data ($\chi^2 = 6.93$, $p = .73$). The significant standardized effect ($-.22$, $p = .05$) indicates that the parent intervention reduced the mother's negative discipline as observed in the family problem solving task, controlling for baseline discipline practices. A consideration, however, is the small amount of variance accounted for in the dependent variable (R square $= .21$).

The univariate means and variances for each of the indicators are shown in Table 12.4. A MANCOVA was used to assess the effect of parent training on improvement in the mean levels for all indicators in

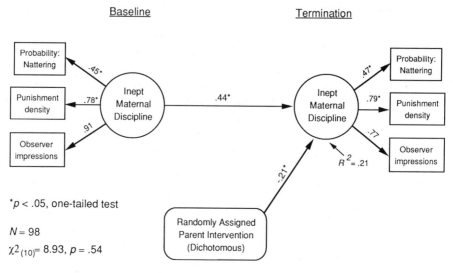

FIGURE 12.3. Short-term impact of family-management (parent focus) intervention on observed parent discipline practices.

the model. Table 12.4 shows the predicted trends of the observer impressions, observed nattering, and punishment density showing improvement with parent training and deterioration in the other intervention conditions. The statistical magnitude of these trends, however, were modest, with only the nattering score ($p < .02$) reaching conventional standards of reliable effects. The multivariate effect (Wilks $\lambda = .94$) was statistically marginal ($p = .12$). Thus the MANCOVA analyses corroborate the SEM analyses in revealing modest effects on mother discipline practices due to random assignment to parent training. Tables 12.5 and 12.6 provide the means for boys and girls separately. In general, the same trends are revealed for boys and girls, with the exception that observer impressions of mother discipline indicate a deterioration for boys and an improvement for girls as a function of parent training. Only the trend of improvement for girls was statistically reliable ($p < .08$).

Child Antisocial Behavior

The second question addressed is the extent negative maternal discipline is associated with change in child antisocial behavior. The model displayed in Figure 12.4 places mother discipline practices at termina-

TABLE 12.4. Mean Level Changes in Indicators for Child Behavior and Mother Negative Discipline (All Children)

| | Parent training | | | | No parent training | | | | Univariate effects |
| | Baseline | | Termination | | Baseline | | Termination | | |
	$\bar{X}$	(SD)	$\bar{X}$	(SD)	$\bar{X}$	(SD)	$\bar{X}$	(SD)	
Child antisocial									
Teacher report	.28	(.39)	.28	(.31)	.28	(.39)	.34	(.41)	$p < .05$
Parent report	.19	(.13)	.15	(.11)	.18	(.13)	.14	(.13)	Not significant
n	43				44				
MANCOVA Wilks $\lambda = .94$, $p = .10$									
Observed mother negative discipline									
Observer impressions	1.71	(.90)	1.56	(.58)	1.57	(.67)	1.70	(.77)	$p < .20$
Nattering	.06	(.08)	.04	(.05)	.06	(.11)	.08	(.09)	$p < .13$
Punishment density	−.11	(1.09)	.01	(.79)	.12	(.88)	−.15	(.91)	$p < .13$
n	50				47				
MANCOVA Wilks $\lambda = .94$, $p = .12$									

TABLE 12.5. Mean Level Changes in Indicators for Child Behavior and Mother Negative Discipline (Boys)

| | Parent training | | | | No parent training | | | | Univariate effects |
| | Baseline | | Termination | | Baseline | | Termination | | |
	$\overline{X}$	(SD)	$\overline{X}$	(SD)	$\overline{X}$	(SD)	$\overline{X}$	(SD)	
Child antisocial									
Teacher report	.50	(.53)	.39	(.34)	.36	(.48)	.49	(.48)	$p < .03$
Parent report	.39	(.34)	.14	(.12)	.18	(.15)	.15	(.14)	Not significant
n	18				35				
MANCOVA Wilks $\lambda = .89$, $p = .09$									
Observed mother negative discipline									
Observer impressions	1.60	(.76)	1.70	(.72)	.170	(.76)	1.78	(.86)	Not significant
Nattering	.07	(.11)	.04	(.04)	.07	(.11)	.08	(.10)	Not significant
Punishment density	−.14	(.87)	.03	(.91)	.04	(.99)	−.17	(1.01)	Not significant
n	21				23				
MANCOVA Wilks $\lambda = .92$, $p = .35$									

TABLE 12.6. Mean Level Changes in Indicators for Child Behavior and Mother Negative Discipline (Girls)

	Parent training				No parent training				Univariate effects
	Baseline		Termination		Baseline		Termination		
	$\overline{X}$	(SD)	$\overline{X}$	(SD)	$\overline{X}$	(SD)	$\overline{X}$	(SD)	
Child antisocial									
Teacher report	.20	(.33)	.19	(.27)	.18	(.24)	.16	(.21)	Not significant
Parent report	.15	(.11)	.15	(.10)	.18	(.24)	.12	(.11)	$p < .03$
n			25				20		
MANCOVA Wilks $\lambda = .88$, $p = .08$									
Observed mother negative discipline									
Observer impressions	1.79	(.99)	1.46	(.43)	1.45	(.56)	1.63	(.68)	$p < .08$
Nattering	.05	(.05)	.05	(.05)	.07	(.15)	.08	(.09)	Not significant
Punishment density	−.10	(1.24)	.03	(.71)	.19	(.77)	−.14	(.81)	Not significant
n			29				24		
MANCOVA Wilks $\lambda = .92$, $p = .27$									

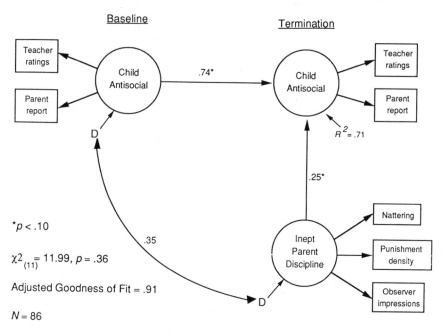

FIGURE 12.4. Short-term impact process model.

tion as a proximal determinant of the child's antisocial behavior. Again, correlated longitudinal measurement error terms were statistically reliable for parent and teacher reports of child antisocial behavior from baseline and termination. Despite the estimation of these error terms, there was a high level of stability in child antisocial behavior from baseline to termination ($B = 0.74$, $p < .05$). As hypothesized, negative discipline competed with the stability to account for unique variance in termination estimates of child antisocial behavior, showing a standardized β of .25 ($p < .05$). The combination of negative discipline and baseline Child Antisocial Behavior accounted for 71% of the variance in the child's problem behavior at the end of the intervention.

The means and variances for each of the collapsed intervention conditions are shown in Tables 12.4, and for boys and girls in Tables 12.5 and 12.6. There was a marginally significant multivariate effect for parent training (Wilks $\lambda = .94$, $p = .10$). The univariate trends differ depending on which outcome variable is considered, and for boys and girls considered separately. For teacher ratings of child antisocial behavior, there was a statistically reliable impact for the parent intervention at the univariate level ($p = .05$), considering boys and girls together. Again, there was a modest trend for the teacher ratings of children whose parents were involved in the parent intervention to improve, compared to those not directly involved to become worse. That is particularly important in that teachers were completely ignorant as to which intervention a child was receiving. When considering boys and girls separately, the improvements in teacher ratings of antisocial behavior was statistically reliable for boys only ($p = .03$).

Parent telephone reports of antisocial behavior improved in families regardless of what intervention they received without regard to gender of the child. The analysis of boys and girls, however, revealed that there was greater improvement in parent-reported antisocial behavior in girls associated with not receiving parent training, compared to those receiving parent training. This result is counter to the expectation that parent training is associated with improvements in child antisocial behavior.

DISCUSSION

Summary

The model originally presented by Patterson (1986) explicitly states that the impact of parenting training on child antisocial behavior is mediated by changes in discipline practices. The findings within this chapter represent a third stage of development for the coercion model of antisocial behavior. The first step was the testing of correlational (Patterson, 1986; Patterson, Reid, & Dishion, 1992) and longitudinal models (Patterson, Crosby, & Vuichinich, in preparation), the second step focused on associating changes in discipline with changes in child antisocial behavior (Forgatch, 1990), and the third is experimental manipulation.

Several small gains were accomplished in the ATP field experiment. These include: (1) the replication of the coercion model to a sample of male and female adolescents defined as at risk; (2) generalizability of a brief videotaped family interaction task in defining the mother discipline constructs; and (3) determining that the parent training technology can be successively administered in groups for families with at-risk young adolescents and resulting in improvements in mother discipline practices which mediated improvements in the children's antisocial behavior at school. Although the range of impact was not dramatic, the formulation of the negative discipline construct was based on previous research (Dishion, 1990; Patterson, Reid, &

Dishion, 1992), and therefore can be considered truly an a priori hypothesis put at risk for rejection in the Popperian sense.

In two respects, we claim that the experimental design provided a conservative test. First, we used a structured research intervention curricula and minimized individualization of the intervention program for families. Research on the effectiveness of marital therapy (Jacobson et al., in press) comparing a structured research intervention with an individualized and flexible intervention (based on the same treatment model) suggested the superiority of the latter. Second, some data indicate that videotape material, by themselves, might be modestly effective in improving parenting practices (Webster-Stratton, Kolpacoff, & Hollinsworth, 1988). This finding implies that the self-directed condition was a conservative contrast condition. Again, a control group is needed, and, as of this writing, is being collected. It may well be that these at-risk families would show more negative outcomes than the self-directed families due to not receiving any supportive interventions.

Reductions in child antisocial behavior were observed across gender and their level of problem behavior by the end of the intervention was associated with observed parent discipline practices at termination. These models support the hypothesis that improvement in child problem behavior is mediated by improvements in parent discipline practices. The most impressive effect was the impact of the parent intervention on teacher ratings of child antisocial behavior at school. This finding is especially important as an indication that parenting practices are etiologically significant to the boy's social adaption in school, a critical social field for all children (Kellam, 1990). Teacher ratings of antisocial behavior showed that problem behavior in school is more prevalent for boys than girls. When analyzing boys and girls separately the effect was statistically reliable only for boys

Measurement-Theory Dialectic

It is not until recently that prevention and intervention researchers used developmental models to guide intervention and evaluation designs, in an effort to test such models and better understand the mediational process between intervention and outcome (Judd & Kenny, 1982). SEM provides a robust and sensitive statistical tool (Dwyer, 1983) for assessing the viability of a model as a guide to preventive interventions. Interpretations of intervention outcomes when modeled provide information as to the fit of the measurement hypotheses, the generalizability of a developmental model, and the efficacy of the intervention technology. This comprehensive statistical approach fits within the framework and objectives of what Kellam (1990) has called experimental epidemiology.

Experimental field studies provide a basis for deriving strong inferences regarding the causal accuracy of developmental models. Rarely, however, do researchers take the measurement problems we encounter seriously. In fact, we often slip out of null findings by blaming the measures used (Meehl, 1954). We suspect that the measure-theory relation requires deeper exploration, and that failed measurement may be informative to theory-building efforts. For example, it is theoretically interesting that parents tend to be biased toward perceiving improvement following involvement in almost any intervention. This consistent finding raises questions about the origins and role of parental perceptions of child behavior. It seems likely that the parent's immediate social context is critically important in determining the kinds of child behavior to which they attend, their sense of the normalcy of the behavior, and level of distress (vis-à-vis social support) concerning their children's functioning.

We think the biases associated with global reports addresses the strength of a social interactional approach to studying social adaption. Although we agree that primary raters (e.g., teachers, peers, and parents) in the child's key social fields reflect the child's adaptation in those settings (Kellam, 1990), the ratings are also reflecting characteristics of the settings that are independent of the child's behavior. Therefore, it is necessary to assess directly the child's behavior with these key social agents to understand both process and context surrounding adaption and maladaption. From a social interactional perspective (Patterson & Reid, 1984; Patterson, Reid, & Dishion, 1992), child behavior is functional at the microsocial level and theory building, at a minimum, needs to focus on understanding processes that are actually formative to the response styles children display in various settings. Dedicated studies on measurement of process and context, although seemingly mundane, would greatly enhance the robustness of a prevention science, which must ultimately be tied to theory building and testing through measurement and intervention.

We share the view expressed by Fiske (1986) that measurement and theorizing behavioral sciences must move away from the macrolevel, theorizing vague constructs or the exclusive use of global reports. An advantage of direct observation research is that it allows for the researchers to obtain more control over the measurement process with clear and circumscribed specification of the theoretical constructs. Fiske (1986) recommends defining constructs relative to the method of measurement used, for example, Observed Mother Negative Discipline. Constructs, such as Child Antisocial, that consist of ratings from different agents experiencing the child in different settings, and each containing unique biases, are probably less useful to a prevention science. In this chapter, for example, parent and teacher ratings of the child's antisocial behavior were impacted somewhat differently by the parent intervention. This finding might serve as an inducement to consider the child's antisocial behavior in the home and school separately, including direct observations as well as ratings from key social agents within each setting. Such data would provide a basis for detailing the generalizability of impact for any given intervention strategy.

These findings suggest that much of the basic interpersonal process at the individual difference level is fairly robust to setting influences and can be assessed in structured tasks designed to organize naturalistic behavior. Naturalistic behavior is best elicited by asking people to discuss or do things relevant to their mutual lives, topics that elicit emotional responses similar to those felt outside the laboratory. In assessing family problem solving (Forgatch, Fetrow, & Lathrop, 1985) parents and child discuss topics that have been identified as currently relevant and "hot" in their families. A similar approach used to assess peer interaction with adolescent boys was successful in identifying interpersonal transactions with friends that show substantial predictive validity (Dishion, 1990). It is our current sense that observation technology is at a stage to make it feasible to include such measures in prevention trials and longitudinal studies. Such control over the measurement process may lead to exciting progress in theory.

Future Directions

The ATP is a secondary prevention program for at-risk early adolescents, attempting to reduce their level of problem behavior, risk for substance abuse, and depression. The program leans heavily on the coercion model of antisocial behavior for guidance, where it is hypothesized that long-term reductions in early adolescent problem behavior can be obtained by improving parenting practices. We see these analyses of the short-term impact as promising estimates of the utility of the model for prevention activity. In addition to the findings reported in this chapter, analyses of the effectiveness of the Teen Focus intervention revealed statistically reliable reductions in the child's report of depressed mood (Dishion, Ray, & Kavanagh, 1990). In contrast, the Parent Focus intervention had no direct impact on children's depression. We hope that the Parent and Teen Focus interventions dovetail to address children's needs in two interrelated realms:

Psychological Well Being and Social Adaption (Kellam, 1990). Long-term follow-up data, however, are needed before firm conclusions can be drawn as to the preventive utility of the parent or teen interventions. As of this writing, such data are available on only half of the sample of 119 families.

ACKNOWLEDGMENTS

The data collection and intervention activity was supported by a grant from the National Institute of Drug Abuse (NIDA) to Thomas J. Dishion titled "Social Learning Treatment of Early Adolescent Drug Abuse" (#DA 05304) and a subsequent NIDA grant entitled "Multicomponent Prevention of Adolescent Substance (Ab)use." (#DA 07031). Support for the data analyses comprising this chapter was supported by a Prevention Research Center Grant for the Prevention of Conduct Problems awarded to Dr. John Reid (#MH 46690). The ATP staff, Gene Brown, Karen Creighton, Annette Estes, and Patty Harrington, are gratefully acknowledged for their dedication to meeting deadlines with limited resources and uncertain futures. Carol Kimball is appreciated for her efforts on the project and for the preparation of this manuscript.

REFERENCES

Achenbach, T. M., & Edelbrock, C. (1986). *Manual for the teacher's report form and teacher version of the Child Behavior Profile*. Burlington: University of Vermont Press.

Bakeman, R., & Gottman, J. M. (1986). *Observing interaction: An introduction to sequential analysis*. New York: Cambridge Univeresity Press.

Barkley, R. A., Karlsson, J., Strzeleck, E., & Murphy, J. V. (1984). Effects of age and Ritalin dosage on the mother–child interactions of hyperactive children. *Journal of Consulting and Clinical Psychology, 52*(5), 750–758.

Baumrind, D. (1985). Familial antecedents of adolescent drug use: A developmental perspective. In C. L. Jones & R. J. Battjes (Eds.), *Etiology of drug abuse: Implications for prevention* (DHHS Publication No. ADM 87-1335, pp. 13–44). Washington, DC: U.S. Government Printing Office.

Biglan, A., Glasgow, R. E., & Singer, G. (1990). The need for a science of larger social units: A contextual approach. *Behavior Therapy, 32*, 195–215.

Block, J., Block, J. H., & Keyes, S. (1988). Longitudinally foretelling drug usage in adolescence: Early childhood personality and environmental precursors. *Child Development, 59*, 336–355.

Bronfenbrenner, U. (1989). Ecological systems theory. In R. Vasta (Ed.), *Annals of child development: Vol. 6. Six theories of child development: Revised formulations and current issues* (pp. 187–249). London: Jai Press.

Bry, B. H., McKeon, P., & Pandina, R. J. (1982). Extent of drug use as a function of number of risk factors. *Journal of Abnormal Psychology, 91*(4), 273–279.

Campbell, D. T., & Fiske, D. W. (1959). Conversant and discriminant validation of the multitrait and multimethod matrix. *Psychological Bulletin, 56,* 81–105.

Campbell, D. T., & Stanley, J. C. (1963). *Experimental and quasi-experimental designs for research.* Chicago, IL: Rand McNally College Publishing.

Capaldi, D., & Patterson, G. R. (1989). *Psychometric properties of fourteen latent constructs from the Oregon Youth Study.* New York: Springer-Verlag.

Caspi, A., & Elder, G. H., Jr. (1988). Emergent family patterns: The intergenerational construction of problem behavior and relationships. In R. A. Hinde & J. Stevenson-Hinde (Eds.), *Relationships within families: Mutual influences* (pp. 218–240). Oxford: Clarendon.

Coie, J. D., & Kupersmidt, J. B. (1983). A behavioral analysis of emerging social status in boys' groups. *Child Development, 54,* 1400–1416.

Dishion, T. J. (1990). Peer context of troublesome behavior in children and adolescents. In P. Leone (Ed.), *Understanding troubled and troublesome youth* (pp. 128–153). Beverly Hills, CA: Sage.

Dishion, T. J., Gardner, K., Patterson, G. R., Reid, J. B., Spyrou, S., & Thibodeaux, S. (1983). *The Family Process Code: A multidimensional system for observing family interaction.* Unpublished technical report. (Available at Oregon Social Learning Center, 207 East Fifth Avenue, Suite 202, Eugene, OR 97401.)

Dishion, T. J., & Loeber, R. (1985). Male adolescent marijuana and alcohol use: The role of parents and peers revisited. *American Journal of Drug and Alcohol Abuse, 11,* 11–25.

Dishion, T. J., Moore, K. J., Prescott, A., & Kavanagh, K. (1990). *Teen Focus: A behavior change curriculum for young adolescents.* (Available at Independent Video Services, 401 East 10th Avenue, Suite 160, Eugene, OR 97401.)

Dishion, T. J., Patterson, G. R., Stoolmiller, M., & Skinner, M. (1991). Family, school, and behavioral antecedents to early adolescent involvement with antisocial peers. *Developmental Psychology, 27,* 172–180.

Dishion, T. J., & Ray, J. (1991, November). *The development and ecology of substance use in adolescent boys.* Paper presented at the annual meeting of the American Association of Psychology, San Francisco.

Dishion, T. J., Ray, J., & Kavanagh, K. (1990, November). *The impact of a peer intervention (Teen Focus) on early adolescent affective adjustment: A case for secondary prevention.* Paper presented at the annual meeting for the Association for the Advancement of Behavior Therapy, San Francisco.

Dishion, T. J., Reid, J. B., & Patterson, G. R. (1988). Empirical guidelines for a family intervention for adolescent drug use. *Journal of Chemical Dependency Treatment, 1*(2), 189–214.

Dodge, K. A. (1983). Behavioral antecedents: A peer social status. *Child Development, 54,* 1386–1399.

Dwyer, J. H. (1983). *Statistical models for the social and behavior sciences.* New York: Oxford University Press.

Elder, G. H., Van Nguyen, T., & Caspi, A. (1985). Linking family hardship to children's lives. *Child Development, 56*, 361–375.

Elliott, D. S., Huizinga, D., & Ageton, S. S. (1985). *Explaining delinquency and drug use.* Beverly Hills, CA: Sage.

Fiske, D. W. (1986). Specificity of method and knowledge in social science. In D. W. Fiske & R. A. Shweder (Eds.), *Metatheory in social science* (pp. 61–82). Chicago: University of Chicago Press.

Fiske, D. W. (1987). Construct invalidity comes from method effects. *Educational and Psychological Measurement, 47*, 285–306.

Forgatch, M. S. (1991). The clinical science vortex: Developing a theory of antisocial behavior. In D. J. Pepler & K. Rubin (Eds.), *The development and creation of childhood aggression* (pp. 291–315). Hillsdale, NJ: Erlbaum.

Forgatch, M. S., & Toobert, D. J. (1979). A cost effective parent training program for use with normal preschool children. *Journal of Pediatric Psychology, 4*, 129–145.

Holleran, P. A., Littman, D. C., Freund, R. D., & Schmaling, D. B. (1982). A signal detection approach to social perception: Identification of negative and positive behaviors by parents of normal and problem children. *Journal of Abnormal Child Psychology, 10*, 549–557.

Huba, G. J., & Bentler, P. M. (1982). On the usefulness of latent variable causal modeling in testing theories of naturally occurring events: A rejoinder to Martin. *Journal of Personality and Social Psychology, 43*(3), 604–611.

Jacobson, N. S., Schmaling, K. B., Holtzworth-Muroe, A., Katt, J. L., Wood, L. F., & Follette, V. M. (in press). *Behavior Research & Therapy.*

Judd, C. M., & Kenny, D. A. (1982). Process analysis: Estimating mediation in treatment evaluations. *Evaluation Review, 5*(5), 602–619.

Kavanagh, K., & Dishion, T. J. (1990). *Parent Focus: A skill enhancement curriculum for parents of young adolescents.* Eugene, OR: Independent Video Services.

Kellam, S. G., Brown, C. H., Rubin, B. R., & Ensminger, M. E. (1983). Paths leading to teenage psychiatric symptoms and substance use: Developmental epidemiological studies in Woodlawn. In S. R. Guze, F. J. Earns, & J. E. Barretts (Eds.), *Childhood psychopathology and development* (pp. 17–47). New York: Raven Press.

Loeber, R., & Dishion, T. J. (1983). Early predictors of male delinquency: A review. *Psychological Bulletin, 94*, 68–99.

McCord, J. (1979). Some child-rearing antecedents of criminal behavior in adult men. *Journal of Personality and Social Psychology, 37*(9), 1477–1486.

McCord, W., McCord, J., & Howard, A. (1963). Family interaction as antecedent to the direction of male aggressiveness. *Journal of Abnormal and Social Psychology, 66*(3), 239–242.

McLloyd, V. (1990). The impact of economic hardship on black families and children: Psychological distress, parenting, and socio-emotional development. *Child Development, 61*, 311–346.

Meehl, P. E. (1978). Theoretical risks and tabular asterisks: Sir Karl, Sir Ronald, and the slow progress of soft psychology. *Journal of Consulting and Clinical Psychology, 46*(4), 806–834.

Miller, F. (1990, June). *Alienation and attachment among adolescents*. Paper presented at the Workshop on Gender Issues in the Development of Antisocial Behavior, Cambridge, MA.

Miller, W. R., & Brown, J. M. (1991). Self-regulation as a conceptual basis for the prevention and treatment of addictive behaviors. In N. Heather, W. R. Mill, & J. Greeley (Eds.), *Self-control and addictive behaviors* (pp. 1–82). New York: Pergamon Press.

Patterson, G. R. (1982). *Coercive family process*. Eugene, OR: Castalia.

Patterson, G. R. (1985). Beyond technology: The next stage in developing an empirical base for parent training. In L. L'Abate (Ed.), *Handbook of family psychology and therapy* (Vol. 2, pp. 1344–1379). Homewood, IL: Dorsey.

Patterson, G. R. (1986). Performance models for antisocial boys. *American Psychologist, 41*, 432–444.

Patterson, G. R., & Bank, L. (1987). When is a nomological network a construct? In D. R. Peterson & D. B. Fishman (Eds.), *Assessment for decision* (pp. 249–279). New Brunswick, NJ: Rutgers University Press.

Patterson, G. R., Chamberlain, P., & Reid, J. R. (1982). A comparative evaluation of parent training procedures. *Behavior Therapy, 3*, 638–650.

Patterson, G. R., Reid, J. B., & Dishion, T. J. (1992). *Antisocial boys*. Eugene, OR: Castalia.

Reid, J. B. (Ed.). (1978). *A social learning approach to family intervention: 2. Observation in home settings*. Eugene, OR: Castalia.

Rutter, M. (1983). Stress, coping, and development: Some issues and some questions. In N. Garmezy & M. Rutter (Eds.), *Stress, coping, and development in children* (pp. 1–41). New York: McGraw-Hill.

Scarr, S., & McCartney, K. (1983). How people make their own environments: A theory of genotype to environment effects. *Child Development, 54*, 424–435.

Walker, H. M., Shinn, M. R., O'Neill, R. E., & Ramsey, E. (1987). A longitudinal assessment of the development of antisocial behavior in boys: Rationale, methodology, and first year results. *Remedial and Special Education, 8*(4), 7–16.

Walter, H. I., & Gilmore, S. K. (1973). Placebo versus social learning effects in parent training procedures designed to alter the behaviors of aggressive boys. *Behavior Therapy, 4*, 361–377.

Wampold, B. E. (1989). Kappa as a measure of pattern in sequential data. *Quality and Quantity, 22*, 19–35.

Webster-Stratton, C. (1984). Randomized trail of two parent-training programs for families with conduct-disordered children. *Journal of Consulting and Clinical Psychology, 52*, 666–678.

Webster-Stratton, C., Kolpacoff, M., & Hollinsworth, T. (1988). Self-administered videotape therapy for families with conduct problem children: Comparison with two cost-effective treatments and a control group. *Journal of Consulting and Clinical Psychology, 56*, 558–566.

Wilson, H. (1980). Parental supervision: A neglected aspect of delinquency. *British Journal of Criminology, 20*(3), 203–235.

CHAPTER 13

◆ ——— ◆

Sociomoral Reasoning in Behavior-Disordered Adolescents:
Cognitive and Behavioral Change

JACK ARBUTHNOT

On December 4, 1990, Jay Bias, age 20, was shopping in a jewelry store when he became involved in an argument with two men. They invited him to step outside, but Jay declined. The men, however, apparently waited outside the store: when Jay left, they shot him twice in the back. He later died at the same hospital where his older brother, basketball star Len Bias, had died from a cocaine overdose in 1986.

Students at the Beltsville, Maryland, high school that the Bias brothers had attended were understandably upset and frustrated. "There's a total disregard for life, for respect," said one. "Jay was shot for no reason. It makes me scared that there's this much violence," said another. Reggie Walton, associate director of the National Drug Control Policy, observed that "Jay's death is a troubling commentary of what is taking place in many communities: The deterioration of our values and morals and a lack of remorse" (Squitieri & Kelley, 1990).

Tom Squitieri, a reporter for the national daily newspaper *USA Today*, interviewed me for the article he wrote about young Jay Bias's murder. Why, he wanted to know, do crimes of this type happen, and why do they seem to be increasing at such an alarming rate? Why do some adolescents have violent, even murderous, reactions over a perceived insult or an argument. Why do some kill for someone's high-fashion running shoes? Granted, violence has always been a problem, but why is it becoming so much more frequent—even casual—among our youth?

The answers to these questions do not come easily, for the phenomenon is no doubt multidetermined and complex. Yet while each case is idiosyncratic, we can speculate about the larger forces at work. Jay Bias died because of the unchecked anger of two men. The speculative part concerns why this anger was so uncontrolled, so easily translated into the taking of a life over what most of us would consider a trivial matter.

The vast majority of people, regardless of income, education, occupation, neighborhood, subculture, peer pressure, childhood traumas, or altered states of consciousness do not kill those with whom they disagree. Even those few who are tempted to kill usually change their minds once they have left the immediate highly arousing situation and pause to think. So Jay Bias's killing was not a "crime of passion" in the usual sense. Neither was the killing of a young boy for his Air Jordan running shoes, nor the gunning down of five innocent school children waiting at a bus stop during a drug turf war. Most of us do not even contemplate such acts, but even if we do plan a murder in our minds in a moment of pique, we easily and quickly separate our fantasy desire from our actual behavior. Evidently something in our socialization has given us the needed capacities and motivations to restrain ourselves from acting violently. And equally evident—at least to some theorists—is the fact that other individuals have *not* been so socialized and therefore lack those abilities and motivations.

THE MATRIX OF BEHAVIOR

However briefly, offenders against individuals and society engage in some cognitive process before acting. Antisocial behavior (whether it be misbehaving in class, stealing someone's property, or lashing out violently against an adversary) occurs when the quantity and/or quality of these cognitions is limited or inadequate.

While prevalent sociological thought ignores such cognitive processes in antisocial acts among juveniles, psychologists (and social policy experts) must attend to these cognitive deficits, their etiology, and their amelioration. As I have argued elsewhere (Arbuthnot, 1990; Arbuthnot & Gordon, 1988; Arbuthnot, Gordon, & Jurkovic, 1987), cognitions about social behavioral choices reflect not only one's logical reasoning capacities, but also a number of other cognitive factors, including the reasoner's sociomoral worldview, empathic capacities, emotions and motivations, will, and perceptions of the behavioral context.

How is it that most individuals come to act in a fashion that we and others think is "right" or "proper"? Is it enough that we are taught "the rules"? Certainly not, if one can rationalize that the rules apply to others, but not to oneself. Is it enough to know the possible consequences of one's choices? Again, not if one feels immune to or exempt from those consequences. The failures of the classic Hartshorne and May studies (1928) underscore the simplicity of the "knowledge-of-rules-governs-behavior" model. Rather, most of us act in accordance with our larger view of what is fair or just in a given situation—that is, we evaluate choices in light of some internal sociomoral worldview.

In the cognitive-developmental approach to moral development espoused by Piaget, and elaborated by Kohlberg (1969, 1984), individuals interact with their social environment and actively construct a model of it. This model is affected both by experience and by one's general cognitive capacities (which, themselves, are expanded through experience, within certain biologically determined limits). The quality of one's moral worldview is thus determined in large measure by the quality of one's social interactions and the cognitive disequilibrium aroused by them. Limited role-taking opportunities and an unchallenging moral and intellectual environment will result in lack of growth beyond the most elementary views of the moral world and one's place within it. Moral reasoning, as a consequence, will be limited to narrow, individualistic perspectives, will lack coordination with the views of others, will be poorly differentiated and integrated internally, and will remain logically unsophisticated.

Kohlberg's work, and that of a number of his disciples, has delineated a series of qualitatively identifiable stages through which moral reasoning may develop, given sufficient stimulation and the capacity for growth (see Table 13.1).[1] These stages appear to be invariant and universal. The defining characteristic of the stages is the structure of the reasoning employed, rather than the content about which one reasons. The "why" of a choice (e.g., one should not steal "because then others would feel free to steal from you," or "because it would violate the legitimate property rights of another and, if unchecked, would result in chaos for the social system") is stage

1. Readers interested in the relationship between Kohlberg's developmental psychology model of moral reasoning development and various philosophical models of morality are directed to Kohlberg (1971, 1984).

TABLE 13.1. Kohlberg's Stages of Sociomoral Reasoning

Level	Stage	Law issue	Life issue
I. Preconventional Social perspective is centered around the self. Events are perceived in terms of physical dimensions or consequences. General lack of awareness of purpose of rules or conventions. An egocentric perspective.	1. Heteronomous morality Equates right behavior with concrete rules backed by power and punishment. Concern with size and importance of damage and/or participants.	Laws are seen as simple labels. Breaking laws results in punishment.	Does not see life as ultimate value. No more important than, say, property.
	2. Individual utilitarianism Right behavior is that which serves one's own interests. Aware of others' needs in an elementary fashion but not of others' rights. Fairness is strict, rigid, concrete. Reciprocal agreements are pragmatic.	Laws are seen as the intentions of the lawmakers. There may be loss to the self if they are broken.	Life is of value because each person wants to live. It cannot be replaced, as can property.
II. Conventional Social perspective is centered on groups or (later) society. Con-	3. Mutual interpersonal expectations Right behavior is the "good"	Laws relate to prosocial motives and conduct. Breaking laws is selfish	People should care for others and their lives. One is not good or human if one

Social perspective	What is right	Laws	Value of life
cern for the opinions of others, for doing one's duty, and for rules to regulate desired behavior. A member-of-society perspective.	that is approved by significant others. Concern for expectations of others, for proper in-role behavior, and good motives.	and deceitful, and people will think badly of you.	doesn't. People have more feeling for life than property.
	4. Social system and conscience Right behavior is meeting the agreed-upon obligations of the society, following rules to preserve order, contributing to the good of society and its institutions.	Laws protect specific rights, practices, and institutions necessary for the social system. To break laws is to undermine various rights, engender disrespect for law, and lead to instability.	Life is valuable because of divine creation and its inherent sacredness. Or it is valuable as a basic right of people.
III. Principled, or postconventional Social perspective is prior-to-society. Human interactions should be based on principles of justice. Human rights and respect for individual dignity are universal.	**5. Social contract and universal ethical principles** Right behavior is determined by mutual trust and respect and by the contract one accepts as a member of society. The greatest good for the greatest number. Or, rights flow from universally applicable principles of fairness and justice.	Laws protect basic human rights against infringement by others or by society's institutions. Breaking laws is generally unacceptable since they derive from common agreement. Laws may (and perhaps must) be broken if they violate fundamental rights.	Logically and morally, life must take priority as a right, since all other rights only make sense as derivatives from this basic right.

characteristic, while the choice itself (e.g., "shall I steal or not?") is generally not stage-specific.

In this view, then, morality is not a characteristic of a given behavior, but of the underlying reasoning that results in a behavior. Unauthorized use of a motor vehicle, in and of itself, is neither moral nor immoral. If done for a joy ride, it may be adjudged immoral. If done to save a life, it would be a moral act (on the basis of the value of life outweighing the value of property).

MORAL REASONING AND MORAL BEHAVIOR

The literature on the relationship between moral reasoning and anti-social and criminal behavior is clear and consistent—especially for juveniles. Nearly all studies on delinquents have found their reasoning to be largely limited to Stages 1 and 2, at least on production measures[2] (Arbuthnot, Gordon, & Jurkovic, 1987; Blasi, 1980; Gibbs, 1987; Jennings, Kilkenny, & Kohlberg, 1983). Similarly, moral reasoning stage also has been found to be related to a variety of other behaviors, including honesty, altruism, conformity, classroom behaviors, resistance to temptation, honoring contracts, aggression, sexual activities, generosity, cheating, guilty feelings, and political behaviors (Blasi, 1980), and teacher ratings of student behavior problems (Bear & Richards, 1981).

That antisocial behavior is more characteristic of preconventional than higher stage reasoning should come as no surprise, for at these stages one's reasoning is limited to personal considerations and satisfaction of egocentric concerns. Preconventional reasoners are not yet able to coordinate personal and societal goals in evaluating a behavioral choice. Damon (1977) has found that children at this stage confuse fairness with their own desires: "I should get it because I want to have it" (p. 75). Lickona (1983) has noted the following about early Stage 2 reasoning: "kids' energy tends to go into asserting *their* needs and desires and making the world accommodate to them. They have a supersensitive Unfairness Detector when it comes to finding all the ways that people are unfair to them. But they have a big blind spot when it comes to seeing all the ways *they* aren't fair to others" (p. 149). Further, failing to advance beyond Stage 2 is probably nor-

---

2. Production measures are those in which the respondent must generate or construct a response (as in an essay exam) rather than merely recognize a response (as in a multiple-choice exam).

mative for youth who live and function in a Stage 2 world (family, friends, and neighborhood), where selfishness is rewarded, kindness and thoughtfulness is mocked, prosocial role-taking opportunities are scarce, and there is a general absence of higher-stage mentors to challenge one's reasoning.

The relationship between sociomoral worldview and antisocial behavior becomes even clearer when one considers the probable reasons for the offender's developmental delay. Antisocial youth are disproportionately likely to have suffered parenting styles described as arbitrary, inconsistent, physically harsh, authoritarian, disharmonious, power assertive, lacking in explanations, and neglectful (Farrington, 1978; Gordon & Arbuthnot, 1987; Hoffman & Saltzstein, 1967; Snyder & Patterson, 1987; Welsh, 1976). Empirical studies have shown mothers (matched on race and IQ) of delinquents (matched on race, age, and IQ) to have lower moral reasoning stages than mothers of matched nondelinquents (Hudgins & Prentice, 1973). And Jurkovic and Prentice (1974) found dynamics among delinquents' families to be higher in conflict, dominance, and hostility, and lower in warmth and complexity. They observed these same differences as a function of preconventional versus conventional moral reasoning in the children.

Gibbs (1991) argues that antisocial youth are also particularly prone to self-centered cognitive distortions, having noted this phenomenon anecdotally in his work with incarcerated delinquents. By way of example, Gibbs asked what he thought was a rhetorical question during a moral dilemma discussion about who was to blame in a situation involving a car theft. The response was that the owner, having left the keys in the car, was a careless, stupid fool who deserved to be ripped off. Similarly, aggressive boys gratuitously attribute hostile intentions to their victims (Dodge, 1980). And Sykes and Matza (1957) have also noted the tendency of delinquents to blame others for their own transgressions ("They had it coming to them" and "Everybody's picking on me."): "By a subtle alchemy, the delinquent moves himself into the position of avenger and the victim is transformed into a wrongdoer. . . . [He justifies] vandalism as revenge on an ['unfair'] teacher or school official [and] thefts from a 'crooked' store owner. . . . By attacking others, the wrongfulness of his own behavior is more easily repressed or lost from view" (p. 668).

With the advance to Stage 3 early conventional reasoning, one becomes capable of taking the viewpoint of a significant group (such as family, friends, and teachers) when examining the desirability of a behavioral choice. To have the capacity to examine one's own thoughts and behaviors from the perspective of valued others enables the cognitive experiences of disapproval and guilt, which act for most individuals as a buffer against antisocial behavior. Gibbs (1987) describes Stage 3 mutualistic thinking as

> less subvertible to antisocial behavior since it features role reversal . . . and empathic role taking. . . . Furthermore, one anticipates adverse self-judgment for transgressing against the values of a relationship. . . . Hence, taking advantage of another individual is not ethically permissable even given the "right" narrow calculations and interests. (p. 305)

TREATMENT IMPLICATIONS

Prior to the project on which this chapter is focused, a number of intervention studies (Gibbs, Arnold, Ahlborn, & Cheesman, 1984; Jennings et al., 1983; Rosenkoetter, Landman, & Mazak, 1980; Séguin-Tremblay & Kiely, 1979; Ventis, 1976) had shown that delinquent and behavior-disordered antisocial youth are not necessarily limited (in a developmental sense) to preconventional reasoning stages. A significant proportion of such youth acquired some Stage 3 structures in response to intensive long-term Socratic dilemma discussion in which participants challenge and are challenged by the reasoning of others, including reasoning one stage higher than their own (see Arbuthnot & Faust, 1981, and the "Procedures and Techniques" section of this chapter).

However, prior to the intervention described here, there had been no demonstration that the enhancement of sociomoral reasoning structures would lead to positive changes in antisocial behavior. This was clearly a critical juncture in the cognitive-developmental literature. To establish that the facilitation of the development of the cognitive processes involved in the evaluation and resolution of moral issues would in turn lead to less antisocial behavior would indeed be a major step forward in both developmental theory and in the more practical aspects of juvenile justice and rehabilitation (although one might more profitably speak here of "habilitation").

The program described below was made possible by the vision of a juvenile court judge (the late Robert Strode), who had grown increasingly discouraged by the growing numbers of youths coming before him, many of whom seemed to have been preceded by older brothers and sisters, cousins, uncles, and even parents. To break the generational cycle, Judge Strode instituted an in-home, behavioral-systems-oriented, family therapy program (Gordon, Arbuthnot, Gustafson, & McGreen, 1988). However, Judge Strode also wanted to do something in the schools to prevent current high-risk youth from getting into trouble. To address this desire, we established the sociomoral reasoning development program.

RESEARCH OVERVIEW

Participants

The participants in the initial intervention study were 35 male and 13 female Caucasian adolescents, ranging in age from 13 to 17 ($M =$ 14.5), and in grades 7 through 10 in the four school districts in one rural county. The location was Appalachian (southeastern) Ohio, a region often characterized as relatively high in unemployment, poverty, and cultural deprivation. All were nominated by teachers as being seriously "behavior disordered" on the basis of histories of unruliness, aggression, impulsivity, disruptiveness, and so forth, as well as having specific predictors of high risk for delinquency, such as stealing, lying, vandalism, and setting fires (Glueck & Glueck, 1950; Patterson, 1982). The 48 students were rank-ordered on the basis of teacher ratings and then, by coin toss within successive pairs, assigned to either a treatment group, or a waiting-list control condition (a subsequent study included an attention control group).

Assessments

The moral reasoning stage of all students was assessed during the third week of the intervention, again at its conclusion, and again at 1-year follow-up. Stage scores were derived from individual oral interviews using the standard Kohlberg Moral Judgment Interview and scoring manuals (Colby et al., 1982). (Scoring was done blindly by an individual trained in the Kohlberg method, with high reliability and interrater agreements.) The interview consists of dilemmas in which the rights or interests of a protagonist are in conflict with those of another, or with other rights or interests. The respondent is asked a series of questions about what the protagonist in the situation *should* or *ought* to do (as opposed to what the protagonist actually *will* do, or what the respondent would do), and *why*. This is followed by a series of about a dozen or so probe questions that seek more reasoning about various aspects of the dilemma as well as variations on the dilemma (e.g., what should X do if Y? What if Y'? What if not Y?). Each dilemma is designed to assess reasoning about specific moral norms or issues, such as the value of life, reasons for following laws, property rights, obligations, trust, and the like. Different dilemmas were used at posttest and follow-up, but the same norms or issues were assessed.

Two types of scores were derived. First, a "global" stage score was determined, which reflects the respondent's dominant (or major) stage and possibly a secondary (or minor) stage. For example, a global score of 2(3) would mean a respondent used at least 50% Stage 2 reasoning, and at least 25% Stage 3 reasoning. Second, a "moral maturity score" was calculated. This score is psychometrically more precise than the global score, ranging from 100 to 500, with 100 reflecting pure Stage 1 reasoning, and 500 indicating pure Stage 5 thought. The global score of 2(3), as in the example above, would encompass moral maturity scores ranging from 225–249.

Pretest scores on the Moral Judgment Interview ranged from middle Stage 1 (164) to early Stage 2 (229), with the average close to Stage 2 (211; *s.d.* = 28). The distribution of global scores[3] was as follows: 1/2 = 4%; 2(1) = 23%; 2 = 50%; 2(3) = 11%; and 2/3 = 8%. These scores are typical of those found for delinquents, and are lower than those typically found for nondelinquents in this age group (see, e.g., Jennings et al., 1983).

All participants were also rated by teachers on an ad hoc School Adjustment Index consisting of 44 items pertaining to the frequency of occurrence of a wide variety of behaviors, attitudes, and traits counterbalanced for desirability (e.g., disruptive, shows consideration, destructive, performs assigned tasks, fighting, able to tolerate frustration, etc.). (Split half reliability was .98.)

In addition, archival data on a number of dimensions was obtained from school and court records, including disciplinary referrals (trips to the principal's office, corporal punishment, in-school and after school detentions, and expulsions), school absenteeism and tardiness, school grades, and police or court contacts.

Procedures and Techniques

The project began with a meeting of all teachers, staff, and administrators in each of the four schools. They were given a brief overview of cognitive-developmental theory, its links with antisocial behavior, the techniques of intervention, and the promise of behavioral change. Each was then asked to nominate the one student in their classes who

---

3. A "1/2" signifies equal Stage 1 and Stage 2 reasoning; "2(1)" signifies dominant Stage 2 reasoning but with at least 25% Stage 1 reasoning; "2(3)" signifies dominant Stage 2 reasoning but with at least 25% Stage 3 reasoning; "2/3" signifies equal Stage 2 and Stage 3 reasoning.

consistently presented the most serious behavior problems and was the greatest challenge to the teacher's skills and patience. All nominees were then rated on the School Adjustment Index by the nominating teacher. (In retrospect, this part of the procedure was probably an error, mitigating against detecting change. These teachers most likely had strong negative impressions of their nominees, producing a negative halo effect in their ratings. They may also have been resistant to detecting positive changes. More neutral raters would have been desirable.)

We then held a meeting in each school of all the nominees, at which I gave a somewhat simplified overview of the same information I gave to the teachers, including the concrete benefits available to them (including improved reasoning and communication skills resulting in better academic performance, fewer problems with teachers, and fewer difficulties with the law). Examples of the discussion format, dilemmas, and other activities were provided, as was a brief dilemma discussion. Students were also told that not all would be able to be in the program right away, due to limited time and resources, but that all who were interested, and who obtained informed parental consent, would eventually be accepted. Of the 64 nominees, 48 returned parent permission slips (75%).

Within each of four schools, nominees were rank-ordered on the basis of their School Adjustment Index scores. They were then grouped into sequential pairs (e.g., the two with the highest scores, the two with the next highest scores, etc.). Within pairs, students were assigned to treatment or control groups on the basis of a coin toss. A total of four treatment and four control groups were thereby created. Mean scores on the School Adjustment Index did not differ across schools or conditions. Groups ranged in size from 5 to 8. Sexes were mixed. In one instance, when a treatment group had only one girl, another was recruited from the control group to join her (she was targeted at random and asked if she would join the other group; she agreed).

Treatment groups met once a week for a 45-minute class period for 16 to 20 weeks (duration varied as a function of exam weeks and vacation periods). The group discussions were led by one of two male group leaders (myself and an advanced doctoral student with extensive training in both moral development theory and techniques).

We spent the first two sessions building rapport, getting to know one another, and modeling a caring and respectful approach to the group members. We paid particular attention to demonstrating warmth, humor, directness, and clarity of expression. Several exercises were used to promote feelings of openness, group identity and cohesion, safety, acceptance, confidentiality, and a respect for the others' right to express their views.

During both the third and the final week of the program, the participants' were individually interviewed on the Moral Judgment Interview. Between these two assessments of moral reasoning stage, students participated in the weekly dilemma discussion sessions ($n = 12$–16).

The moral dilemma discussions were run according to the principals espoused in Arbuthnot and Faust (1981), consisting primarily of guided moral dilemma discussions using the Blatt and Kohlberg "+1 stage" method of disequilibrium induction. Basically, this meant that during the course of a session, each student's reasoning was challenged by reasoning one stage higher than his or her own. Under preferred circumstances, this higher challenge would come from higher-stage peers. However, since nearly all of our participants were Stage 2 reasoners, we had nonpreferred circumstances, requiring "+1" reasoning to be supplied by the group leader.

The group leader played a number of roles. He always came to the session with two or more dilemmas, each with minor modifications in case there was too little disagreement to produce a lively discussion. The leader sat in a circle with the group, initiated discussion, and kept things moving along. He interrupted to steer discussions back onto the issues of the day, to ask a prompting question, to draw a member into the discussion, or to challenge a position with a response at the next higher stage of reasoning.

In addition to dilemma discussions, we used both planned and spontaneous role plays in some sessions, a technique also espoused in Arbuthnot and Faust (1981).

Dilemmas were chosen on the basis of both their intrinsic interest for this age group and subculture, and for their appropriateness in stimulating transition from Stage 2 to Stage 3 reasoning. Dilemmas were drawn from four different sources: (1) the sound-filmstrip series, *Relationships and Values*, from Guidance Associates (1976); a book of moral dilemmas designed for the Kohlberg approach by Ladenburg, Ladenburg, and Scharf (1978); my own files of real-life dilemmas as reported in various media; and, increasingly as the program proceeded, the participants' own lives (in family, peer group, and school situations).

During the first third of the program, the dilemmas were highly structured, usually the Guidance Associates sound filmstrips. During the second third of the program, the Guidance Associates dilemmas were used at the beginning of the session, but then the leader would change the dilemma to one having similar issues but with a content and setting appropriate to the participants' daily lives. During the final third of the program, the students brought in their own dilemmas. During these last weeks, the participants were encouraged to assume responsibilities for leading portions of the group sessions.

Throughout the discussions, the leader challenged the participants to examine the reasoning of others, to anticipate consequences, and to see the dilemma from the viewpoint of all of the characters as well as the community at large. This was usually accomplished by using a number of different questioning techniques. These included:

1. *Perception-checking questions*: "Ken, would you summarize for us the problem Bill faces?"
2. *Clarification-of-meaning questions*: "When you say, 'It just isn't fair,' what do you mean by 'fair'?"
3. *Reason-seeking questions*: "John, can you tell us why you believe that's the best choice?"
4. *Role-switch questions*: "Alan, suppose it was your dad's store from which Jill took the blouse. How would you feel then?"
5. *Universal-consequences questions*: "You say stores expect to lose merchandise, and they make enough profit to cover it. Well, suppose everyone just took things from stores whenever they wanted to. Then what? What would happen to the stores?"
6. *Issue-related questions* "Kari, under what conditions do you think it would be justifiable to break a promise?"
7. *Participation questions*: "George, what do you think of what Kari just said?"

It would have been naive on our part to assume that we could spend all of each session only on discussions of moral dilemmas. Having worked with this population in other contexts, we were prepared for a number of diverting experiences, mostly behavior problems within the groups. When these occurred, we took pains to turn them into growth-enhancing opportunities—that is, into focused discussions (and modeling) of respect for privacy, individual dignity, self-control, and the unfair egocentrism of wasting the group's time. Our techniques in dealing with disruptions included not only the cognitive-developmental focus of Kohlberg on moral reasoning, but also Dreikurs's (1964) use of logical consequences for mistaken goals.

We also spent two sessions about a third of the way into the program on listening and communication skills. It became obvious early on that our participants, because of their cultural deprivation as well as cognitive immaturity, had considerable difficulty paying attention to what others had to say, often missing the messages entirely.

And they had trouble expressing themselves without provoking defensiveness or antagonism. To remediate these problems, we spent two sessions on active listening and sending "I" messages. Each concept was carefully and concretely explained, and numerous examples given. We then engaged in dilemma discussions deliberately chosen to evoke a divergence of opinion (one with conflicting Stage 2 perspectives). As each dysfunctional communication or response occurred, we stopped and analyzed what had happened, including group members' affective reactions and comprehension. The group leader then modeled alternate techniques, followed by questioning to elicit reactions and comprehension. Improvements were discussed, then group members were invited to offer still other effective "I" message statements. A good deal of praise and encouragement was used throughout.

Group members often raised issues from their own lives during discussion—some true, some exaggerated, and others no doubt fictitious. Often these were attention-seeking ploys. Such instances required judgment calls on the part of the group leader. On the one hand, we recognized the needs of the students to receive attention, both from us and from the other group members. (The self-esteem levels of these youth was very low.) We tried to give all members as much attention as possible. On the other hand, we did not wish to reinforce either exaggeration or prevarication. Thus, in most cases, we tried to turn the comments into a discussion of the underlying issue or to direct discussion back to the main topic if the comments were frivolous.

When students revealed ongoing behaviors that would be illegal or dangerous (to themselves or others), we directed appropriate questions (e.g., role-switch or universal consequences; see above) to the discloser and the larger group. We made every effort to abide by our assurances to the group of confidentiality, but also let them know that if we feared for their welfare or safety, we might need to take appropriate steps after consulting with the participants involved.

On three occasions we did speak privately with participants, but felt further action was unnecessary. For example, one girl, age 14, told the group about her exploits during regular Saturday night "parties" with a group of men in their 20s. She was the only girl at these events, held at an abandoned strip mine. She would become heavily intoxicated and was allowed to drive a car on "joy rides." The group challenged her to explore the possible serious consequences for her, including accidental injury or death for her, the others, or for innocent people on the road (Stage 3 concerns). (Some members raised Stage 2 issues about consequences if her parents found out.) The group leader spoke with her in private about the circumstances leading to her decisions (family problems and apparent parental indifference to her drinking), and other possible consequences not raised in the group, including health problems, disease, pregnancy, and the like. She had not considered these issues, having focused until this time only on the attention, pleasures, and thrills involved. She seemed to welcome our interest in her welfare, and promised to think about the issues we had raised. She proudly informed us in the next few weeks of her success in avoiding this group of men.

Outcomes of the Program

Before discussing the formal outcomes of this intervention, we should point out that the students very much enjoyed the program. Attendance was high. Participants' friends often approached us to seek admission into the program. The principal, several teachers, and even some parents commented on the students' enthusiasm for the program and their improved attitudes at school and at home.

Our interests in outcomes from the intervention lay along two dimensions, the cognitive versus behavioral, and the immediate versus enduring. We were fairly certain that we could produce changes in moral reasoning level, although there had been no prior developmental efforts with this exact population: culturally deprived, behaviorally disordered adolescents. The greater target, however, was the behavioral dimension, both for theoretical as well as practical considerations. While we expected a congruence of behavior with cognitive change, our confidence before the sponsoring juvenile court judge and the various school officials was purely theoretical.

Second, assuming that we could produce a behavior change, would it persist after our departure? Maintenance of change is a common problem for many interventions. Nonetheless, we were confident that since our intervention would produce *structural* change, as opposed to mere *attitudinal* change or behavioral compliance, that future behaviors would derive from and be congruent with newly acquired sociomoral worldviews. Mitigating against such persistence, however, was the fact that we were not intervening at a systems level—that is, these youth would continue to live in powerfully influential social settings (family, peer, and school) that would remain largely unchanged. Of course, with more mature perspectives and behaviors, our participants' social stimulus value would change, and hence members of these social systems should gradually shift in their expectations and responses to the participants. Such a change in response to the participants' use of new reasoning structures should both encourage further use and provide an atmosphere more conducive to the exchange of ideas. Therefore, while we eagerly awaited the immediate outcome data, we were far more excited about what we would find 1 year later.

For the immediate posttest data, a series of analyses of covariance (covarying pretest scores) showed all comparisons to be significant except teacher ratings and absenteeism.[4] Stage of sociomoral reasoning for intervention students increased on the average about half a stage, a highly significant change. In contrast, there was a slight decline for those in the control condition.

The two primary indicators of antisocial behavior, disciplinary referrals to the school office and police or court contacts, both showed significant declines for treatment students, and slight increases for control students. The students who participated in the program were sent to the principals' offices, picked up by the police, or had to appear in court so infrequently that their scores approached zero.

Of four related school behaviors, two showed significant improvements for treatment students. Tardiness declined, in contrast to the control students' increase, and grades in English and humanities classes improved while those of the control students declined. Both teacher ratings and absenteeism showed improvement, but these changes were not statistically significant. Teacher ratings are perhaps resistant to change for antisocial youth who are likely to engender strongly negative perceptions.

We were, of course, quite pleased with these group comparison data. However, to further assess the cognition-behavior link in this project, we computed correlations between individual change scores on the moral maturity scores and the outcome measures. Reverse stepwise multiple regression analyses on the correlation matrix showed all to be highly significant, producing a final adjusted squared multiple correlation of .90. Thus, change in sociomoral reasoning was highly related to changes in behavior.

A year after the completion of the intervention, we obtained follow-up data for students in two of the four schools. (There was no difference on pretest scores between this subsample and those not included.) These data are illustrated in Figure 13.1.

The moral maturity scores of the two groups remained significantly different, and continued to diverge (the interaction term was significant). It would appear, then, that having stimulated cognitive growth and fostered a questioning approach to values issues, matura-

4. For the reader interested in details of analyses and results, please see Arbuthnot and Gordon (1986). Further, in a subsequent study, an attention control group was included. It did not differ from the waiting-list control on any outcome measure.

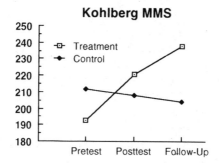

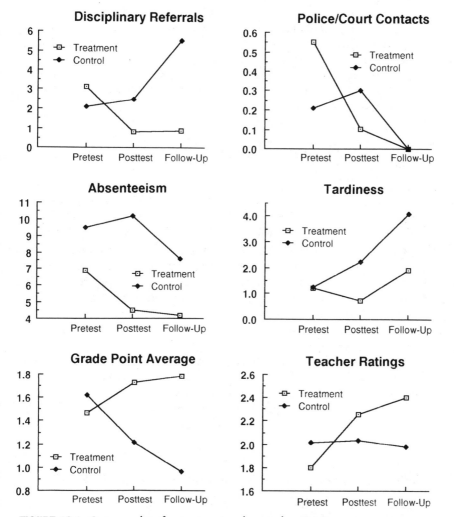

FIGURE 13.1. Outcome data for treatment and control groups.

tion in the moral realm can continue even without deliberate disequilibrating experiences.

For the primary behavioral indicators, the improvements shown by the intervention group were maintained over time. (Floor effects prevented further improvement.) In contrast, in-school behavior problems among the control group students seriously escalated, more than doubling. Police and court contacts for both groups had declined to zero at follow-up.

Other in-school outcome measures showed highly significant differences between the two groups at the 1-year follow-up. Teacher ratings diverged, with a significant interaction effect. Tardiness continued to differ significantly. Absenteeism rates became significant (in contrast to the nonsignificant trend at the immediate posttest). Grades also continued to diverge, with the intervention group showing a continued improvement, while the control group showed a continuing decline.

And, as was the case for the immediate follow-up, changes in moral reasoning scores were strongly tied to all behavioral outcomes.

SIGNIFICANCE AND IMPLICATIONS

The research goals of this project were achieved with a high degree of statistical significance. It was convincingly shown that the average level of maturity of sociomoral reasoning of this population of rural, culturally deprived, antisocial youth can be appreciably improved through an intervention based on guided dilemma discussion. It was further apparent that while not all participants showed increases in moral reasoning scores, changes among those who did were associated with improvements in a number of in-school and out-of-school behaviors. Finally, both the cognitive and behavior changes persisted over a 1-year follow-up period, and on most measures the two groups continued to diverge.

A number of issues were raised by the results of this intervention. First, why did it work? Second, why did it not work for all participants? Third, what are the limiting factors on its widespread use in the schools and the juvenile justice system? And fourth, how do the results of this intervention fit within the larger debate about rehabilitation and "what works"?

Why Does the Cognitive-Developmental Approach Work?

As was argued in the introduction to this chapter, intentional human behavior—whether prosocial or antisocial—is preceded by a decision-making process. While many antisocial acts appear not to have engaged even the most basic moral perspectives of the actor, we nonetheless maintain that such behaviors do take place within a sociomoral framework. A major difficulty for victims (individual or societal) is the actor's *inability* in many cases to utilize a conventional, let alone a principled, moral worldview. The killers of Jay Bias took a very casual view of the importance of Jay's life. It was all too easy for them to avenge an "insult to honor" by taking an extreme action. While we may express disgust at their claim to honor, it is *their* perspective that we need to understand, and from which we need to analyze this tragic act.

A preconventional sociomoral perspective permits a variety of antisocial and destructive behaviors to occur simply because such a worldview not only permits them to occur but lends them a "logical" appropriateness, and may make such acts a requirement to avoid oneself becoming a future victim of another's preconventional act. This will be especially true in situations that trigger or evoke antisocial behaviors: criminal acts, dangerous circumstances, adrenaline-producing situations, real or perceived threats, peer pressure, and the like.

> The predisposition to offend may have its roots in affective attitudes/ feelings and cognitive/moral backwardness, but it only manifests itself as behaviour in particular settings. . . . There are criminogenic situations in society, as there always have been, but not everyone when confronted with those situations behaves criminally. . . . So we have two major factors affecting our decision-maker: his internal cognitive and affective "map" or level of development, and the social, economic, and personal situations he finds himself in. (Duguid, 1981, p. 5)

Unfortunately, the actor's perceptions of the context of behavior may not be the same as ours. In fact, many criminal offenders do not perceive themselves as blameworthy for their actions—in their own minds, they were "victims of the situation," left with no other choice. This "externalizing" is characteristic of the preconventional perspective.

A good example of this perspective can be found in the person of David Harris, a career criminal instrumental as an "eyewitness" in the wrongful conviction of Randall Dale Adams for the murder of a Dallas policeman (for which crime Adams faced execution, served 12 years in prison, and was released only as a result of Harris's admission in a documentary film called *The Thin Blue Line* that he, not Adams, shot the policeman). Harris committed a number of other serious crimes, including murder. In one instance, he broke into a home, locked a woman's male partner in the bathroom, and then brutally raped the woman. As he left the building with the woman as a hostage, the man (who had managed to escape) gave chase, and Harris shot him. He said in an interview in *The Thin Blue Line* that the man's death was his own fault, that the man shouldn't have come after them.

The cognitive dynamics of this scenario exhibit classic preconventional reasoning. What is right is what protects the self. There is no influence here of mutualistic or third-person thinking. There is no empathic role taking. There is no guilt or adverse self-judgment. In fact, conventional (Stage 3) morality is held in contempt. As Duguid (1981) notes,

> Goodness, justice, humility, honesty and similar qualities are mere hypocrisy or the attributes of a fool. This surfaces in a kind of anaesthetized sensibility toward violence, a defense of violence as simply a tool of the trade, and the criminal's all-too-frequent stance toward the victim as someone who simply gets in the way. In this world of "us and them" the relationship is inevitably hostile." (p. 3)

So, why does the facilitation of sociomoral reasoning, the enhancement of a more differentiated and coordinated social perspective, the development of a tie to others in a sense of community, the acquisition of the capacity for self-disapproval, *why* do these result in less antisocial behavior? Because the behavior can now be evaluated in a larger context than short-term self-interest.

Gibbs (1987, 1991) has suggested that our results were due to more than the development of higher-stage moral reasoning alone—that our additional training in communication and listening skills and emphasis on empathy contributed to our behavioral outcomes and differentiated our intervention from those of Niles (1986) and Gibbs et al. (1984), which found reasoning change with delinquents, but no associated behavioral effects. We do not dispute this charge. On the contrary, our dilemma discussions were far from intellectually sterile treatments of logical or illogical conclusions. We made every attempt to link values perspectives to the impact of choices on others, as well as on oneself in a longer time perspective. We emphasized the consequences for the community, and the community's reactions to both antisocial and prosocial actors. We invited (and modeled) caring responses.

In fact, it is our position (Arbuthnot, 1990) that the acquisition of higher sociomoral reasoning abilities alone, while necessary, is not sufficient for moral behavior. Rather, one must also consider the influence of the context of the behavior, one's affective or emotional state, and the will to act consistently with one's judgment. In this light, the work of Vicente Garrido (Garrido, Redondo, & Perez, 1989; Garrido Genovés, 1990) with incarcerated delinquents in Spain further underscores the advantages to be gained by combining sociomoral reasoning development with related social and interpersonal skills.

We can rarely have an influence over contextual variables, though we can promote more accurate perceptions and more thorough analyses of contextual variables. We may have little influence over an actor's emotions, but we can enhance the actor's sensitivity to and caring about the emotions of others. In this regard, we have found affective empathy, but not cognitive empathy (role-taking ability), to be related to delinquency (Kaplan & Arbuthnot, 1984). One may logically see the implications of various choices, yet lack the will to act consistently with higher moral perspectives. This sense of will, we believe, derives from one's sense of connectedness to a "community" which, in turn, cares about the actor. We could not, of course, alter the larger community in which our students lived. However, we could offer a model of what such a community can be.

Why Did Some Participants Mature in Their Reasoning while Others Did Not?

There are a variety of speculations one can offer for the differential effectiveness of the moral reasoning development intervention. First, the medicine may be correct, but the dosage or treatment duration may have been insufficient. Second, there is ample evidence that one's more general logical reasoning capacities set upper limits to the growth of moral reasoning. Beginning formal operations,[5] for example, are necessary for Stage 3 moral thought (Arbuthnot, Sparling,

---

5. In beginning formal operation thought one observes not only explicit, but implicit, understanding of reciprocity—as in verbal as well as concrete seriation problems—and also a coordination of reciprocity with inversion. In the realm of social cognition, this enables Stage 3 moral reasoning, with mutual role-taking perspectives recursively organized to ensure complementarity of expectations, including the viewpoint of an impartial third party. For example, Kohlberg argues that the Golden Rule can be first understood at Stage 3, via coordination of inversion and reciprocity (i.e., the negation of some undesired action on the basis of being able to simultaneously, or serially, take the perspective of both parties). Stage 3 also involves the coordination of the relationship between reward and goodness with that between goodness and the actor. In combination, the Stage 3 reasoner now views morality not as a function of particular individuals' interests (Stage 2), but from the perspective of interpersonal relations, with integrated and coordinated needs and views. This, in turn, permits a distinction between what one does, or wants to do, and what one *ought* to do.

Faust, & Key, 1983; Walker, 1980). It is quite likely that many participants in our program were not yet capable of this level of reasoning. Third, there may well be motivational factors that we have not yet identified that affect one's response to disequilibrium.

What Are the Limiting Factors on the Sociomoral Reasoning Development Approach?

We have discussed elsewhere (Arbuthnot & Gordon, 1988) what we see as essential elements for the dissemination of cognitively based sociomoral reasoning development programs. Among the more important are a theoretically sound intervention; a champion of the approach within the administering organization; interventionists with good "clinical" skills and a caring attitude; careful adherence to the intervention model; support from the sponsoring organization in terms of time, materials, and other resources; adequate time for the intervention to be effective; and training and continuing supervision for the interventionists by an outside expert.

Training should include a thorough understanding of the theoretical model as well as skill in the use of intervention techniques. In our case, discussion leaders were thoroughly conversant with Kohlberg's model, had extensive experience working with groups of adolescents, and had many hours of supervised training with the intervention materials and techniques. Further, it is important to have continuing on-site supervision of actual sessions (or tapes of them), especially early in the intervention to assess and modify techniques to assure fidelity to the model. It is not sufficient to rely on group leaders' self-reports, since they may erroneously be convinced that their behaviors are consistent with their knowledge. For other caveats regarding successful versus unsuccessful moral reasoning interventions, the reader is referred to Arbuthnot et al. (1987).

How Does the Sociomoral Reasoning Approach Fit within the Larger "Rehabilitation" Debate?

A number of important papers have been published recently that have addressed the general question of "what works" in corrections, and the importance of cognitively based programs in this context (e.g., Andrews et al., 1990; Gendreau & Ross, 1987; Ross & Fabiano, 1985; Ross & Gendreau, 1980). Owing largely to less-than-carefully-reasoned reviews (such as that of Martinson, 1974, which concluded that "nothing works"), the field of rehabilitation during the 1970s and early 1980s was largely cast aside by political conservatives and liberals alike, with the result that subsequent sentencing reforms (emphasizing "law and order," determinant sentences, and "warehousing") largely undercut the role of rehabilitative efforts in the criminal justice system.

However, recent reviews of controlled studies (and even Martinson, 1979, in a little-read revision of his views) have found that criminal sanctions are only minimally related to recidivism. Further, such highly touted and frequently used approaches as unstructured group counseling, relationship-oriented milieu therapies, and traditional psychodynamic and nondirective client-centered therapies are ineffective, and may well be counterproductive. What "works" are programs that deliver services to higher-risk cases, target criminogenic needs, and use styles and modes of treatment (e.g., cognitive and behavioral) that are congruent with recipients' needs and learning styles (Andrews et al., 1990).

Interventions for antisocial youth and criminal offenders that fail to include cognitive development of sociomoral reasoning perspectives, empathy, cognitive control, and ties to community are, I believe, inherently limited and do not address the underlying factors within the individual that permit immoral, illegal, and inhuman behavior.

One may well find statistical relationships that suggest that antisocial behavior is associated with feelings of relative deprivation, immersion in specific subcultures, acceptance of deviant life-styles, lack of adequate supervision, a broken family during childhood, latent hostility, or diets high in sugar or artificial additives. What, then, are the logical treatment modalities? Economic reform, job training, neighborhood "renewal," outreach programs, wilderness experiences, diversions (e.g., build a neighborhood recreation center), scaring children "straight," foster care, psychotherapy to help unruly adolescents adjust to chaotic families and threatening neighborhoods, incarceration to teach fear of consequences or modify institutional behaviors through token economies, nutrition classes, among other options. The record of such treatments is not encouraging.

The overall failure of most approaches for correcting or preventing antisocial behavior, I believe, lies in their failure to address directly the adolescent's worldview. An improved neighborhood economy or housing project may alter the circumstances in which choices are made, but fails to enhance the process of choosing. Sending a teenager on an Outward Bound experience may develop some survival skills and perhaps even increase his or her self-esteem. But learning to rappel down a cliff has little relevance for resisting the temptations of street crime and substance abuse. Being "scared" by the unpleasant realities of prison life as related by "big-time losers" may serve only to stiffen one's resolve to be clever enough not to get caught. Psychotherapies may develop insight into the pressures impinging upon one, but rarely will they address or correct the unfairness or injustice of such pressures or remove them. Prompting an institutionalized adolescent felon to make his bed or attend class on time in order to earn points or privileges is immediately perceived as a meaningless, manipulative, and trivial program inviting subversion—which inadvertently "reinforces" cheating, lying, and insincerity. And while some may "straighten up" to avoid reincarceration, others wear their institutionalization as a badge of honor and "graduate" with enhanced criminologic skills.

Antisocial behavior is permitted by a worldview that approves of such actions, that does not evoke a judgment process that condemns such choices. To change such behaviors in the short run it may be sufficient to threaten negative consequences. But in the longer time frame, and in the broader array of incipient choices, resistance requires internal and generalizable controls. It is indeed rare for one to choose to behave in a manner not approved by one's *own moral judgment*. While behavioral choices may be subjected to powerful situational influences (e.g., fear of bodily harm or loss), the presence of *empathy* and *will* and *courage* can restore choice consistent with judgment.

From where do such cognitive abilities come? Unfortunately, the evidence is quite clear that moral *judgment* is much more difficult to acquire than mere moral *belief*. The latter is the stuff of parental demand and ministerial pleading. It is easy to subscribe to a moral belief—for example, "Do unto others as you would have them do unto you." Yet it is another matter for one to invoke the moral principles that underlie such teachings when making a behavioral choice. To the cognitively immature reasoner (e.g., Stage 2), the Golden Rule provides justification for self-indulgence ("I'd better get mine, 'cause if I don't somebody else will.") Indeed, it is not until Stage 3 reasoning structures are achieved that the prescriptive nature of the Golden Rule is understood—that there is a moral "should" involved that is based in hypothetical reciprocity in acts of fairness. This worldview cannot emerge absent empathy and reciprocal role taking.

One cannot, then, *instruct* a child to be fair or moral. (Were it so easy, preachers could simply read the Ten Commandments once, quit the pulpit, and go play golf.) Nor can one produce a sense of fairness or respect for the rights of others through threat or intimidation or bribery or psychotherapy (else prison officials could follow the preachers). A sense of fairness and a felt duty to behave fairly emerge out of the individual's experiences. It is cognitively *constructed* in an active sense. If one lacks an understanding of fair play as a part of one's larger worldview, it can (for many) be developed through structured experiences that compel the individual to examine and reconcile his or her views with those of others and with the hypothetical consequences of universal adoption of the individual's point of view.

Moral behavior, then, is the result of cognitive development in combination with examined experience. Cognitive development, with certain limitations, can be stimulated and facilitated through structured activities. Experience can be examined in light of newly acquired cognitive capacities. It is this author's belief that interventions for juvenile and adult offenders that fail to address the offenders' sociomoral worldview are condemned to limited success, if any, in producing prosocial behavioral choices. Imprisonment may temporarily forestall the repetition of murderous acts by the killers of Jay Bias, but what effect will it have on their views of the morality of murder and their desire to act as responsible members of a just community?

REFERENCES

Andrews, D. A., Zinger, I., Hoge, R. D., Bonta, J., Gendreau, P., & Cullen, F. T. (1990). Does correctional treatment work: A clinically relevant and psychologically informed meta-analysis. *Criminology, 28*, 369–404.

Arbuthnot, J. (1990). The matrix of behavior: Reason, ethics, emotion, will, and context. In S. Duguid (Ed.), *Yearbook of correctional education* (pp. 45–62). Burnaby, B.C., Canada: Institute for the Humanities, Simon Fraser University.

Arbuthnot, J., & Faust, D. (1981). *Teaching moral reasoning: Theory and practice.* New York: Harper and Row.

Arbuthnot, J., & Gordon, D. A. (1986). Behavioral and cognitive effects of a moral reasoning development intervention for high-risk behavior-disordered adolescents. *Journal of Consulting and Clinical Psychology, 54*, 208–216.

Arbuthnot, J., & Gordon, D. A. (1988). Disseminating effective interventions for juvenile delinquents: Cognitively-based sociomoral reasoning development programs. *Journal of Correctional Education, 39*, 48–52.

Arbuthnot, J., Gordon, D. A., & Jurkovic, G. (1987). Personality. In H. Quay (Ed.), *Handbook of juvenile delinquency* (pp. 139–182). New York: Wiley.

Arbuthnot, J., Gustafson, K., Kaplan-Reiss, P., Gotthardt, J., Swanson, H., & Gordon, D. (1987). When sociomoral reasoning development interventions fail: Some commonalities and non-commonalities. *Moral Education Forum, 12*, 25–28.

Arbuthnot, J., Sparling, Y., Faust, D., & Key, W. (1983). Logical and moral reasoning in preadolescent children. *Psychological Reports, 52,* 209–210.

Bear, G. G., & Richards, H. C. (1981). Moral reasoning and conduct problems in the classroom. *Journal of Educational Psychology, 73,* 644–670.

Blasi, A. (1980). Bridging moral cognition and moral action: A critical review of the literature. *Psychological Bulletin, 88,* 1–45.

Colby, A., Kohlberg, L., Gibbs, J., Candee D., Speicher-Dubin, B., Hewer, A., Kauffman, K., & Power, C. (1982). *Standard Form scoring manual, Forms A and B.* Cambridge, MA: Center for Moral Education.

Damon, W. (1977). *The social world of the child.* San Francisco: Jossey-Bass.

Dodge, K. A. (1980). Social cognition and children's aggressive behavior. *Child Development, 51,* 162–170.

Dreikurs, R. (1964). *Children: The challenge.* New York: Dutton.

Duguid, S. (1981). Prison education and criminal choice: The context of decision-making. *Canadian Journal of Criminology, 23,* 421–438.

Farrington, D. P. (1978). The family backgrounds of aggressive youth. In L. A. Hersov & M. Berger (Eds.), *Aggression and antisocial behavior in childhood and adolescence.* Oxford, England: Pergamon Press.

Garrido, V., Redondo, S., & Perez, E. (1989). El tratamiento de delincuentes institucionalizados: El programa de competencia psicosocial en la prision de jovenes la Trinidad de Barcelona. *Delincuencia/Delinquency, 1,* 37–57.

Garrido Genovés, V. (1990, July). *The cognitive model in the treatment of Spanish offenders: Theory and practice.* Address presented to the 45th International Conference of the Correctional Education Association, Vancouver, B.C.

Gendreau, P., & Ross, R. R. (1987). Revivification of rehabilitation: Evidence from the 1980s. *Justice Quarterly, 4,* 349–408.

Gibbs, J. C. (1987). Social processes in delinquency: The need to facilitate empathy as well as sociomoral reasoning. In W. M. Kurtines & J. L. Gewirtz (Eds.), *Moral development through social interaction* (pp. 301–321). New York: Wiley.

Gibbs, J. C. (1991). Sociomoral developmental delay and cognitive distortion: Implications for the treatment of antisocial youth. In W. M. Kurtines & J. L. Gewirtz (Eds.), *Handbook of moral behavior and development, Vol. 3: Application* (pp. 95–110). Los Angeles: Erlbaum.

Gibbs, J. C., Arnold, K. D., Ahlborn, H. H., & Cheesman, F. L. (1984). Facilitation of sociomoral reasoning in delinquents. *Journal of Consulting and Clinical Psychology, 52,* 37–45.

Gordon, D. A., & Arbuthnot, J. (1987). Individual, group, and family interventions. In H. Quay (Ed.), *Handbook of juvenile delinquency* (pp. 290–324). New York: Wiley.

Gordon, D. A., Arbuthnot, J., Gustafson, K., & McGreen, P. (1988). In-home behavioral systems family therapy with adjudicated delinquents. *American Journal of Family Therapy, 16,* 243–255.

Glueck, S., & Glueck, E. (1950). *Unraveling juvenile delinquency.* Cambridge: Harvard University Press.

Guidance Associates (Producer). (1976). *Relationships and values* [Sound-film-strip]. Mt. Kisko, NY.

Hartshorne, H., & May, M. A. (1928). *Studies in the nature of character.* New York: Macmillan.

Hoffman, M. L., & Saltzstein, H. D. (1967). Parental discipline and the child's moral development. *Journal of Personality and Social Psychology, 5,* 45–47.

Hudgins, W., & Prentice, N. M. (1973). Moral judgment in delinquent and nondelinquent adolescents and their mothers. *Journal of Abnormal Psychology, 82,* 145–152.

Jennings, W. S., Kilkenny, R., & Kohlberg, L. (1983). Moral development theory and practice for youthful and adult offenders. In W. S. Laufer & J. M. Day (Eds.), *Personality theory, moral development, and criminal behavior* (pp. 281–355). Toronto, Canada: Lexington Books.

Jurkovic, G. J., & Prentice, N. M. (1974). Dimensions of moral interaction and moral judgment in delinquent and nondelinquent families. *Journal of Consulting and Clinical Psychology, 42,* 256–262.

Kaplan, P. J., & Arbuthnot, J. (1984). Affective empathy and cognitive role-taking in delinquent and non-delinquent youth. *Adolescence, 20,* 323–333.

Kohlberg, L. (1969). Stage and sequence: The cognitive-developmental approach to socialization. In D. Goslin (Ed.), *Handbook of socialization theory and research* (pp. 347–480). Chicago: Rand McNally.

Kohlberg, L. (1971). From is to ought: How to commit the naturalistic fallacy and get away with it in the study of moral development. In L. Kohlberg, *Cognitive development and epistemology* (pp. 151–235). New York: Academic Press.

Kohlberg, L. (1984). *Essays on moral development: Vol. 1. The philosophy of moral development.* San Francisco: Harper and Row.

Kohlberg, L. (1984). *Essays on moral development: Vol. 2. The psychology of moral development.* San Francisco: Harper and Row.

Ladenburg, T., Ladenburg, M., & Scharf, P. (1978). *Moral education.* Davis, CA: Responsible Action.

Lickona, T. (1983). *Raising good children.* Toronto, Canada: Bantam.

Martinson, R. (1974). What works? Questions and answers about prison reform. *Public Interest, 35,* 22–54.

Martinson, R. (1979). New findings, new views: A note of caution regarding prison reform. *Hofstra Law Review, 7,* 243–258.

Niles, W. J. (1986). Effects of a moral development discussion group on delinquent and predelinquent boys. *Journal of Counseling Psychology, 33,* 45–51.

Patterson, G. R. (1982). *Coercive family process.* Eugene, OR: Castalia.

Rosenkoetter, L., Landman, S., & Mazak, S. (1980). Use of moral discussion as an intervention with delinquents. *Psychological Reports, 16,* 91–94.

Ross, R. R., & Fabiano, E. (1985). *Time to think: A cognitive model of delinquency prevention and offender rehabilitation.* Johnson City, TN: Institute of Social Sciences and Arts.

Ross, R., & Gendreau, P. (1980). *Effective correctional treatment.* Toronto, Canada: Butterworths.

Séguin-Tremblay, G., & Kiely, M. (1979). Dévelopment du judgment moral chez l'adolescente en rééducation. *Canadian Journal of Behavioral Science, 11,* 32–44.

Snyder, J., & Patterson, G. R. (1987). Family interaction and delinquent behavior. In H. C. Quay (Ed.), *Handbook of delinquency* (pp. 216–243). New York: Wiley.

Squitieri, T., & Kelley, J. (1990, December 4). Bias' slaying reflects 'disregard for life.' *USA Today,* p. 3A.

Sykes, G. M., & Matza, D. (1957). Techniques of neutralization: A theory of delinquency. *American Sociological Review, 22,* 664–670.

Ventis, W. L. (1976). *Moral development in delinquent and non-delinquent males and its enhancement.* Paper presented at the annual meeting of the Southeastern Psychological Association, Williamsburg, VA.

Walker, L. J. (1980). Cognitive and perspective-taking prerequisites for moral development. *Child Development, 51,* 131–139.

Welsh, R. S. (1976). Severe parental punishment and delinquency: A developmental theory. *Journal of Clinical Child Psychology, 5,* 17–21.

CHAPTER 14

◆ ──────── ◆

Theory-Guided Investigation:
Three Field Experiments

DENISE C. GOTTFREDSON
GARY D. GOTTFREDSON

This chapter describes three field experiments examining the efficacy of approaches to delinquency prevention based on three different causal theories. These experiments demonstrate that field studies are useful tools for testing theory, despite obstacles that can limit their utility.

Each of the three experiments was developed and evaluated using a structured method for researcher-practitioner collaboration—Program Development Evaluation (PDE; G. Gottfredson, 1984a)—that was devised to attain the scientists' aim of strong tests of theories and the practitioners' aim of effective programs. Using the PDE method, we worked with practitioners developing three programs to elaborate the rationales underlying each, refine them by introducing theory and research, and hew program activities as closely as possible to the emergent program theories.

The three programs resulting from this collaboration correspond to different academic theories of crime, and their results reflect on these theories. In the following discussion, the experiments are first described and their results analyzed, then instructive features of some obstacles inherent in using experiments to test theory are examined to draw lessons for improving the utility of future research.

THREE INTERVENTION PROGRAMS

This section describes three programs with different approaches to reducing delinquent behavior among high-risk adolescents.

Positive Action Through Holistic Education

Positive Action Through Holistic Education (Project PATHE) was implemented in seven secondary schools (for students approximately ages 11 through 17) in Charleston, South Carolina, between fall 1980 and spring 1983. It was a comprehensive school improvement program that simultaneously altered school organization and management and intervened directly with high-risk youths. Elsewhere D. Gottfredson (1986) reported that the broad changes in the discipline, resources, and management of the school that were directed to the entire school population appeared to be effective for increasing social bonding to the school and reducing disorder. Here we focus on the portion of the program intended to reduce delinquency and increase learning for high-risk students.

The program called for diagnosis of student needs, prescription of services to meet those needs, and frequent monitoring of student progress. School specialists carried out these activities with approximately 10% of the student population in each school. The target population was identified through teacher referrals and screening of academic and behavior records. The specialists were usually experienced teachers, but some were assistant principals or guidance counselors.

The specialists were provided with information about each target student's school experiences. This information included standardized achievement test scores in detailed skill areas, school grades by subject, and attendance and disciplinary records. Specialists met with each student—and sometimes with the student's parents and teachers—to establish behavioral objectives. Academic objectives, conduct objectives, or both were defined for each student, and the specialists devised an individualized treatment program directed at those objectives. These programs most often included counseling and tutoring services, and usually extracurricular activities as well. These activities included peer counseling and rap sessions during which students were expected to discuss topics of concern in a constructive environment, participation in a student leadership team that involved students directly in planning for and implementing school change, field trips, and other extracurricular activities and clubs. In addition, specialists worked with students' teachers to recommend instructional strategies, and they referred students and their families to other community services.

The target students were closely monitored. For a period of either 1 or 2 years, specialists recorded daily attendance, and they were immediately informed of any disciplinary incident involving a target student. Specialists called a target student's parents after three absences and met with the student and his or her parents following disciplinary incidents. They also received each target student's grades and test scores throughout the project. Target students had an average of about two contacts per month with the specialists or a project activity, although this average masks high involvement by some students and low involvement by others. The prevention services provided were more intensive, systematic, and enduring than the services that schools are typically able to provide.

The services were intended to increase attachments to the school specialists and commitment to school by increasing success experiences in school. Services were intended to provide rewarding school experiences for students who had usually found school unrewarding and to ameliorate the negative self-perceptions of these high-risk youths.

Positive Action Through Holistic Education attempted to provide a "stake in conformity" within the school setting for youths whose previous school experiences had not promoted such a social bond. The program's emphasis on increasing student attachments and commitment to school and on integrating youths at especially high risk of delinquency and drop-out into ongoing social activities in the school make it consistent with the social control (Hirschi, 1969) perspective, according to which social bonds (attachments to others, commitments to conventional goals, and beliefs in the validity of rules) provide restraints against delinquent activities. Individuals who are bonded to the social order are restrained from delinquent behavior, according to social control theory.

Student Training Through Urban Strategies

Student Training Through Urban Strategies (Project STATUS) operated in one junior (student ages 12 through 14) and one senior (student ages 15 through 17) high school in Pasadena, California, from fall 1980 through spring 1983. The Student Training Through Urban Strategies intervention for high-risk youths was a combined English and social studies class with a coordinated law-related education curriculum.

The yearlong alternative class contained five units. Each unit introduced youths to a different institution in American society. The first seventh grade unit explored the school; it focused on the functions of school rules, school decision-making processes, rule enforcement, and students' rights and responsibilities as school citizens. The second unit explored human nature and interpersonal relations; it focused on informal codes of conduct and how these codes are translated into more formal rules for behavior. The third unit examined the role of the family from personal, sociological, and legal perspectives. The fourth unit explored social contracts and their basis in the need for order in society. The fifth unit covered the criminal justice system, including issues of justice, fairness, and equity; it built on prior units to show how informal contracts and the need for order are expressed as laws. The high school curriculum substituted units on the job market and life planning for the units on human nature and the family.

Instruction entailed active participation. Field experiences included visits to a variety of community organizations and agencies. Guests were frequently asked to speak to students on topics related to the curriculum. Structured role-plays and simulations were common. Students carried out research, both independently and in small groups, and reported their results to the class. Teachers were trained to use (1) student teams for tutoring and support, (2) rewards for both individual and group progress, and (3) individualized learning plans.

The English and social studies classes were scheduled together in a 2-hour block to increase flexibility and coordination. The curriculum called for frequently combining the two classes to allow for activities (such as field trips and work with community volunteers) that required more than 1 hour's time. The English and social studies teachers worked as a team: when a particular theme was covered in social studies, the same theme was explored in the literature used in the English class.

Although the program contained elements that made it consistent with several theories of delinquency, its underlying philosophy was most consistent with the strain or opportunity perspective (Cloward & Ohlin, 1960), especially as applied to the condition of adolescents in contemporary society (Coleman, 1961). According to this perspective, the status of youths isolates them from productive experiences with major social institutions. The isolation of youths in a relatively sterile, book-learning environment robs them of the opportunity to grow and experience the world in a meaningful way. According to this perspective, youths are alienated from their natural enthusiasm for learning when they are forced to focus on curriculum materials that are largely irrelevant to their lives. The Student Training Through Urban Strategies program attempted to decrease alienation by providing a "high-interest" curriculum and participatory instructional methods, by helping students gain an appreciation for the function of law in society, and by fostering the growth of new student roles as participating citizens. This high-relevance curriculum was also expected to increase the likelihood of academic success for the participants.

The intervention was also based on the theory that education about law, the justice system, the role of the government, and the responsibilities of individuals will develop moral reasoning and produce law-abiding citizens. It was intended to promote student understanding of society and its system of laws by showing students how they could function effectively within the law; by clarifying students' attitudes, values, and perceptions regarding law and our legal system; and by developing students' critical-thinking abilities and problem-solving skills. Through increased involvement in the school and community, adolescents were expected to see the school as an institution of legitimate authority and to believe that the institution's rules were fair.

Peer Culture Development

The Peer Culture Development (PCD) intervention involved daily group counseling meetings for a 15-week period for secondary school students (ages 14 through 17) in three Chicago public high schools from fall 1980 through spring 1983. The classes were offered as a course for which students received social studies credits. Peer Culture Development is based on the popular Guided Group Interaction (GGI; Bixby & McCorkle, 1951; McCorkle, 1952) model, which assumes that delinquents will learn to conform to conventional social rules by gaining more social rewards through conformity than through nonconformity.

This model is often used in preventive and rehabilitative settings for delinquents or persons at risk for engaging in delinquent activities. It has been used in community-based residential treatment programs (Empey & Erickson, 1974; Empey & Lubeck, 1971; McCorkle, Elias, & Bixby, 1957), in institutional correctional programs (Knight, 1969, 1970), and in school-based prevention programs (Boehm, 1976, 1977; Boehm & Larsen, 1978; Malcom & Young, 1976; M&E Associates, 1980). G. Gottfredson's (1987) review concluded that the earlier evidence for the efficacy of programs across these settings is unconvincing.

The Peer Culture Development program was delivered to classes of 15 students of a single sex. The classes were heterogeneous with respect to ethnic group, age, socioeconomic status, and conduct.

Special attention was given to composing the groups to include approximately equal numbers of students in trouble in school and students expected to provide positive role models. Project personnel were also careful to compose the groups of equal numbers of positive leaders (youths who were nominated as demonstrating leadership skills and conventional socialization) and negative leaders (youths who were nominated as demonstrating leadership skills and delinquent socialization). All Peer Culture Development participants were volunteers, although teachers and peers often referred troublesome students to the program.

All Peer Culture Development classes taught and closely adhered to the same basic tenets: (1) You do not have a right to hurt others; (2) You do not have a right to hurt yourself; and (3) You have an obligation to help others. The Peer Culture Development group leader helped students examine the problems in their lives in relation to these tenets, and helped the group encourage individuals to take responsibility for their problems and behaviors. The leaders were charged with helping students assess possible solutions to the problems in light of the basic principles.

The group began by sharing life histories. Once familiarity was established and trust began to build, the daily structure changed. Sessions began with students reporting problems they were having. Then the group consensually awarded the meeting to the student with the most serious problem. A problem-solving discussion ensued, after which the Peer Culture Development teacher summarized the salient points of the session.

Although the leader had the ultimate authority and responsibility for ensuring faithful implementation, the students themselves were primarily responsible for initiating, conducting, and properly using the process. Students quickly learned how to monitor the process. Group development was facilitated by including about five students with prior group experience in each group.

The Peer Culture Development rationale implies that delinquency occurs because many students do not believe in conventional rules, and instead subscribe to subcultural values such as seeking excitement, gaining immediate gratification, being tough, showing off, and displaying racial biases. According to the program theory, these values fail to encourage commitment to conventional goals and allow youths to shirk responsibility for their actions. The subculture is maintained because youths are seldom confronted with demands to be responsible for their actions, and because they lack conventional role models in their environments.

The Peer Culture Development intervention was intended to provide confrontation and examination of undesirable behavior and antisocial beliefs under the guidance of conventional role models. It aimed to alter peer interaction during the counseling sessions to bring about a lasting reduction in the amount of negative peer influence experienced by the youths.

The intervention is most consistent with Miller's (1958) subcultural perspective on delinquency. According to Miller, socialization in the lower-class culture centers around the "focal concerns" of trouble, toughness, smartness, excitement, fate, and autonomy. According to Miller, delinquent behavior is a natural by-product of action oriented to the lower-class subculture.

The Peer Culture Development intervention is also consistent with the differential association perspective on delinquency (Sutherland & Cressey, 1974). According to this perspective, delinquency results when individuals experience an excess of definitions favorable to law violation. Individuals learn these definitions, as well as techniques, motivations, and rationalizations for law violation, through association with delinquent peers. Peer Culture Development's emphasis on ensuring the presence of positive models in the group and on castigating members for delinquent self-revelations were attempts to alter the balance of definitions experienced by the youths.

EVALUATING THE THREE PROGRAMS

Directors of each of these three programs collaborated with us to implement their programs as experiments. This section explains these arrangements.

Random assignment from pools of eligible students to treatment and control conditions was attempted in each of the three programs. For the Positive Action Through Holistic Education experiment (D. Gottfredson, 1986), high-risk students identified through teacher referrals and the examination of academic and behavior records were randomly assigned to treatment and control conditions. Postrandomization checks indicated that the randomization resulted in equivalent treatment and control groups. In all, 468 treatment and 401 control students were assigned to the groups and participated in the experiment.

The Peer Culture Development evaluation (G. Gottfredson, 1987) involved random assignment of pools of eligible volunteer students to treatment and control conditions. The randomization was done separately for pools of male and female students in each of the following four categories: (1) negative leaders, (2) positive leaders, (3) students in trouble, and (4) conventional students. Experienced students who helped to run the groups were not included in the evaluation. Postrandomization checks showed no significant or substantial differences between the experimental and control students on any of eight personal characteristics. In all, 184 experimental and 176 control students were randomly assigned and participated in the experiment.

Random assignment was also attempted in each of the two schools implementing Student Training Through Urban Strategies. Pools of students eligible for the options class were developed through school staff and self-nominations. Researchers randomly assigned students to each experimental condition, but scheduling difficulties prevented the randomization from being fully implemented. Nonequivalent treatment and control groups resulted: Postscheduling checks showed that for the junior high school, the treatment and comparison groups were equivalent on gender, race, prior academic achievement, and socioeconomic status. The treatment students were two months older than the comparison students, however, and this difference was nearly significant ($p = .06$). For the senior high school, the groups were equivalent on prior academic achievement, age, and socioeconomic status. But the treatment group had significantly more females and more African-American students than did the comparison group. D. Gottfredson and Cook (1986) describe the experimental design in more detail and show results of postrandomization checks. In all, 120 treatment and 127 comparison students participated in the experiment.

Treatment and control students in the three programs were assessed each spring with a standard survey designed to measure delinquent behavior and the theoretical variables targeted by all of the programs. The psychometric properties of most of the measures are shown by G. Gottfredson (1984b). Measures from school and justice system records augment the self-reports. These are not parallel across projects.

Briefly, delinquent behavior was measured by student self-reports of delinquent behavior and drug involvement in the last year and by counts of police or court contacts and school suspensions.

Peer influence was a focus of the Peer Culture Development program only. It was measured by student self-reports of negative peer influence. School success/failure experiences were targeted by the Student Training Through Urban Strategies and Positive Action Through Holistic Education programs. These experiences were measured by students' reports of the rewards and punishments they experienced in school, the grades they earned in the last semester, and their actual grades from school records.

The remaining theoretical variables are collected under the heading "stakes in conformity." Positive Action Through Holistic Education focused on increasing affective attachment to others in the school, improving self-concept, and increasing commitment to conventional goals such as obtaining a high school degree and going on to college. Student Training Through Urban Strategies focused on reducing alienation. Student Training Through Urban Strategies and Peer Culture Development both tried to increase belief in the validity of rules. Attachment was measured by student self-reports of positive regard for teachers and others in the school and caring about the opinions of others in the school. Positive self-concept was measured by students' reports that they liked themselves and saw themselves as persons of worth. Commitment to school was measured by school attendance and expectations to continue schooling. Alienation was measured by the Social Integration scale which included students' reports of their sense of belonging in the school. Belief was measured by student self-reports of their belief in laws and their perceptions of themselves as law-abiding citizens.

RESULTS

A summary (abstracted from the original research reports) of the treatment-control group differences for the three programs appears in Table 14.1. The columns for Positive Action Through Holistic Education and Peer Culture Development are based on comparisons of treatment and control group means using analysis of variance. For Student Training Through Urban Strategies, the table summarizes results from analyses of covariance that controlled for each pretreatment measure for which significant treatment and control group differences were found.

Table 14.1 shows that the Positive Action Through Holistic Education treatment had little effect on delinquent behavior. (Effect sizes[1] for these measures range from 0.0 to 0.02, except for the difference favoring the control group on drug involvement—$ES = 0.23$—which is attributable to one high school in which the program was not well implemented and in which the treatment had a negative effect.)

1. For Positive Action Through Holistic Education and Student Training Through Urban Strategies, effect sizes (ES's) are equal to the difference between the means for the treatment and control groups divided by the standard deviation for the control group.

TABLE 14.1. Summary of Treatment and Control Group Differences for Three Experiments

Outcome measure	PATHE	PCD	STATUS Junior high	Senior high
Delinquent behavior				
Self-reported serious delinquency	0	−	+	++
Self-reported drug involvement	−−	−−	++	++
Official contacts	0	−	+	+
School suspensions	−	−	−	−
Delinquent associates				
Negative Peer Influence	−	−	++	++
School success/Failure experiences				
Self-reported grades	+	+	++	++
Grades from records, 82–83	+	−	++	++
Promotion rate, 82–83	+	NA	NA	NA
Promotion rate, 81–82	++	NA	NA	NA
Graduation rate, 81–82	++	NA	NA	NA
School rewards	+	+	+	++
School punishments	−	−	++	++
Stakes in conformity				
Belief in rules	0	−	−	−
Attachment to school	−	−	++	++
Social integration	−	+	+	++
Nonattendance	+	−	+	+
Educational expectations	−	+	−	+
Positive self-concept	+	0	+	++

Note. A plus sign indicates that the treatment-control group difference favored the treatment group. A minus sign indicates that the difference favored the control group. A zero indicates that no difference was found. Double plus or minus signs denote statistical significance at the $p < .05$ level or better. PATHE = Positive Action Through Holistic Education; PCD = Peer Culture Development; STATUS = Student Training Through Urban Strategies; NA = Not available.

The results summarized in Table 14.1 favor Positive Action Through Holistic Education treatment students on several measures of academic success (ES's range from 0.03 to 0.68), and these differences are statistically significant for promotion to the next grade and graduation in spring 1982. The treatment had no significant effect on delinquent associates ($ES = 0.05$) or stakes in conformity (ES's range from −0.09 to 0.06). Any increases in academic success were not accompanied by significant increases in attachment or commitment to school, or in the treatment students' self-concepts.

The Peer Culture Development program was also unsuccessful in reducing delinquent behavior. Indeed, it appears to have had an adverse effect. Treatment students reported more drug use ($p < .02$;

$\eta = 0.19$) and more serious delinquency ($p < .06$; $\eta = .17$). Police contacts and suspensions were also greater for treatment students (η's $= 0.04$ and 0.06). The two theoretical variables targeted by the Peer Culture Development program—belief and negative peer influence—also favored the control students, although these differences were not significant (η's $= 0.14$ and 0.08).

The remaining columns of Table 14.1 summarize the results for Student Training Through Urban Strategies. The treatment students reported significantly less drug involvement than the comparison students in both schools (ES's $= -0.42$ and -0.35). The self-report of serious delinquency also favored treatment students in both schools (ES's $= -0.33$ and -0.42), but was statistically significant only in the high school. Lower rates of contact with the court were also evident for treatment students in both schools (ES's $= -0.07$ and -0.18), although the difference was not statistically significant.

The program reduced negative peer influence (ES's $= -0.53$ and -0.47) and resulted in greater academic success (ES's range from 0.08 to 1.07 and average 0.62) among treatment students in both schools. The measures of stakes in conformity also favored the alternative class students in both schools, although the effects were larger for the high school. All measures except belief (ES's $= -0.04$ and -0.25) and Educational Expectations for the junior high students (ES's $= -0.27$) favored the treatment students. Effect sizes for the other social bonding measures ranged from 0.10 to 0.47 in the junior high and 0.38 to 0.75 in the senior high school. When statistical controls were applied, the high school treatment students remained significantly less alienated, were more attached to school, and had more positive self-concepts. The junior high school treatment students also were significantly more attached to school.

In summary: The program that attempted to reduce delinquency by counseling and tutoring to improve attachment, commitment, academic success, and self-concept failed to reduce delinquency or to change any of the theoretical variables it targeted (except perhaps academic achievement). The program that tried to reduce delinquency by altering beliefs in the validity of conventional rules and by promoting positive peer influence through peer group intervention also failed to reduce delinquency or to change the targeted theoretical variables. The program that altered curriculum and instructional methods to decrease alienation, increase academic success, and increase belief in law and society did reduce delinquency. It decreased alienation and increased academic success, but did not alter belief in conventional rules.

DISCUSSION

Contributions to Theory

Each of these experiments can help to refine thinking about delinquency causation. The Positive Action Through Holistic Education experiment has implications for the design of programs targeting social bonding. The results of the experiment did not disconfirm the theory on which the intervention rested because the intervention was not successful at altering most of the theoretical variables of interest: attachment, commitment, and self-concept. Stronger interventions will be required to alter these intervening variables.

The experiment did result in slight increases in academic success for the targeted students. Many theories of delinquency, including social control theory (Hirschi, 1969) and its derivatives (Elliott, Huizinga, & Ageton, 1985; Hawkins, Catelano, & Miller, in press) predict that increasing school success will reduce delinquency by increasing social bonding. The Positive Action Through Holistic Education results provide little support for this prediction. Possible explanations for the pattern of results observed include: (1) social bonding is not malleable during the secondary school years—that is, increasing school success at an earlier age might increase bonding, but by secondary school bonding is difficult to alter; (2) social bonding is malleable during this time period, but the improvements in school success observed in Positive Action Through Holistic Education were not large enough to increase bonding; or (3) social bonding is malleable during this time period, but is determined by variables other than school success.

Of these possibilities, we can tentatively reject (1) based on the Student Training Through Urban Strategies results, which implied that attachment to school did respond to experimental manipulation.

Results from the Peer Culture Development experiment also do not allow a rejection of the theory underlying the program because the program did not alter the targeted theoretical variables: belief systems and patterns of peer influence. The apparent failure to alter these intermediate outcomes came as a surprise because observations in the Peer Culture Development classes suggested that *at least during the classroom period* participating youths voiced belief in conventional rules and applied prosocial pressure to their peers. Possibly, the students altered their behavior during the class under adult influence. We have no evidence that the newly acquired behaviors extended beyond the classroom.

The experiment revealed that, whatever effect negative peer influence and subcultural belief systems may have on delinquent behavior, this Guided Group Interaction–type treatment was unsuccessful in altering these intervening variables. The only apparently successful tests of Guided Group Interaction–based programs have been tests in which other potential influences have been combined with the Guided Group Interaction treatment, introducing ambiguity about causal influences.

The Student Training Through Urban Strategies results suggest that a strong school-based program that changes the way youths are educated in school *can* reduce delinquency.[2] But what is the mechanism? The study design does not lend itself to confident interpretations of the essential features of the program, but some speculation is possible.

The results seem at least partly to support the social control, strain, and differential-association-social-learning perspectives. The intervention increased school success and attachment to school and reduced negative peer influence. It also reduced alienation and altered self-concepts in the high school. We cannot be sure what combination of these variables, if any, was responsible for the reductions in delinquency.

Student Training Through Urban Strategies increased school success experiences and attachment to school. Recall that Positive Action Through Holistic Education increased school success experiences (slightly) but did not increase attachment to school. These discrepant results may be due to differences in the strength of the programs: The Positive Action Through Holistic Education program maintained the traditional school structures and processes and provided "add-on" services to high-risk youths. But the Student Training Through Urban Strategies program altered the school structure and traditional processes in major ways. These alterations changed the daily experience of the youths, transforming them from passive recipients of educational material to active participants in the production of knowledge. Patterns of interaction with other students were also altered through the use of cooperative learning.

The increased school success observed in the Student Training Through Urban Strategies experiment was not accompanied by an

---

2. Of course, the Student Training Through Urban Strategies design was weak compared to those of the two true experiments described, and the results may reflect unmeasured and uncontrolled preexisting differences between the treatment and comparison groups. The observation that the program effects were also strong in the junior high school, where the groups appeared to be nearly equivalent, argues against spuriousness. Also, a nonexperimental evaluation of law-related education programs (Hunter, 1987; Law-Related Education Evaluation Project, 1981) found evidence that an intervention similar to the one described in this chapter reduced delinquent behavior when it succeeded at altering the key theoretical variables it targeted.

increase in commitment to future educational goals. These results lend more support to an attachment-delinquency link than to a commitment-delinquency link.

The Student Training Through Urban Strategies results also suggest that altering belief in rules or laws is not necessary for reducing delinquency. Student Training Through Urban Strategies may have worked not because it increased belief in the validity of laws but because it increased school success, liking for school, or positive peer influence. In any event, replications would be required to make any confident interpretations of these results.

Contributions to Theory-Testing Methodology

Field experiments to test academic theories of delinquency causation are difficult undertakings. Two sources of difficulty are common to measurement-based and field-based theory-testing research. These are imprecise theory statements and difficulty in constructing unique and unambiguous operationalizations of the constructs of each theory. Special problems arise, however, when theory is translated into practice in field experiments.

Common Problems

Scientists often fail to agree on how a theoretical statement should be operationalized. Some influential theorists neither suggest operations for their theoretical constructs nor state the constructs and relations in clear enough language to guide others in translating the theoretical statements into operational measures. Differential association theory is perhaps most often criticized for its lack of specificity (Cressey, 1969), but the problem is widespread. For example, strain theory is the subject of an ongoing debate over whether the theory is intended to apply to the behavior of individuals, groups, or both (Agnew, 1987; Bernard, 1987a, 1987b).

Even when theories are more carefully stated (e.g., Hirschi, 1969), ambiguities exist regarding some fine points—the timing and stability of the theoretical variables, for instance. Control theorists have not clearly specified the stage of life during which social bonds are developed or whether social bonds are characterized by stability over time or by temporal fluctuations. Perhaps the social bond is established early in life and is not malleable during adolescence. Perhaps it is malleable during adolescence, but is extremely sensitive to short-term fluctuation in the environment. These features of theoretical constructs should guide the design of studies to test the theories—the age of the study participants, frequency of measurement, for example. In the absence of clear theoretical statements, theory testers may be inclined to let the convenience or characteristics of available data dictate research designs.

The problem of imprecise theory is exacerbated in comparisons of competing theories. In the work described in this chapter, for example, we were unable to measure the social control belief construct distinctly from the subcultural socialization concept of "focal concerns." Confusion about the measurement of social control and differential association constructs abounds. For instance, Elliott, Huizinga, and Ageton (1985) noted that the same measure had been used in research as an operationalization of belief in the validity of norms (control theory) and as socialization within the delinquent peer group (learning theory). They proceeded to use that same measure to operationalize yet another theoretical construct: bonding to delinquent peers. Theories cannot be compared if they cannot be distinguished at the measurement level.

Problems Specific to Field Tests

Although field experimentation can increase the internal validity of tests of theory by introducing randomization to experimental conditions, it introduces another layer of difficulty in operationalizing theory by requiring a marriage of theory and practice. Scientists often have limited influence on the practitioners who implement the tests. Even when key decision-makers in an organization agree to alter policies and practices to enable the test of theory, myriad obstacles can undermine the test. Political interference, cultural incompatibilities, and unanticipated difficulties of a technical nature (e.g., the intervention takes longer than expected or the staff need more training than anticipated) are among the many obstacles that can thwart implementation of an agreed-upon design.

One of the biggest problems for field-based theory testing is the difficulty in getting practitioners to stick with the theory for the duration of the test. Practitioners are fickle (or scientists are inflexible) when it comes to causal theories. Whereas scientists have little difficulty focusing on a particular set of causal variables, practitioners are more likely to adopt a "bag-of-tricks" approach to problem solving—that is, to try one approach after another until they hit upon one that seems to work. They can be quick to abandon an approach that does not seem right, and quick to modify a program with the latest new idea about what works. Field tests of theory are often possible only when scientists recognize a "window of opportunity" during which practitioners are committed to an idea that happens to accord with a theory of interest.

Scientists also need to recognize that a "pure" test of an interesting theory will usually be difficult to achieve. For example, the Positive Action Through Holistic Education experiment described above targeted theoretical variables of interest (e.g., attachment to school and commitment to conventional goals). But the practitioners who owned the program believed that self-esteem is as important a contributor to delinquency as is social bonding. Hence many of the activities focused on helping the students to improve their self-images. This focus on self-esteem reduced the clarity of the test of social control theory, but it was a compromise necessary in order to conduct the test at all.

Obtaining both researcher and practitioner concord to the theory underlying an intervention is essential to the conduct of field-based theory testing. Understanding of and commitment to the theory will insulate the test, at least for a while, against fads and other pressures to do something different. Practitioner commitment to the theory can be secured using a method (PDE) that involves practitioners and scientists in a collaborative theory-generation exercise. The resulting theory will sometimes differ from the academic theory of most direct interest to the scientist, but it is likely to have much in common with the theory—and it will have a higher chance of being implemented.

Problems related to program strength (Sechrest, West, Phillips, Redner, and Yeaton, 1979) also beset field research. Program components that an organization is able to implement may be too weak to exert powerful influence on the theoretical variables of interest. In both of the ineffective experimental manipulations described in this chapter (Peer Culture Development and Positive Action Through Holistic Education), hindsight implies that the interventions may not have been of sufficient strength.

Was it reasonable to expect that offering additional counseling and tutoring services approximately once every 2 weeks to adolescents at high risk for drop-out and delinquency would produce increased social bonding? Probably not. A more plausible intervention to increase social bonding among this population might be a restructuring of the classroom environment during the early elementary years to reallocate instructional resources so that the youths with the greatest skill deficits receive more intensive assistance targeted at their specific deficiencies.

Was it reasonable to expect that a Guided Group Interaction–type classroom intervention would change the peer culture of urban high school students? Probably not. Research on the development of deviant peer groups suggests that certain youths are rejected by prosocial peers at an early age, and that these rejected youth gravitate to deviant peer groups (Coie, 1990). In light of this evidence, interventions to build social skills at an early age and that rehearse young people in controlling themselves seem more plausible than do interventions that attempt to alter the content of peer interactions in adolescence.

Unfortunately, the social service and educational agencies whose missions it is to address social problems have limited resources, and they have to settle for intervening within their means. The Positive Action Through Holistic Education and Peer Culture Development interventions are examples of unusually strong and well-focused delinquency prevention programs. They were far stronger than the intervention strategies typically found in community-based and educational agencies in the absence of generous federal funding. The problem of weak program designs is likely to continue to hinder attempts to achieve strong field tests of theory.

CONCLUSION

This chapter reviewed three experiments to illustrate the use of field experiments to test theory. Although experience implies that field experiments can be used to test theory, several conditions must be met to advance science through this mechanism. These conditions are (1) clear theoretical statements; (2) unambiguous operationalizations of the key theoretical variables; (3) distinct measurement of program outcomes (e.g., delinquency), theoretical causal variables (e.g., belief in the validity of rules, association with delinquent peers), and the strength and fidelity of implementation of the program components (without which it is impossible to separate implementation breakdown from disconfirmation of the theory); (4) experimental design that enables confident causal conclusions; (5) practitioner commitment to the theory being tested; (6) replication (because no single experiment is likely to provide an unambiguous test of a theory); and (7) strong program design consistent with the theory to be tested.

ACKNOWLEDGMENTS

The research reported in this paper was supported in part by grant no. 82-JS-AX-0037 from the National Institute for Juvenile Justice and Delinquency Prevention and grant no. R117R90002 from the Office for Educational Research and Improvement to the Johns Hopkins University.

REFERENCES

Agnew, R. (1987). On "Testing structural strain theories." *Journal of Research in Crime and Delinquency, 24,* 281–286.

Bernard, T. J. (1987a). Testing structural strain theories. *Journal of Research in Crime and Delinquency, 24,* 262–280.

Bernard, T. J. (1987b). Reply to Agnew. *Journal of Research in Crime and Delinquency, 24,* 287–290.

Bixby, F. L., & McCorkle, L. W. (1951). Guided group interaction and correctional work. *American Sociological Review, 16,* 455–459.

Boehm, R. G. (1976). *Peer group counseling: A school based juvenile diversion program.* St. Louis: Gateway Information Systems.

Boehm, R. G. (1977). *An evaluation of the Berrien County school-based delinquency prevention/diversion program: Peer group counseling (P.G.C.).* Berrien County, MI: Probate and Juvenile Court Services.

Boehm, R. G., & Larsen, R. D. (1978). *An evaluation of peer group counseling in Berrien County, Michigan 1977–78. Michigan Office of Criminal Justice Programs.* Berrien County, MI: Probate and Juvenile Court Services.

Cloward, R. A., & Ohlin, L. E. (1960). *Delinquency and opportunity: A theory of delinquent gangs.* New York: Free Press.

Coie, J. D. (1990). Towards a theory of peer rejection. In S. R. Asher & J. D. Coie (Eds.), *Peer rejection in childhood.* New York: Cambridge University Press.

Coleman, J. S. (1961). *The adolescent society.* New York: Free Press of Glencoe.

Cressey, D. R. (1969). Epidemiology and individual conduct. In D. R. Cressey & D. A. Ward (Eds.), *Delinquency, crime and social process.* New York: Harper and Row.

Elliott, D. S., Huizinga, D., & Ageton, S. S. (1985). *Explaining delinquency and drug use.* Beverly Hills, CA: Sage.

Empey, L. T., & Erickson, M. L. (1974). *The Provo experiment: Evaluating community control of delinquency.* Lexington, MA: Lexington Books.

Empey, L. T., & Lubeck, S. G. (1971). *The Silverlake experiment: Testing delinquency theory and community interventions.* Chicago: Aldine.

Gottfredson, D. C. (1986). An empirical test of school-based environmental and individual interventions to reduce the risk of delinquent behavior. *Criminology, 24,* 705–731.

Gottfredson, D. C., & Cook, M. S. (1986, October). *Increasing school relevance and student decisionmaking: Effective strategies for reducing delinquency?* Paper presented at the annual meeting of the American Society of Criminology, Atlanta.

Gottfredson, G. D. (1984a). A theory-ridden approach to program evaluation. *American Psychologist, 39*(10), 1101–1112.

Gottfredson, G. D. (1984b). *Effective School Battery: User's manual.* Odessa, FL: Psychological Assessment Resources.

Gottfredson, G. D. (1987). Peer group interventions to reduce the risk of delinquent behavior: A selective review and a new evaluation. *Criminology, 25*(3), 671–714.

Hawkins, J. D., Catalano, R. F., & Miller, J. Y. (in press). Risk and protective factors for alcohol and other drug problems in adolescence and early adulthood: Implications for substance abuse prevention. *Psychological Bulletin.*

Hirschi, T. (1969). *Causes of delinquency.* Berkeley and Los Angeles: University of California Press.

Hunter, R. M. (1987). Law-related educational practice and delinquency theory. *International Journal of Social Education, 2*(2), 52–64.

Knight, D. (1969). *The Marshall program assessment of a short-term institutional treatment program: 1. Parole outcome and background characteristics* (Report No. 56). Sacramento: California Youth Authority.

Knight, D. (1970). *The Marshall program assessment of a short-term institutional treatment program: 2. Amenability to confrontive peer-group treatment* (Report No. 59). Sacramento: California Youth Authority.

Law-Related Education Evaluation Project. (1981). *Law-related education evaluation project: Final report, phase II, year 1.* Boulder, CO: Center for Action Research.

Malcom, P. J., & Young, I. C. (1976). *Evaluation: Positive peer culture program* (Instruction Research Report No. 1975-10). Omaha, NE: Department of Human-Community Relations Services, Omaha Public Schools.

M & E Associates (1980). *Peer culture development, Chicago: Final report.* Chicago, IL: Author.

McCorkle, L. W. (1952). Group therapy in the treatment of offenders. *Federal Probation, 16,* 22–27.

McCorkle, L. W., Elias, A., & Bixby, F. L. (1957). *The Highfields story.* New York: Holt.

Miller, W. B. (1958). Lower class culture as a generating milieu of gang delinquency. *Journal of Social Issues, 14,* 5–19.

Sechrest, L., West, S. G., Phillips, M. A., Redner, R., & Yeaton, W. (1979). Introduction. In L. Sechrest, S. G. West, M. A. Phillips, R. Redner, & W. Yeaton (Eds.), *Evaluation studies review annual* (Vol. 4, pp. 15–35). Beverly Hills, CA: Sage.

Sutherland, E. H., & Cressey, D. R. (1974). *Principles of criminology* (7th ed.). Philadelphia: Lippincott.

◆ ——— ◆

CHAPTER 15

Intensive Supervision of Status Offenders:
Evidence on Continuity of Treatment Effects for Juveniles and a "Hawthorne Effect" for Counselors

KENNETH C. LAND
PATRICIA L. MCCALL
JAY R. WILLIAMS

Prior to the passage of the federal Juvenile Justice and Delinquency Prevention Act in 1974, status offenders (also termed undisciplined juveniles or undisciplined youths) in many U.S. states—North Carolina, in particular—had been subjected to commitment to state training schools and detention in local jails.[1] Part of the deinstitutionalization movement of the past 2 decades, this act tied the receipt of federal funds for juvenile justice programs to the removal of status offenders from institutions that treat juveniles and/or adults who violate the criminal code.

The response in North Carolina has been a sequence of governmental acts to address to the needs of its status offender population in

1. By statutory definition, a *status offender* in North Carolina is a juvenile less than 16 years of age who (1) has run away from home (i.e., is a *runaway*), (2) is unlawfully absent from school (i.e., is a *truant*), (3) is regularly disobedient to her/his parent, guardian, or custodian and beyond their disciplinary control (i.e., is *ungovernable*), or (4) is regularly found in places where it is unlawful for a juvenile to be.

the juvenile court. In 1977, the North Carolina Legislature enacted House Bill 456, which eliminated, as a dispositional alternative, commitment of status offenders to the state training schools. This bill also provided for appropriation of funds to create community-based programs to respond to the needs of the juvenile population. In its 1987 legislative session, the North Carolina Legislature appropriated funds to continue for 2 years an intensive juvenile probation program established in 1985 and to expand it to include, on an experimental basis, the intensive protective supervision of status offenders. The appropriation also included provision for an independent study and evaluation of the intensive protective supervision program.

The appropriation was approved and the project—henceforth known as the North Carolina Court Counselors' Intensive Protective Supervision Project (IPSP)—was implemented on 1 November 1987, under the direction of the Juvenile Services Division of the Administrative Office of the Courts, State of North Carolina. As compared to regular procedures for juvenile court protective supervision of status offenders, intensive protective supervision involves more extensive and proactive contact between the court counselor, the status offender, and the status offender's family. The basic idea is that through the intensive supervision and provision of professional services to status offenders it may be possible to decrease the rate of occurrence of additional status offenses and the likelihood that the youths will commit more serious delinquent offenses.

From October 1987 through November 1988 responsibilities for project-evaluation research design, implementation, and reporting belonged to members of the staff of the National Center for Juvenile Justice in Pittsburgh, Pennsylvania. From December 1988 through May 1991 the present authors were responsible for a continuing evaluation.[2] In each case, the evaluators were independent of, and external to, the project management staff of the Juvenile Services Division of the North Carolina Administrative Office of the Courts.

Results of our evaluation of the operation and outcome of the IPSP through May 1989 were published in Land, McCall, and Williams (1990). Based on a statistical and field-based evaluation, these results suggested that intensive supervision was quite successful in achieving some of its goals for those undisciplined youths who had not previously been charged with delinquent offenses.

This chapter updates and extends our previously published evaluation report on the IPSP. The next section offers a brief description

2. Land and McCall worked on the evaluation project through May 1991; Williams through May 1990.

of the design of the project and its youth clients. The third section updates our statistical analysis of outcomes of the IPSP for those youths who were treated during the first year-and-a-half of the project, including both supervision-period and cumulative (supervision period plus 1-year follow-up) results. The fourth section describes outcomes of the project for those youths who were treated during the second year-and-a-half of the IPSP. The fifth section reports our conclusions.

Without trying to give the full detail of our analyses, suffice it to say that we continue to find evidence that the intensive supervision of status offenders "worked" during the early part of the IPSP. But we also find that the impacts of the intensive treatment deteriorated during the later phases of the IPSP. We assess the plausibility of various hypotheses to explain these findings.

DESCRIPTION OF THE PROJECT

A detailed description of the Intensive Protective Supervision Project was published in Land et al. (1990). The essentials will be reviewed here.

Project Goals

The general mission of the experimental project was to evaluate and address the reasons for continued undisciplined acts toward the end of reducing such negative behavior and increasing constructive behaviors. Specific objectives were that the juvenile clients not become delinquent, that undisciplined acts cease, and that the juvenile display more socially acceptable behaviors.

Expected Treatment Impacts

The IPSP is predicated on the proposition that, by the time a juvenile has come under the court's jurisdiction for status offenses, he or she almost surely has a substantial prior history of "continued" undisciplined acts. Moreover, an implicit "delinquent careers" model underlies the IPSP, that is, a model in which juveniles charged with status offenses are more likely to commit delinquent acts than are juveniles who have not been charged with either status or delinquent offenses but less likely to commit delinquent acts than are juveniles who have been charged with delinquent offenses or both delinquent and status offenses.

Land et al. (1990) surveyed a number of extant studies of status offenders to ascertain the extent to which this model is plausible. Based on this review, they concluded that the following general bounds on the per-year prospective probabilities of delinquent offenses (i.e., both felony and misdemeanor violations as distinct from status offenses) are reasonable as a baseline for youths not in an intensive treatment program: for an initial delinquent charge for youths not previously charged with either status or delinquent offenses, 5% to 15%; for youths previously charged only with status offenses, 20% to 40%; for youths previously charged with delinquent or both delinquent and status offenses, 40% to 60%.

Land et al. (1990) also reviewed previous research to formulate expectations about the likelihood of success of the IPSP in achieving its stated objectives. They noted that the controversial exchange of R. Martinson and T. Palmer over Martinson's mid-1970s review of evaluation studies of correctional programs (Martinson, 1974; Palmer, 1975, 1978) resulted in the conclusion that intensive probation supervision for younger offenders works in the sense of reducing the probability of additional serious offenses. The subject of these studies was the *intensive probation* of juveniles who had committed more serious offenses and had been adjudicated delinquent rather than the *intensive protective supervision* of status offenders (there are no evaluation studies of the latter). Nonetheless, Land et al. (1990) argued that the latter might be expected—because of structural similarities in the treatment procedures—to have impacts on the probability of subsequent delinquent offenses similar to the former. But they also noted previous research evidence (Walker, 1989, p. 213) of a "goldfish bowl" effect, the tendency of officials in charge of intensive probation to be more aware of "technical violations" of the conditions of the probation because of the more extensive contact involved in intensive as compared to regular probation and the corresponding tendency to cite the clients for technical violations of the conditions of probation. In the context of the IPSP, this goldfish effect could result in an apparent failure of the intensive treatment procedure to reduce the rate of continued status offenses of juveniles compared to that of juveniles in regular protective supervision.

Project Sites and Experimental Design

From the outset, the IPSP was designed to serve juvenile clients on a randomly assigned basis at multiple sites in North Carolina. Four juvenile court sites participated in the project from 1 November 1987 through May 1991: Wake County/Raleigh, Guilford County/Greensboro, Cabarrus and Rowan Counties/Concord, and Salisbury and Buncombe County/Asheville. Beginning 1 November 1989, the project and its evaluation were expanded to four new sites: New Hanover County/Wilmington, Alamance County/Graham, Wilkes County/ Wilkesboro, and Gaston County/Gastonia. These sites were chosen to satisfy several criteria, including both urban and rural representation, sufficient professional service resources within the district to support the project, support of the juvenile court judges within the district, and strong enthusiasm and leadership within the district for the project.

Any youth adjudicated undisciplined in the experimental sites during the operative period of the project who received a protective supervision disposition and who was not already under the court's supervision for a delinquent or undisciplined offense was a potential client of the IPSP. Potential clients were put into a pool from which experimental and control groups were randomly assigned. The experimental (treated) group was assigned to intensive protective supervision (IPS); the control (comparison) group was assigned to regular protective supervision (RPS). Field observations suggest that the random assignment procedure, which was described in great detail in the project manual, was administered correctly.

It was recognized by IPSP supervisors that vacancies could occur within the experimental and control groups from time to time due to a number of possible factors:

- The client *successfully completed* the assigned (intensive or regular) supervision program;
- The client *aged-out* in the sense of being in the program the maximum allowable time (1 year, although extensions occasionally are granted by a juvenile court judge) or having reached age 16;
- The client was *adjudicated delinquent* on a subsequent petition resulting in a change of status;
- The client *moved out* of the district; or
- There was *self-exclusion* due either to the client's or her/his family's refusal to continue participation or to the judge's determination that the client should be discontinued in the program because of her/his lack of cooperation.[3]

3. Attrition due to client youths moving out of the district in which they were assigned to protective supervision might reasonably be expected to vary randomly between the experimental and control groups. The possibility of attrition due to self-exclusion, however, raises the question of whether there was differential attrition

When vacancies occurred for any of these reasons, the corresponding cases were closed and the random selection process for replacements resumed.

Intensive Treatment Procedures

As compared to regular procedures for juvenile court protective supervision of status offenders, IPS involves more extensive and proactive contact between the IPS counselor, the status offender, and the status offender's family. Caseloads are much lower: no more that 10 concurrent cases as compared to 35 to 50 in RPS. Because of their reduced caseload, IPS counselors have more time available to work with the family and not just the youth, and to deal with situations (including crisis intervention) as they develop. In addition, IPS counselors were given authority to contract for professional evaluation and service delivery (e.g., by a child psychologist or a family therapist).

The core idea of IPS is that through intensive supervision and the provision of professional analytic or therapeutic services (such as cognitive or counseling services) to status offenders and their families, it may be possible to decrease the rate of occurrence of additional undisciplined acts as well as the likelihood that the youths will commit more serious (delinquent) offenses. The IPS treatment procedure ideally comprises a six-step process: (1) initial testing and evaluation (after random assignment) by the IPS counselor through meeting(s) with the juvenile and her/his parent(s) or guardian(s); (2) external evaluation by an expert (e.g., child psychologist or mental health expert) to identify areas of need and service providers; (3) an interdisciplinary team meeting (chaired by the IPS counselor) to discuss the case and its services; (4) development of a service plan, including selection of the most important desired behavioral changes (e.g., more consistent school attendance, improved interactions with family members), behavioral objectives (e.g., reduce the number of truancy periods, reduce the number of incidents that the youth curses and/or yells at her/his mother), and identification of resources to achieve these objectives; (5) service delivery and monthly updates; and (6) case closing through one of the outcomes identified above.

Information from field observations of the IPSP reported in Land

---

between the experimental and control groups—which could bias inferences about treatment effects. Both statistical and field-based data reported in Land et al. (1990) and in Land and McCall (1991) suggest that differential attrition due to self-exclusion was not a problem in the IPSP.

et al. (1990) suggests that these ideal procedures were reasonably well approximated in practice. IPS counselors came to view assessment as an ongoing process with needs and objectives changing as they became intensively involved in a case. Objectives changed because close scrutiny of a youth's family often revealed more dysfunction than was originally identified. For example, by spending more time with the youth and visiting in the home, the counselor could discover a parent's alcoholism that might have been kept hidden if the counselor had visited less frequently.

The actual delivery of services typically involved some combination of professionals/specialists (e.g., for individual and/or family counseling/therapy or assistance with school-related problems) and home visits by the IPS counselors. After initial frequent home visits (often on a daily basis), counselors reported that, on average, they made one or two home visits per week for each client. Counselors reported that the advantage of these more frequent visits (than in RPS) is that it allows them to understand critical aspects of the juvenile client's behavior more quickly by observing the juveniles and their families in the home setting. In the home visits, the IPS counselors (1) check on the progress of their clients, (2) observe family conditions that may facilitate or hinder client progress, (3) broker community services to the clients and their families, (4) provide support to the parents to encourage them to take control of their families (called "empowering"), and (5) model appropriate behaviors for the clients and their families. In sum, the frequent home visits and family counseling orientation makes the approach of the IPS counselors uniquely different from the casework of the RPS counselors.

Intensive Counselors

IPS counselors were selected on the basis of willingness to work intensively with a chronic status offender caseload. Initially, counselors at the four original sites were given training only with respect to the rules and forms of the project and its evaluation. Because of the perceived regularity of occurrence of a relationship of family dysfunction to status offending behavior (noted above), however, IPS counselors came to believe that the program's intervention often must be family-focused, intensive, and quickly dispatched. This perception led the IPS counselors at the initial four experimental sites to request training in family therapy techniques. In response, training in "structural family therapy" was provided on two occasions, May 1988 and December 1988.

Project Clients

A detailed statistical description of demographic and court-related characteristics of the youth clients (assigned to both experimental and control groups) assigned to the IPSP was given in Land et al. (1990). Although more than twice as many youths were assigned to the program by its end in May 1991, the frequency distributions of these client characteristics remained much the same. In particular, the *modal youth* who participated in the program was a *female* (about 70% of the total), *age 14 at assignment* to protective supervision (about 40% of the total with roughly 30% less than age 14 and 30% greater than age 14 at assignment), *nonblack* (about 70% of the total), and referred to the court for *runaway* behavior (about 53%, with truancy accounting for about 31%, and ungovernable behavior account for 16% of the total). About 80% of the youths had no prior court referrals for *status offenses*, 13% had one previous referral, and the remainder had two or three prior referrals. By comparison, about 90% had no prior court referrals for *delinquent violations*, 7% had one previous referral, and 2% had two or three such prior referrals.

Of juveniles who participated in the IPSP, approximately equal numbers were assigned to the experimental and control groups—as one would expect if the random assignment procedure were functioning properly. Also, the frequency distributions of the youths by the foregoing demographic and court-related characteristics are roughly equivalent between the two groups. The only significant exceptions to this statement are that there were slightly more youths in the experimental group who had two or more prior court referrals for status offenses and similarly who had two or more delinquent offenses. In brief, the experimental group appears to have had slightly more relatively "tough" cases than the control group.

TREATMENT EFFECTS DURING THE EARLY PERIOD OF THE PROJECT

Supervision-Period Effects

To evaluate the extent to which the IPSP achieved its objectives *during the period under which its client youths were assigned to protective supervision*, measurements on three outcome variables were available for youths in both the experimental (IPS) or control (RPS) groups. The first of these, denoted DELOFF, was computed as the percentage of cases in the group that had one or more referrals to the juvenile court for delinquent acts during the supervision period. The second, denoted STATOFF, refers to the percentage of cases in the group that had one or more status offenses reported during the supervision period. A third outcome variable, denoted SUCCESS, refers to the percentage of cases in the group for which the counselor's judgment was that "overall" the client successfully completed the supervision period. Note that these summary judgments were based not only on such externally applied criteria as whether a youth client was charged with a delinquent or status offense but also on many other dimensions of cooperation and progress during the period of protective supervision. Indeed, field observations suggested that some court counselors judged "any significant progress whatsoever" in achieving the behavioral objectives of the service plan on the part of a youth under protective supervision as constituting "success."

Before examining data based on these variables, we should note that our analyses of the delinquency and status outcome variables are based on the presumptions that juvenile court referrals of these offenses either have been accurately and completely reported for youths who participated in both the experimental and control groups, or, if the records are incomplete, that they do not reflect a differential bias toward either group. That is, if offense reports are missing, we presumed that they are missing in a random fashion for both groups. We have no way of knowing with certainty whether this is a valid presumption; indeed, it probably is impossible to know in some absolute sense. On the other hand, efforts were made by Administrative Office of the Courts personnel to ensure an accurate and complete reporting of all offense reports for youths in the IPSP, and field observations did not give any cause to suspect differential bias. Accordingly, in the absence of information to the contrary, we believe that the inferences made below are not artifacts of differential reporting.

With respect to each of these outcome variables, Table 15.1 reports estimates of mean effects of the experimental versus control treatment for the "early" period of the IPSP—namely, cases that had participated in the program and that were closed (for any of the reasons for case closure listed above) in approximately the first year-and-a-half (between November 1987 and June 1989).[4] In addition to

4. The means (percentages) and mean differences reported in Panel A of Table 15.1 differ slightly from those previously published in Panel A of Table 4 of Land et al. (1990) due to the presence of three additional cases in the control group of the present table and to some corrections of the data files that have been made since publication of our original research report. However, these differences do not alter the substantive inferences previously made for the outcome variables.

TABLE 15.1. Period of Supervision Means (Percentages) on Seven Outcome Variables for Cases Closed by June 1989—Experimental and Control Groups Compared

Outcome variables	Means in experimental group	Means in control group	Differences of means	t-statistics (one-tailed p values)
	A: Original outcome measures			
DELOFF	7.1	25.9	−18.8	−2.59 (p < .01)
STATOFF	26.2	27.8	−1.6	−0.17 (p > .25)
SUCCESS	65.0	45.3	−19.7	1.92 (p < .05)
	B: Breakdowns of original outcome measures			
Felony	0.0	1.9	−1.9	−1.00 (p < .20)
Nonfelony	7.1	24.1	−16.9	−2.38 (p < .01)
Runaway	21.4	22.2	−0.8	−0.09 (p > .25)
Truancy	7.1	9.3	−2.1	−0.37 (p > .25)
n	42	54		

the group means and mean differences (experimental minus control), the table also displays the corresponding t statistics for the difference-of-means tests and an indication of the corresponding levels of statistical significance (on a one-tailed test because directional hypotheses have been specified). Because the randomization of assignment has made the experimental and control groups approximately statistically equivalent except for the treatment, mean differences that are not attributable to chance variability can be attributed to the effects of treatment.

Previously, Land et al. (1990) noted that the experimental treatment of the IPSP appeared to "work" only for those youths in the program who had not been referred to the juvenile court for delinquent acts prior to being assigned to protective supervision. All subsequent observations and analyses during the period of the IPSP were consistent with this conclusion. Accordingly, the three outcome variables in Panel A of Table 15.1 (and all subsequent comparisons discussed in this chapter) are defined for youths who meet this criterion.

As the results presented in Table 15.1 indicates, 7.1% of the 42 closed cases in the experimental group (IPS) were referred to the juvenile court for one or more delinquent offenses (DELOFF) versus 25.9% of the 54 closed control-group (RPS) cases. This yields a mean difference of 18.8% between the two groups, a difference that is well beyond the .01 level of statistical significance on a one-tailed test. By comparison, the mean difference of the two groups on the status offense variable (STATOFF) is less than 2 percentage points, which is not statistically significant. Regarding the court counselor's judgments of whether a client youth successfully completed the protective supervision period (SUCCESS), however, the experimental group scores 65% successful versus about 45% of the control group. This yields a mean difference of 19.7%, which is statistically significant at the one-tailed .05 level.

Because of the possibility of heterogeneity in the outcome measures of Panel A of Table 15.1, Panel B reports experimental and control group comparisons for more refined outcome measures. In particular, the DELOFF outcome variable is disaggregated into Felony and Nonfelony categories in Panel B, where offenses in the former are statutorially defined criminal violations and the latter includes misdemeanors, traffic offenses, and violations of city ordinances (the majority are misdemeanors). Similarly, Panel B disaggregates the STATOFF outcome variable into Runaway and Truancy categories.

An examination of the results in Table 15.1 shows that the primary effect of the treatment procedure on delinquent offenses was concentrated in the Nonfelony category. Rates of referrals for Felony offenses are very low for both the experimental and control groups, although the difference of means is in favor of the experimental group. By comparison, the lack of a significant difference between the two groups for the STATOFF outcome variable noted above also applies to each of the components (Runaway and Truancy) in Panel B. Again, however, the differences of means in these outcome categories show that the experimental group had slightly lower status offense recidivism rates during protective supervision.

In brief, the results reported above indicate that, during the early period of the IPSP, the treatment (IPS) procedures had the desired outcomes of reducing the probability that a youth client would be referred to the juvenile court for a delinquent (nonfelony) act while under protective supervision and increasing the probability that the youth would be judged by the court counselor as having successfully completed the protective supervision program. On the other hand, although the direction of mean differences is in favor of IPS relative to RPS for two status offense types (runaways and truants), IPS is not significantly more effective overall than RPS in reducing the probability that a client youth will be cited for a status offense while under supervision.

Cumulative Effects

Note that the results reported above pertain only to outcomes during the period of protective supervision. In her discussion of Land et al. (1990), which similarly was limited to supervision-period outcomes, McCord (1990) noted this limitation and the fact that previous studies of a variety of behavior modification programs have shown that benefits from treatments often fade when treatment ends. McCord (1990, p. 614) then raised the possibility that "youths assigned to IPS have merely delayed their antisocial activities" and called for a longer-term follow-up evaluation of the effectiveness of intensive protective supervision. Table 15.2 responds to McCord's suggestion by exhibiting the means (percentages), mean differences, and t-statistics parallel to those of Table 15.1 for a *cumulative period of evaluation* that includes the period of protective supervision for each youth client plus a 1-year follow-up period after her/his case closing date.

It can be seen that the results contained in Table 15.2 are broadly similar to those reported in Table 15.1. First, in Panel A the treatment (IPS) group continued to display a delinquent offense referral rate (DELOFF) substantially and significantly lower than that of the control (RPS) group, but the status offense recidivism rates (STATOFF) of the two groups were of comparable levels. Second, in Panel B the treatment impacts on the delinquent offense rate continued to be concentrated in the Nonfelony category. Third, the cumulative Runaway recidivism rates of the two groups continue to be of the same order of magnitude. But the experimental group shows a cumulative Truancy recidivism rate that is considerably lower (but not statistically significant) than does the control group. Thus, while not reaching conventional levels of statistical significance, IPS appears to have a cumulative effect on one of the status offense categories that is in the direction of a lower rate of offending—the objective of the IPSP.

TREATMENT EFFECTS DURING THE LATER PERIOD OF THE PROJECT

Deterioration of the Treatment Effects

Our story would be simple if the evaluation results ended with Tables 15.1 and 15.2. We would conclude that, relative to regular protective

TABLE 15.2. Cumulative Means (Percentages) on Seven Outcome Variables (for Period of Supervision and 1 Year after Closing Date) for Cases Closed by June 1989—Experimental and Control Groups Compared

Outcome variables	Means in experimental group	Means in control group	Differences of means	t-statistics (one-tailed p values)
A: Original outcome measures				
DELOFF	14.3	35.2	−20.9	−2.45 ($p < .01$)
STATOFF	31.0	35.2	−4.2	−0.43 ($p > .25$)
B: Breakdowns of original outcome measures				
Felony	2.4	3.7	−1.3	−0.38 ($p > .25$)
Nonfelony	11.9	31.5	−19.6	−2.40 ($p < .01$)
Runaway	26.2	25.9	0.3	0.03 ($p > .25$)
Truancy	7.1	13.0	−5.8	−0.95 ($p > .20$)
n	42	54		

supervision, intensive protective supervision appears to have the desired effects on the delinquency and success outcome variables during the period of supervision and that the effects on delinquency appear not to fade after treatment ends. However, we continued to evaluate the outcomes of the IPSP as it progressed through the second and third years and moved beyond the original four experimental sites to encompass four additional sites (beginning in November 1989). During this "later" period of the project, we noted evidence of a tendency toward deterioration of the effectiveness of the experimental treatment in periodic updates of outcome data. Specifically, relative to RPS, IPS seemed to have been more effective for youth clients who were under protective supervision during the first year-and-a-half of the project (roughly November 1987 to June 1989) than for those who were under supervision during the second year-and-a-half (roughly June 1989 through December 1990).[5] In other words, mean differences

5. Although the full period of the IPSP was 3½ years (from November 1987 through May 1991), the "early" and "late" periods compared in this chapter encompass only the 3-year period from November 1987 through December 1990. This is due to the fact that the full period of the project had not been monitored as of the writing date of this

TABLE 15.3. Cross-Tabulations of Delinquent Offense Outcome Variable by Experimental vs. Control Group for Four Original Sites Only: Early (First Year and a Half) and Late (Second Year and a Half) Comparison

Outcome variable	Experimental	Control
Early		
No delinquent offenses	27	17
	(90.0%)	(56.7%)
One or more delinquent offenses	3	13
	(10.0%)	(43.3%)
Total	30	30
Late		
No delinqent offenses	19	18
	(63.3%)	(60.0%)
One or more delinquent offenses	11	12
	(36.7%)	(40.0%)
Total	30	30

on the outcome variables were larger for the "early" project participants than for the "late" participants.

One mode of analysis of these changes is displayed in Table 15.3 which contains cross-tabulations of the DELOFF outcome variable (supervision-period only) for the first 30 closed cases in each of the experimental and control groups in the top panel and for the last 30 closed cases in each group in the bottom panel (to maximize comparability, only cases from the four original experimental sites are included in the table). As all of the 60 cases in the top panel were under protective supervision during the first year-and-a-half of the project and all 60 cases in the bottom panel similarly were under supervision during the second year-and-a-half, these cross-tabulations are appropriate for assessing "early" versus "late" effectiveness of IPS relative to RPS.

The top panel of Table 15.3 indicates that, relative to the goal of reducing delinquent court referrals of youths under protective supervision, the experimental treatment was quite effective during the early period of the project: the ratio of youths who completed supervision with no delinquent referrals to those with one or more referrals was 9.0 (90% to 10%) in the early experimental group as compared to 1.31 (56.7% to 43.3%) in the early control group. By contrast, the

chapter in spring 1991. Because only a relatively small number of additional cases remained to be closed between January and May 1991, however, this will not have much impact on the final outcomes of the project.

corresponding ratio in the late experimental group was 1.72 (63.3% to 36.7%) and that in the late control group was 1.5 (60% to 40%). While not included in Table 15.3, cross-tabulations of the SUCCESS outcome variable showed similar patterns of change for "early" versus "late" comparisons.

These changes in outcome ratios are due both to an increase in the effectiveness of the control (RPS) treatment and a decline in the effectiveness of the experimental (IPS) treatment over the full 3 years of the project.

The decreased delinquent offending rate in the control group is consistent with field-based observations and interviews in early 1990. These observations and interviews suggested a "trickle-down effect" in that some RPS counselors were attempting to use "experimental" methods in their work. Some diffusion of knowledge about these procedures (through professional diagnosis, team meetings, behavioral objectives, family therapy, etc.) across the IPS and RPS counselor lines apparently was inevitable, as both types of counselors worked within the same juvenile court facilities in the experimental sites. After the first 2 years of the project, in fact, all counselors at some sites began using "behavioral objectives" as an approach to dealing with their youth clients. In addition, during the springs of 1989 and 1990, the Administrative Office of the Courts held regional workshops at various locations around the state for all juvenile court counselors. At these workshops counselors (including RPS counselors) were able to choose from a variety of sessions on various analytic and therapeutic techniques, including sessions on "structural family therapy." Thus, it is possible that some RPS counselors received training in family therapy techniques similar to those in which the IPS counselors were schooled.

The increased delinquent offending rate in the experimental group in the "late" period of the IPSP could be due to one or more of several factors, such as:

1. Staffing changes among the IPS counselors at two of the original four sites;
2. Changes in the characteristics of the youths assigned to protective supervision from the "early" to the "late" period of the project, including a greater awareness of (and discounting about the "seriousness" of) the Intensive Protective Supervision treatment procedures among juvenile status offending populations in experimental site areas;
3. Some decline in enthusiasm among the IPS counselors as the novelty of the IPS process declined and the program became a

routinized part of the juvenile court bureaucracy (an outcome not unheard of in human services experiments); and/or
4. Other systematic factors of which we are not aware.

It is, of course, impossible to rule out hypothesis 4, and we do not have a sufficiently rich body of data on the IPSP to definitively assess hypotheses 1, 2, and 3. We can, however, bring some evidence to bear on each of these alternatives.

To examine the possibility that hypothesis 1 could account for the changes observed above, we computed cross-tabulations like those in Table 15.3 for a site (Raleigh) that had stable and experienced staffing of the IPS counselor position throughout the project. Again, effectiveness declined for the "late" experimental period as compared to the "early" period. A further cross-tabulation of outcome variables for all closed cases from two districts with stable staffing throughout the 3-year project period (Raleigh and Asheville) versus two districts that experienced some personnel changes (Greensboro and Concord/Salisbury) suggests that stability in counseling staff might account for a small part of the change in outcome effectiveness but not much.[6]

Our data base for the evaluation does not permit a detailed examination of the plausibility of hypothesis 2. Nonetheless, field reports from chief court counselors in the original four experimental sites suggested that the youth clients of the project during the "late" period were "not different" from those of the "early" period.

To examine the plausibility of hypothesis 3, we note first that, during the first year-and-a-half of the IPSP, intensive counselors at the four original sites received regular visits and communications from the project supervisory staff in the Administrative Office of the Courts as the project was formed, routines were worked out, paperwork was established and explained, and so forth. In addition, during the first year, they received attention and monthly visits from the field staff of the initial project evaluators. Finally, as noted earlier, training of the intensive counselors in "structural family therapy" was provided in May and December 1988. Thus it is possible that all this attention during the formative phase of the IPSP led to a higher level of enthusiasm *and* effectiveness among the intensive counselors, and that when such attention diminished during the "late" period of the project enthusiasm and effectiveness declined.

To further examine this hypothesis, we computed cross-tabulations, displayed in Table 15.4, of the delinquency offense outcome

6. To conserve space, the cross-tabulations mentioned in this paragraph are not reproduced in this chapter, but are available from the authors on request.

TABLE 15.4. Cross-Tabulations of Delinquent Offense Outcome Variable for Four New Sites Only—Experimental and Control Groups Compared

Outcome variable	Experimental	Control
No delinquent offenses	18	18
	(72.0%)	(78.3%)
One or more delinquent offenses	7	5
	(28.0%)	(21.7%)
Total	25	23

variable (supervision-period only) for the 48 closed cases from the four "new" experimental sites: Gastonia, Graham, Wilkesboro, and Wilmington. As noted earlier, these four sites joined the IPSP in November 1989. In addition to instruction on experimental procedures and paperwork, IPS counselors at these four sites received training in "structural family therapy" in two 1-day workshops during January 1990. Because these start-ups occurred after the intensive program had been formed and routinized, however, it is possible that the intensive counselors at these four new sites did not receive the same level and type of attention from project supervisory staff and evaluators as counselors from the original four sites did during the "early" period of the project. If this hypothesis is valid, and if the level and type of attention given to the intensive counselors is important in the effectiveness of intensive supervision, then outcomes at the four new sites should resemble those at the four original sites in the "late" rather than the "early" period.

It can be seen that the results reported in Table 15.4 for the four new sites are entirely consistent with those noted above for the "late" period of the four original sites. That is, the experimental treatment group in Table 15.4 does not exhibit a lower delinquent offense referral rate than that of the control group. Indeed, if anything, the delinquent offense rate is higher for the experimental group than for the control group. In brief, hypothesis 3 is consistent with the observed ineffectiveness of IPS in the four "new" experimental sites.

A "Hawthorne Effect" for Counselors

In the realm of experiments involving human subjects, the tendency of outcome variables to react to *any change* in attention given to subjects is known as the "Hawthorne effect." This term is derived from the name of the site of a famous "before-and-after" study in which researchers attempted to determine the effects of varying light intensity on the productivity of women assembling small electronic parts (Roethlisberger & Dickson, 1939). It was discovered that any change in the intensity of illumination, positive or negative, produced a rise in worker output. The researchers interpreted this effect as an artifact result of conducting the research.

Nominally, the researchers were studying the effects of variations in illumination levels, but during the research there was continuous observation of work-group members by researchers stationed in the assembly room. Roethlisberger and Dickson concluded that the workers inferred from all of this attention that the firm was interested in their personal welfare. In response, the workers developed high work-group morale and increased productivity accordingly. Because productivity increased throughout the duration of the study (about 3½ years) even after workplace illumination eventually was decreased, the researchers concluded that the workers' increased productivity could not be a response to variations in the levels of lighting, but instead was due to the continuous presence of the researchers themselves.

The Hawthorne effect may be present in any study involving human subjects. Conventional randomized research designs attempt to control for the Hawthorne effect on *experimental subjects* by use of a "control group," as in the IPSP. However, as Rossi and Freeman (1989, p. 248) note, in evaluation research experiments *every* aspect of the intervention delivery system, *including the personnel who deliver the treatment process*, can affect the outcome of the intervention. In particular, based on the cross-tabulation results noted above, it may be the case that the Hawthorne effect affected the "early" versus "late" outcomes of the IPSP, not through the experimental subjects (the youth clients), but rather at another level, that of the intensive counselors. In other words, whereas the original Hawthorne effect referred to effects on the behavior of the experimental subjects, in the present study it appears that the Hawthorne effect may have operated through the counselors who delivered the intervention to the juvenile clients.

At the level of the intensive counselors themselves, the flip side of the Hawthorne effect is "counselor burnout" or decline in "extra" efforts to "save" the juvenile clients from further status offending and/or delinquent behavior. Because we were not commissioned to study the counselors, we have little direct evidence to assess this possibility. It is plausible, however, that the effects of counselor burnout would be reflected in the assigning of services to the juvenile clients by the counselors, a hypothesis for which we do have data. Significantly, Land and McCall (1991) report that, for the first 100 (i.e., early) cases (50 experimental, 50 control), intensive counselors assigned three or more professional diagnostic and/or therapeutic services to 62% of their cases, whereas regular counselors assigned three or more services to just 24% of their cases. By comparison, for the last 100 (i.e., late) cases (50 experimental, 50 control), they find that intensive counselors assigned this level of services to 42% of cases compared to 28% for the regular counselors.

This documents a slight increase in the number of services assigned by regular counselors as they presumedly attempted to adopt "intensive procedures" during the late period of the project. But, even more dramatically, these figures demonstrate a large drop in the frequency of assignment of services by the intensive counselors. Assuming that these behavioral changes in numbers of services assigned to the juvenile clients or their families reflect changes in intensive counselors efforts to change the behavior of their clients, and that the latter reflect levels of counselor enthusiasm, morale, and commitment to "save" the youths, we conclude that there was indeed some substantial level of counselor burnout in the late period of the IPSP experiment as compared to the early period.

CONCLUSION

It must be concluded that, relative to regular protective supervision, intensive supervision of status offenders was successful in achieving most of its goals during the first year-and-a-half of the IPSP. That is, whether assessed in terms of supervision period only or supervision period plus follow-up outcomes, intensive supervision "worked." However, it must also be concluded that the effectiveness of intensive supervision virtually disappeared during the second year-and-a-half of the project. Whatever the intensive treatment program "had" during the "early" part of the project appears to have been lost during the "late" phase. Put otherwise, it appears that, for intensive protective supervision to continue to be effective, whatever the program "had" during the first year-and-a-half must be recaptured.

Based on our analyses of these project outcomes, it is possible that intensive counselors must receive continuing and periodic "shots" of care and attention in order for intensive supervision to achieve maximum effectiveness. That is, in order for the objectives of intensive supervision to continue to be observed in practice, conditions of care, attention, and training for the counselors—all of which are associated with making the counselors feel "special" and "empowered to make a difference" in the lives of their youth clients and which presumedly reduce and/or protect against "counselor burnout"—may be necessary. Therefore, to achieve these objectives, it may be necessary to create a "perpetual Hawthorne effect" for the intensive counselors.

This conclusion raises a number of questions that should be followed up in subsequent research on correctional treatment. For instance, can evidence of similar Hawthorne effects on counselors be found in other intensive supervision or probation experiments? Is it possible to "institutionalize" Hawthorne effects for counselors? Or will the counselors' effectiveness inevitably deteriorate over time as they become inured to the efforts of correctional management to provide periodic stimulation? Finally, is it possible that the effectiveness of *regular* protective supervision or probation counselors could be increased by the provision of care, attention, and training? Numerous experimental efforts should be evoked by these questions.

ACKNOWLEDGMENT

The research reported here was supported, in part, by the North Carolina Administrative Office of the Courts, Juvenile Services Division. The authors, however, bear sole responsibility for the analysis and conclusions reported.

REFERENCES

Land, K. C., & McCall, P. L. (1991). The North Carolina Court Counselor's Intensive Protective Supervision Experiment, Phase III: Final evaluation report. Durham, NC: Department of Sociology, Duke University.

Land, K. C., McCall, P. L., & Williams, J. R. (1990). Something that works in juvenile justice: An evaluation of the North Carolina court counselors' intensive protective supervision randomized experimental project, 1987–1989. *Evaluation Review*, 14(6), 574–606.

Martinson, R. (1974). What works? Questions and answers about prison reform. *Public Interest*, 35(1), 22–54.

McCord, Joan (1990). Comments on "Something that works in juvenile justice." *Evaluation Review*, 14(6), 612–615.

Palmer, T. (1975). Martinson revisited. *Journal of Research on Crime and Delinquency*, 12(1), 133–152.

Palmer, T. (1978). *Correctional intervention and research*. Lexington, MA: Lexington Books.

Roethlisberger, F. J., & Dickson, W. (1939). *Management and the worker*. Cambridge: Harvard University Press.

Rossi, P. H., & Freeman, H. E. (1989). *Evaluation: A systematic approach* (4th ed.). Newbury Park, CA: Sage.

Walker, S. (1989). *Sense and nonsense about crime: A policy guide*. Pacific Grove, CA: Brooks/Cole.

PART V

◆ — ◆

CONCLUSION

◆ ──────── ◆

CHAPTER 16

The Need for Longitudinal–
Experimental Research
on Offending and
Antisocial Behavior

DAVID P. FARRINGTON

This chapter argues that there is a need for longitudinal–experimental research to advance knowledge about the explanation, prevention, and treatment of offending and antisocial behavior. In this type of research, people are followed up for some time (at least 2 or 3 years) with repeated personal contacts, a randomly chosen experimental group is then subjected to an intervention, and subsequent to this intervention all the people are followed up for a further period of at least 2 or 3 years with repeated personal contacts. In order to bring out the merits of the longitudinal–experimental method, I will first discuss the advantages and limitations of the longitudinal and experimental methods separately.

LONGITUDINAL RESEARCH

Advantages

Longitudinal data involve repeated measures of the same people. For example, a sample of individuals may be followed up from birth to age 25, with yearly data collection. In contrast, cross-sectional data involve measures at one time only. For example, 26 different samples of individuals, of each age from just after birth to age 25, may be studied at the same time.

Longitudinal and cross-sectional data can be distinguished from longitudinal and cross-sectional surveys. In particular, longitudinal data can be collected (retrospectively) in a cross-sectional survey. For example, people aged 20 may be asked to report their own offending acts in each of the last 5 years. To the extent that retrospectively collected data are inadequate or invalid (because of faulty memory, retrospective bias, or destruction of old records; see, e.g., Yarrow, Campbell, & Burton, 1970), a prospective longitudinal survey is needed to collect longitudinal data.

In the interests of clarity, the longitudinal survey of one sample from birth to age 25 will be contrasted with the cross-sectional survey of 26 different samples of individuals at each age from birth to age 25 (see also Farrington, 1991b; Farrington, Ohlin, & Wilson, 1986). The main advantages of the longitudinal survey lie in its ability to provide information about the natural history of offending and antisocial behavior, about the extent to which later outcomes are predicted by earlier factors, about developmental or causal sequences, and about the effects of specific events on the course of development.

Longitudinal and cross-sectional surveys can provide information about the "point prevalence" of offending at each age (the number of different offenders), about the frequency of offending at each age (the number of offenses committed by offenders), and hence about the peak ages for prevalence and frequency. However, only the longitudinal survey can provide information about other key features of criminal careers, notably the ages of onset of different types of offending, the ages of desistance, and the lengths of criminal careers (e.g., Blumstein, Cohen, Roth, & Visher, 1986). Establishing ages of onset and desistance requires longitudinal data showing that the behavior did not occur before or after the specified ages. Cross-sectional surveys are inadequate for establishing ages of onset and desistance, because retrospective recall is biased by current conditions. (The points made here about offending apply to other types of antisocial behavior as well.)

Only the longitudinal survey can provide information about cumulative phenomena, such as the cumulative prevalence of offending up to a certain age or the percentage of total crimes that are committed by "chronic offenders" (e.g., Wolfgang, Figlio, & Sellin, 1972). Similarly, only the longitudinal survey can provide information about sequential patterns of criminal careers, such as escalation in seriousness or specialization in types of offending over time (e.g., Farrington, Snyder, & Finnegan, 1988).

The longitudinal survey is needed to investigate stability and continuity over time. For example, individuals may exhibit consistency in their relative ranking as regards frequency or seriousness of offending, or even consistency in the absolute values of frequency or seriousness over time. A longitudinal survey is also necessary to study developmental sequences, as for example, when investigators are interested in the progression from smoking cigarettes to smoking marijuana to using illegal drugs (e.g., Yamaguchi & Kandel, 1984). The longitudinal survey is also needed to throw light on different manifestations of the same underlying theoretical construct, for example, antisocial personality, at different ages (see Farrington, 1991a). Another distinctive use of the longitudinal survey is to investigate to what degree later events can be predicted from earlier events. Information about prediction and about sequences should be useful in determining when it would be most effective to intervene to try to interrupt the development of criminal careers.

Longitudinal surveys are also needed when aggregate trends over time differ from individual trends over time. For example, the prepubertal growth spurt is often seen in individual growth curves but not in aggregate curves, because it occurs at different ages for different individuals (Bell, 1954). Similarly, the age-crime curve seems to be very different for individuals versus groups described in aggregate data. In aggregate data, offending rates show a marked peak in the teenage years, but studies of individuals show that their offending rates stay tolerably constant for as long as they are active offenders (Farrington, 1986). In this latter example, it seems that the marked peak in aggregate data reflects a peak in the prevalence of offenders, not in the frequency of offending. More generally, it is often difficult to know whether changes over time seen in aggregate data reflect changes within individuals or changes in the population at risk (e.g., due to mortality).

Perhaps the greatest importance of the longitudinal survey stems from its ability to compare the same person at different times, and hence to permit within-individual analyses of individual change. The cross-sectional survey allows only the study of variations between individuals, whereas the longitudinal survey allows the study of both *changes within* individuals and *variations between* individuals (see Farrington, 1988).

Causal effects are often inferred from variations between individuals rather than from changes within individuals. For example, a study might demonstrate that males were more likely to be offenders than females, and that this relationship held after controlling statistically for other measured variables. Some researchers would then conclude that gender was a cause of offending. However, drawing conclusions about causes, in other words, about the effect of changes *within* individuals, on the basis of variations *between* individuals, involves a conceptual leap that may not be justifiable. Interindividual differences might not correspond to intraindividual changes. Thus it is crucial to investigate how far these two approaches produce similar indications about the importance of explanatory variables. Also, the cross-sectional (between-individual) study inevitably has low internal validity because of the impossibility of measuring and controlling for all the factors that might influence the dependent variable.

Longitudinal surveys are superior to cross-sectional ones in establishing the time ordering of events. They can demonstrate causal effects by showing that changes in one factor are followed by changes in another factor, or by showing the effects of a specific event by tracking the course of development before and after that event. In studying the impact of specific events, quasi-experimental analyses of longitudinal data are desirable to draw causal conclusions with high internal validity, by eliminating plausible alternative explanations (I will return to this point later in this chapter; for a quasi-experimental study of offending, see Farrington, 1977).

Longitudinal surveys have primarily advanced our knowledge concerning the natural history of offending and antisocial behavior (see Farrington et al., 1986, chapter 2). A great deal has been learned about prevalence (e.g., Farrington, 1986), about onset (e.g., Farrington et al., 1990), about stability or continuity over time (e.g., Farrington, 1990a), and about prediction (e.g., Farrington & Hawkins, 1991). For example, Farrington (1990b) reported that the best childhood predictors of offending by males were (1) socioeconomic deprivation (low family income, large family size, poor housing); (2) poor parental child-rearing conditions (harsh or erratic discipline, parental conflict, poor supervision or monitoring, separation from a parent); (3) family deviance (convicted parent, delinquent sibling, sibling with behavior problems); (4) school problems (low intelligence, low attainment, high delinquency rate school); (5) hyperactivity-impulsivity-attention deficit (high daring, poor concentration, high restlessness); and (6) childhood antisocial behavior (troublesomeness, dishonesty, laziness).

Problems

While longitudinal studies have many advantages, they also have a number of significant limitations. An important limitation of past longitudinal studies was the infrequency of data collection, which often made it difficult to pinpoint causal order. Also, information was often collected from a very limited range of data sources, making it hard to disentangle true relationships between important theoretical constructs from artefactual ones reflecting common response biases. Data must be collected from a variety of sources to establish the reliability and validity of measures. Another problem of past studies was attrition: the loss of subjects for a variety of reasons, principally their own refusal to continue to participate or the researchers' difficulties with locating people. Fortunately, these kinds of problems have largely been overcome in modern longitudinal studies. For example, in the Pittsburgh Youth Study, data were collected from boys, mothers, and teachers every 6 months, and attrition was low (Loeber, Stouthamer-Loeber, Van Kammen, & Farrington, 1991).

Another problem of longitudinal research centers on the distinction between aging, period, and cohort effects (e.g., Baltes, Reese, & Lipsitt, 1980; Glenn, 1977). In developmental research, a cohort is defined as a group of individuals experiencing the same event (often, birth) during the same time period (often, 1 year). Cohort effects follow from membership in one cohort rather than another; for example, persons born at the peak of a "baby bulge" might suffer more intense competition for resources at several ages and in several periods (e.g., Maxim, 1985). Period effects refer to influences specific to a particular time period; for example, a period of high unemployment or economic depression might influence the crime rates of several ages and several cohorts. Aging effects refer to changes that occur with age; for example, aging eventually leads to physical deterioration for all cohorts in all periods. Researchers have only one chance to study any given cohort or period effect, but aging effects can be studied repeatedly and replicated.

Cross-sectional data confound aging and cohort effects, while longitudinal data confound aging and period effects. For example, in cross-sectional data 10 year olds may differ from 20 year olds in cohort composition (e.g., because of immigration, emigration, or deaths) as well as in age, while in longitudinal data people aged 10 in 1980 may differ from the same people aged 20 in 1990 because of changes over the time period as well as in age. Hence, in order to draw conclusions from longitudinal data about the effects of aging, it is necessary to devise some method of disentangling aging and period effects.

There are other difficulties with the single long-term longitudinal survey. Key results may be long delayed, so that a danger exists that theories, methods, instrumentation, and policy concerns may be out of date by the time the key results are published. Researchers often find it difficult to obtain the guarantee of continued funding necessary to encourage forward planning in a long-term project. It may be difficult to persuade leading researchers to devote many years of their lives to one project, and to keep a research team together for a long period. Farrington et al. (1986) and Tonry, Ohlin, and Farrington (1991) proposed to overcome age-period-cohort and time delay problems by using an "accelerated longitudinal design" in which several age cohorts were each followed up for several years.

Testing effects can also be a problem in longitudinal research (Thornberry, 1989). Perhaps the greatest weakness of existing longitudinal studies on offending and antisocial behavior is their lack of attention to questions about effects. Probably because of the focus on passively recording the natural history of development, few researchers have tried to investigate the effects of specific events on the course of development. This is unfortunate because effect studies are important in drawing conclusions about explanation, prevention, and treatment. The best way to investigate effect questions is to carry out a randomized experiment within a longitudinal study; these kinds of experiments will be discussed next.

EXPERIMENTAL RESEARCH

Advantages

An experiment is a systematic attempt to investigate the effect of variations in one factor (the independent variable) on another factor (the dependent variable). The independent variable is under the control of the experimenter; in other words, the experimenter decides which people receive which treatment (I am using the word "treatment" in a broad sense to include all kinds of interventions). The focus here is on randomized experiments, where people are randomly assigned to different treatments. Providing that a large number of people are assigned, randomization ensures that the average person receiving one treatment is likely to be equivalent (on all possible extraneous variables) to the average person receiving another treatment, within the limits of small statistical fluctuations. (Of course, it would be prudent for a researcher to check that this equivalence has indeed been achieved in any given experiment.) Hence, it is possible to isolate and disentangle the effect of the independent variable from the effect of all other extraneous variables (see, e.g., Farrington, 1983).

It is also possible to carry out randomized experiments with other units, such as schools or school classes, or even communities or areas. However, units larger than individuals are seldom so numerous that randomization would ensure equivalence of units in different conditions. In most cases, experiments with large units such as schools or communities should use some form of matching to ensure equivalence of units. Such experiments can be extremely valuable, but my focus in this chapter will be on experiments targeted on individuals.

Experiments are essentially explanatory or pragmatic: they are designed to test causal hypotheses or to evaluate the impact of different preventive interventions or treatments. Although these two aims are not necessarily incompatible, in practice most experiments fall into one or the other of these categories. Because of the difficulty of mounting randomized experiments and carrying them through successfully, such experiments should only be conducted when there is good reason (from prior nonexperimental research) to believe that the hypothesis to be tested is correct or that the treatment will be effective. Conversely, an experiment should not be carried out in the absence of an explicit hypothesis about the effect of an independent variable on a dependent one. (Useful points about experiments are also made in chapter 1 by Lee Robins in this book.)

Technically, a randomized experiment is the best method of testing and eliminating alternative explanations of apparent causal effects (or threats to internal validity; see Campbell & Stanley, 1966; Cook & Campbell, 1979). The major alternative explanations are: (1) history: the observed effect is caused by other independent variables; (2) maturation: the observed effect is part of a preexisting trend; (3) testing: the observed effect is caused by prior testing of the subjects of the research; (4) instrumentation: the observed effect is caused by changes in measurement techniques; (5) regression: the observed effect is caused by statistical regression to the mean by extreme scorers; (6) selection: the observed effect is caused by preexisting differences between the groups being compared; (7) mortality: the observed effect is caused by differential loss from the comparison groups; (8) instability: the observed effect reflects random variation; and (9) causal order: the true causal order is opposite to that hypothesized.

The only one of these alternative explanations that is typically a problem in randomized experiments is mortality, or differential loss of subjects from different experimental conditions. One way of dealing with this problem is to randomize treatments within matched pairs of subjects, and to drop both members of a pair from the experiment if one member is lost for any reason. (This discussion assumes a simple experiment with one independent variable and two experimental conditions; more complex experiments are, of course, possible, but these basic arguments are essentially unaffected by this increase in complexity.)

In contrast, these threats to valid causal inference are a great problem in nonexperimental, especially correlational, research projects. In particular, in correlational research it is impossible to measure all extraneous variables that might influence the presumed dependent variable; hence it is impossible to isolate and disentangle the causal effect of a presumed independent variable convincingly. The impact of extraneous variables is typically controlled by statistical means, but this can never be as satisfactory as experimental control, partly because of the limited number of variables included in most so-called "causal" analyses. Hence, correlational research projects inevitably have low internal validity and a poor ability to demonstrate causal effects unambiguously.

A great deal has been learned from experimental research about the prevention and treatment of offending and antisocial behavior (see Farrington et al., 1986, chapter 3). Early experiments suggested that prevention efforts in schools (e.g., Reckless & Dinitz, 1972) or communities (e.g., McCord, 1978) were ineffective. Similar results were obtained in studies of juvenile diversion (e.g., Severy & Whitaker, 1982), intensive probation (e.g., Lichtman & Smock, 1981), community treatment (e.g., Empey & Lubeck, 1971), group counseling (e.g., Kassebaum, Ward, & Wilner, 1971), therapeutic communities (e.g., Cornish & Clarke, 1975), work release (e.g., Waldo & Chiricos, 1977), and in the "Scared Straight" program designed to deter juveniles from offending (e.g., Finckenauer, 1982). However, more recent experiments have yielded more hopeful results, as is shown by the meta-analyses of Gendreau and Ross (1987) and Lipsey (1988) and indeed in other chapters of this book. Some promising interventions will be recommended later in this chapter.

Problems

Many thorny methodological problems arise in the course of randomized experiments on offending and antisocial behavior. For example, it is hard to ensure that all those in a treatment group actually receive the treatment while all those in a control group do not receive it. There is often some blurring of the distinction between treatment and control groups, leading to an underestimation of the effect of the treatment. Also, as I have already mentioned, differential attrition from treatment and control groups can lead to problems of interpretation. Another difficulty is that subjects and treatment professionals can rarely be kept blind to the experiment; such knowledge about participation in the experiment may bias outcomes or outcome measurement. Common design problems include insufficient statistical power to detect the strength of likely effects and failure to study possible interactions between types of people and types of treatments.

These methodological problems can be overcome by high-quality design and implementation.

In practice, the major problems arising in experiments are often the legal, ethical, and practical difficulties of mounting an experiment and carrying it through successfully. The literature is full of implementation failures and randomization designs that broke down (e.g., Conner, 1977), and many other failures never reached the publication stage. Hence, randomized experiments are more difficult and risky than, for example, correlational research projects.

Typically, it is only possible to study the effect of one or two independent variables, at two or three different levels (different experimental conditions) in a randomized experiment in the field (as opposed to the laboratory). For example, few of the possible causes of offending could in practice be studied experimentally, because few of the important variables associated with offending can be experimentally manipulated. It would be extremely difficult for any independent variable to build up something approximating a dose-response curve using randomized experiments. Hence, a theory of offending that was limited to results obtained in experiments would be extremely inadequate. An interesting question is how far experimental and nonexperimental projects agree about the importance of explanatory variables. The poorer control in nonexperimental research may lead to an overestimation of the importance of certain variables.

Experiments are usually designed to investigate only immediate or short-term causal effects. It is rare to find that subjects have been followed up for more than 1 year after an experiment. However, some experimental interventions may have long-term rather than short-term effects, and in some cases the long-term effects may differ from the short-term ones (e.g., Waldo & Griswold, 1979). More fundamentally, researchers rarely know what is the likely time delay between cause and effect, suggesting that measurements at several different time intervals are desirable. This and other problems of experiments can be overcome in a longitudinal-experimental study, in which experimental interventions are investigated during a long-term longitudinal project, with repeated measurement points.

LONGITUDINAL-EXPERIMENTAL RESEARCH

Advantages

Strictly speaking, every experiment is prospective and longitudinal in nature, since it involves a minimum of two contacts or data collections with the experimental subjects: one consisting of the experimental intervention (the independent variable) and one consisting of the outcome measurement (the dependent variable). However, as already indicated, the time interval covered by the typical experiment is relatively short. I will argue here that what is needed are longitudinal–experimental studies with three elements: (1) several data collections, covering several years; (2) the experimental intervention; and (3) several more data collections, covering several years, afterward. Studies of this kind have rarely been carried out on offending and/or antisocial behavior (excluding studies in which all data collections are from official statistics; I will return to this topic).

Economy is one important advantage of a combined longitudinal–experimental study in comparison with separate longitudinal and experimental projects. It is cheaper to carry out both studies with the same individuals than both with different individuals. The number of individuals and separate data collections (e.g., interviews) is greater in two studies than in one (other things being equal).

More fundamentally, the two types of studies have complementary strengths and weaknesses, and the combined longitudinal–experimental study can build on the strengths of both. For example, the longitudinal study can provide information about the natural history of development, while the experimental study will yield knowledge about the impact of interventions on development. Even if the experimental part cannot be carried through successfully, the longitudinal–experimental study still will have yielded valuable knowledge about the natural history of development, and data for quasi-experimental research on the impact of specific events. Hence, longitudinal–experimental research is less risky than experimental research alone.

Experiments are for testing hypotheses. However, in the combined project, causal hypotheses can be generated in the longitudinal study and then tested on the same individuals in the experimental study. Experiments are the best method of testing the effects of variations in an independent variable on a dependent one, whereas the longitudinal study can investigate the effect of changes in an independent variable on a dependent one. Hence, the combined project can compare the impact of variation with the impact of change, to see if the same results are obtained with the same individuals. This is an important issue, because most findings on offending and antisocial behavior essentially concern variations *between* individuals, whereas most theories and interventions refer to changes *within* individuals. The longitudinal and experimental elements are also complementary in that the experiment can demonstrate (with high internal validity) the effect of only a few independent variables, whereas the longitudinal study can demonstrate (with somewhat lower internal validity, in quasi-experimental analyses) the effect of many independent variables.

Some readers might think that an experimental study with a single pretest measure and a single posttest measure would have many of the advantages of a longitudinal–experimental study, for example, in permitting the comparison of changes within individuals and variation between individuals. However, Tonry et al. (1991, pp. 38–39) have showed how a longitudinal–experimental study was superior to a pretest-posttest study. In essence, the pretest-posttest study cannot distinguish many different outcomes, such as an immediate lasting effect of an intervention, an immediate but short-lived effect, no effect on a pre-existing trend, random oscillation, and a discontinuity in a pre-existing trend.

Some of the advantages of longitudinal–experimental research have been summarized by Blumstein, Cohen, and Farrington (1988). As I have already indicated, the impact of interventions can be better understood in the context of pre-existing trends or developmental sequences, which would help in assessing maturation, instability, and regression effects in before-and-after comparisons. The prior information about subjects would help to verify that comparison groups were equivalent, to set baseline measures, to investigate interactions between types of persons (and their prior histories) and types of treatments, to establish eligibility for inclusion in the experiment, and to estimate the impact of differential attrition from experimental conditions. The long-term follow-up information would show effects of the intervention that were not immediately apparent, facilitate the study of different age-appropriate outcomes over time, make it possible to compare short-term and long-term effects, and enable investigation of the developmental sequences linking them. The experimental intervention could help to distinguish causal or developmental sequences from different manifestations of the same underlying construct (Farrington et al., 1990).

The longitudinal–experimental method has been used most extensively in investigating medical interventions. Many clinical trials involve a long-term follow-up period. For example, in the U.S. Multiple Risk Factor Intervention Trial, 22 clinical centers examined over 360,000 male volunteers aged 35–57 and identified nearly 13,000 with the highest risk of coronary heart disease. The subjects had to undergo three extensive examinations and were then randomized to receive either "special intervention" or "usual care." The former group were seen every 4 months and received personal dietary advice, advice to stop smoking, and drugs to control hypertension (where applicable). A 6-year follow-up showed that the treatment was successful in reducing the risk factors, but that coronary heart disease mortality was only 7% lower (a nonsignificant difference) in the treatment group, largely because men in the control group also reduced their risk factors (Multiple Risk Factor Intervention Trial Research Group, 1982). These kinds of large-scale longitudinal–experimental studies have never been carried out on offending or antisocial behavior.

Problems

A major problem centers on the extent to which the experiment might interfere with the goals of the longitudinal study. In a simple experiment, some of the sample will be ineligible, some will be in the experimental group, and the remainder will be in the control group. Careful thought would need to be given to the proportions in these three groups. After the experimental intervention, it might be inadvisable to draw conclusions about the natural history of offending from the experimental group, since this group would have been treated in an unusual way. The experiment may even increase or decrease attrition from the longitudinal study. Hence, in drawing conclusions about the whole sample, results obtained with the ineligibles and controls will have to be weighted appropriately.

It is less clear that experimental subjects would have to be eliminated in investigations of effect questions using quasi-experimental analyses. If the experimental intervention could be viewed as just another independent variable impinging on the subjects, then investigations of the effect of nonmanipulated independent variables could be based on the whole sample. Of course, it might be interesting to investigate whether the impact of an independent variable differed at different levels of another independent variable (e.g., in experimental and control groups).

It could be argued that each person should receive only one experimental treatment, because of the likely effect of the treatment in making the person different from a control or an ineligible. However, there may be good reasons to investigate the interactive effect of two consecutive treatments. If the "controls" received a special treatment (e.g., being denied something that is usually available in the community), then it might even be argued that they also should not be included in a subsequent experiment. It seems unlikely that more than one or two experiments could be conducted during any longitudinal study.

The passage of time will inevitably cause problems. An experiment that was desirable and feasible at one time (e.g., at the start of a longitudinal study) may be less desirable and feasible some years later because of changes in theory or policy concerns, in methodology, or in practical constraints (e.g., a change in a "gate-keeper" such as a police chief). Also, the subjects of a longitudinal study will move around, and it may be that an experiment can only be conducted in a specific location. Hence, only subjects who are residentially stable (at least by staying in the same metropolitan area) may be eligible to participate in the experiment. For a number of reasons, the eligibility of subjects could change over time, as their personal circumstances changed. Future researchers need to develop ways of overcoming these kinds of problems in future longitudinal-experimental studies. However, it is also important to learn from the experience of existing longitudinal-experimental studies.

EXISTING LONGITUDINAL-EXPERIMENTAL RESEARCH ON OFFENDING AND ANTISOCIAL BEHAVIOR

Very few longitudinal-experimental studies of offending or antisocial behavior have included several years of personal contacts with the subjects both before and after an intervention. Some existing experiments collected official record data for several years before and after an intervention. For example, the Provo experiment (Empey & Erickson, 1972) included information about official offending in the 4 years before and the 4 years after the experiment, showing that the number of recorded offenses was very similar for those in the special community program (based on guided group interaction) and those on probation. More experimental researchers should aim to collect record data for long periods before and after the intervention, where possible.

Several studies have been carried out in which people in an experiment have been followed up, by means of personal contacts and searches of records, for many years afterward. The most important pioneering research of this kind was carried out by McCord (1978). In the Cambridge-Somerville study, the experimental boys received special counseling help between the average ages of 10 and 15, and both experimental and control groups were then followed up for over 30 years. The treatment was ineffectual in preventing offending, since about a quarter of both groups were known to have committed crimes as juveniles, while about two-thirds of both groups had been convicted as adults.

There were two major advantages of the long-term follow-up. One was that later life outcomes could be investigated. For example, more of the experimental group became alcoholics, developed mental illness, suffered from stress-related diseases, and died early. McCord (1978) tried to explain these negative effects by speculating that the intervention might have created a dependency on outside assistance, which in turn led to resentment when the assistance was withdrawn. Alternatively, the treatment program might have generated high expectations that subsequently led to feelings of deprivation when these expectations were not met.. Another possibility was that the treated group might have justified the treatment they received by perceiving themselves as being in need of welfare help. (These adverse effects are further investigated in Joan McCord's chapter in this book.) Whatever the true reason for them, the fact that welfare-oriented programs could end up damaging their clients would not have been so well documented if the follow-up period had been short.

The second major advantage of the long-term follow-up was that many important conclusions could be drawn about the natural history of offending and antisocial behavior from childhood to middle age. McCord's study would not have become so famous if it had been merely an experiment with negative results, however well the experiment had been conducted. The fact that McCord (1979) was able to document the childhood antecedents of adult criminal behavior was extremely important. It is interesting that most of McCord's longitudinal investigations have been carried out with the treated group (because of the extensive information collected on these boys), rather than with the control group. An important methodological question to be investigated in the future is how far natural history results from experimental groups are similar to those from control groups.

Another extremely important experiment with a long-term follow-up is the Perry Preschool Project (Berrueta-Clement, Schweinhart, Barnett, Epstein, & Weikart, 1984), which is also described in more detail in this book. This was essentially a "Head Start" program targeted to disadvantaged black children. The experimental children attended a daily preschool program, backed up by weekly home visits, usually lasting 2 years, covering ages 3 and 4. The aim of the program was to provide intellectual stimulation, to increase cognitive abilities, and to increase later school achievement.

An important feature of this project is that its true significance only became apparent after long-term follow-ups to ages 15 (Schweinhart & Weikart, 1980) and 19 (Berrueta-Clement et al., 1984). As demonstrated in several other Head Start projects, the experimental group initially showed only short-lived gains in intelligence. At age 15, however, they were better on self-reports of offending and of classroom behavior. At age 19, they were less likely to have been arrested, more likely to be employed, more likely to have graduated from high school, and more likely to have received college or vocational training. Hence, the long-term follow-up was necessary to bring out the true beneficial effects of the intervention. The results of this project have had a major impact on American public policy, for example, on Public Law 99-457, which mandates the states to provide health, educational, and social services for high-risk children aged 3–5 (Short, Simeonsson, & Huntington, 1990).

These pioneering examples undoubtedly influenced modern longitudinal–experimental studies of offending and antisocial behavior, of which perhaps the two best current examples are directed by David Hawkins in Seattle (e.g., Hawkins, Von Cleve & Catalano, 1991) and Richard Tremblay in Montreal (e.g., Tremblay et al., 1990). Both of these studies are fully described in this book. Other important intervention projects, such as that directed by Sheppard Kellam in Baltimore (see chapter 8 of this book) may in due course prove to be equally significant longitudinal–experimental studies, but they are not as far advanced at present.

The Hawkins program was aimed to decrease aggressive behavior, delinquency, and substance abuse by promoting social bonding. Importantly, the intervention was targeted simultaneously on teachers and parents. About 500 first grade children in 21 classes in eight schools were randomly assigned to be in experimental or control classes. The parents and teachers of the experimental children received special training designed to encourage reinforcement of socially desirable behavior. The experimental boys proved to be significantly less aggressive in a follow-up than the control boys, and the experimental girls were significantly less self-destructive, anxious, and depressed than the control girls (Hawkins et al., 1991). (Their chapter in this book also shows that the experimental children were less likely to have initiated delinquency and alcohol use by the fifth grade.)

The Tremblay study began with a kindergarten assessment at age 6 that identified about 250 disruptive boys for the experiment. The treated boys received social skills training between ages 7 and 9, while their parents received parent training, and the boys were then followed up every year. By age 12, the treated boys committed less burglary and less theft, and were less likely to get drunk, than the controls. Interestingly, the differences in antisocial behavior between treated and control boys increased as the follow-up progressed (Tremblay et al., 1991).

The Hawkins and Tremblay studies probably represent the "state of the art" of modern longitudinal–experimental studies. However, as I have already mentioned, studies with several years (e.g., three or more) of personal contacts with the subjects both before and after an experimental intervention have rarely been carried out. These types of projects could greatly advance knowledge. Some desirable features of future projects will now be summarized (see also Tonry et al., 1991).

FUTURE LONGITUDINAL-EXPERIMENTAL RESEARCH

Aims

The main aim of one future project should be to advance knowledge about the development of offending and antisocial behavior from birth to the mid-20s, focusing on predatory and violent crimes in large U.S. cities. Much prior criminological research has concentrated on the teenage years when offending is in full flow and has neglected factors leading to onset before the teenage years and factors leading to desistance in the 20s. Also, much prior criminological research has neglected the continuity between predatory and violent crimes such as burglary and robbery and many other types of antisocial behavior, including childhood conduct disorder, teenage drug and alcohol abuse, and adult abuse of spouses and children. Hence, the focus on predatory and violent crimes should naturally be expanded to encompass associated types of antisocial behavior.

Future projects should be particularly concerned with explaining the onset, persistence, and desistance of offending. A comprehensive research program should investigate a wide range of possible influences on these stages of criminal careers, including biological, individual, family, peer, school, and community factors. Previous longitudinal studies have rarely investigated all these different types of factors. If only because of the different ages at which events occur, the factors influencing onset are likely to differ from those influencing persistence, which in turn are likely to differ from those influencing desistance (see Farrington & Hawkins, 1991). For example, family factors may influence onset in the preteenage years, peer group factors may influence the persistence of offending in the teenage years, and employment factors may influence desistance in the 20s.

Prior longitudinal research shows that there is some continuity in antisocial behavior from childhood to adulthood. For example, children with high impulsivity and low empathy at age 2 may tend to show cruelty to animals and other symptoms of conduct disorder at age 8, minor delinquency such as shoplifting at age 12, more serious delinquency such as burglary at age 15, robbery and violence at age 20, and eventually spouse abuse, child abuse, and alcoholism in their 20s and 30s. However, much more needs to be known about these kinds of developmental sequences, and about progressions in antisocial behavior from childhood to adulthood. In particular, it is important to discover why some badly behaved children do not progress into delinquency and crime, what are the most promising intervention strategies to prevent this progression, and at what developmental stages these interventions are likely to be most effective.

Future projects should not aim to test one particular theory but to test hypotheses that can be derived from numerous theories. Many key questions need to be addressed, only some of which can be mentioned very briefly here. For example, delinquents tend to have delinquent peers (e.g., Elliott, Huizinga, & Ageton, 1985), but it is not clear whether this finding merely reflects the fact that delinquency is committed in groups, whether "birds of a feather flock together," or whether delinquent peers facilitate offending in some way. Offenders tend disproportionally to live in socially disorganized areas (e.g., Bursik, 1988), but it is not clear whether this merely reflects the fact that problem people are forced to live in problem areas or whether the problem areas in some way produce the problem people. There is a link between crime and drug abuse (e.g., Ball, Rosen, Flueck, & Nurco, 1981), but it is not clear whether this merely reflects the fact that deviant people tend to engage in both, or whether drug abuse causes crime or crime causes drug abuse. To resolve these and other similar questions about, for example, the effects of marriage or unemployment or sanctions on crime, ambitious longitudinal–experimental research projects are needed.

Designs

As an example of a desirable future research program, Tonry et al. (1991) proposed a design in which seven cohorts, beginning at birth and at ages 3, 6, 9, 12, 15, and 18, were each followed up for 8 years. While these would be the starting ages, the ages of interest would be the year before; for example, the oldest cohort would be first interviewed soon after the 18th birthday and asked about their behavior while aged 17. In order to maximize the yield of frequent and serious offenders, most cohorts would consist of males, except for the birth cohort (which would consist equally of males and females) and the age 12 cohort, which would be supplemented by females and siblings. (For more details, see Tonry et al., 1991.) Some members of the youngest cohort would have data collected prenatally from their mothers, who would be first contacted in the second trimester of pregnancy.

This design ensured a 5-year overlap in age between each adjacent cohort, and 3 years of data collection before and after any given age (except for the youngest and oldest ages). The 8-year follow-up period would permit conclusions about development from the prenatal period to age 25, and after only a 3-year follow-up period it would be possible to draw provisional conclusions about development from the prenatal period to age 20. The validity of these conclusions, and of the methods of data linkage, could be established by the later follow-up data.

Experimental interventions should be included in longitudinal studies to investigate the effectiveness of methods of interrupting the course of development of offending and antisocial behavior. However, in general, these interventions should not occur until after about 3 years of data collection. Information should be collected at least yearly, directly from the subjects themselves and from other informants such as mothers and teachers. Cohort members could be obtained by household sampling of mothers and their biological children (who might as yet be unborn).

In order to investigate community influences on crime in a future project, a target city could be partitioned into about 25 to 50 community areas, classified according to key community features, including crime rates. There could be oversampling in high crime communities, and information could be collected from the cohort members and their families about the communities in which they were living. A project should track changes in communities over time as well as changes in individuals, and investigate how patterns of individual development vary with the community context. Individuals should be followed as they move between communities, to disentangle individual and community influences on crime. This has never been done before in criminology.

Very little existing research relates factors measured prenatally or soon after birth, or in early childhood, to later criminal careers. In birth and early childhood cohorts, the main aim should be to study the development of conduct disorder. Individual factors such as high impulsivity and low intelligence should be measured, as well as peer rejection, adverse family experiences, school underachievement, and the physical health and growth of the child. Biological measures should be taken, including birth weight, resting pulse rate, and testosterone levels in saliva. The focus should be on risk factors for conduct disorder, on critical periods in development, and on the effect of life transitions, for example, from home to preschool or from preschool to school.

One important theory for this age range suggests that there is a difficult temperament (characterized by impulsivity, boredom, low empathy, and irritability), which is apparent in the first year of life and which predicts later conduct disorder (e.g., Garrison & Earls, 1987). Attachment theory is also important; this theory emphasizes the significance of the mother–child relationship in the first 3 years of life, identifying an insecure avoidant relationship as a precursor of conduct disorder (e.g., Erickson, Sroufe, & Egeland, 1985). Social learning theory suggests that harsh or inconsistent parenting produces conduct disorder (e.g., Patterson, 1982). The most important intervention that might be recommended is a preschool program including good health care and nutrition, parent training in child-rearing methods, intellectual stimulation, and social skills training in peer interaction, tackling impulsivity, and low empathy.

In early adolescent cohorts, the main focus should be on the onset of offending, on factors influencing onset, on linkages between onsets of different kinds of antisocial acts, and on the implications of onset features for the development of the later criminal career (Farrington et al., 1990). The aim should be to identify developmental sequences that begin with conduct disorder or minor offending and then escalate into more serious crime, and manipulable factors that are present before the stabilization of antisocial behavior. Numerous criminological theories apply to the teenage years, but they usually aim to explain differences between offenders and nonoffenders rather than to predict the developmental course of offending. Hence, researchers should not be guided by any one existing theory, but should aim to generate new theories that are more applicable to developmental changes within individuals. Individual factors such as impulsivity and intelligence should be measured, as well as biological factors such as the onset of puberty, family factors, peer relationships, school achievement, drug use, interactions with the juvenile justice system, and eventually employment.

Several experimental interventions seem promising for adolescents. In view of research showing that school students can be taught to resist peer influences encouraging smoking, drinking, and marijuana use (e.g., Botvin & Eng, 1982; Evans et al., 1981; Telch, Killen, McAlister, Perry, & Maccoby, 1982), experiments on training teenagers to resist other types of antisocial peer influences can be recommended. Parent management training (e.g., Patterson, 1982), promoting social competence through skills training (e.g., Ladd & Asher, 1985), and promoting academic competence through special tutoring (e.g., Coie & Krehbiel, 1984) can also be suggested.

Study of older teenage cohorts should focus on the persistence or desistance of criminal careers, and on the development of frequent or serious offending. Attempts should be made to investigate the impact of the transition from school to work, of settling down with a wife or cohabitee, of alcohol and drug use, and of the transition from juvenile to criminal justice sanctions. There should be a special focus on social control or bonding to school, marriage, and work, on the development and persistence of peer networks and co-offending, and on links between offending and community disorganization. The major experimental intervention that might be recommended is intensive community supervision based on the work of Greenwood (1986). This involves street contacts with youth on a one-to-one basis, behavioral contracts, and helping to resolve family, school, or employment problems. It is similar in some ways to the "buddy" program described by Clifford O'Donnell in this book (chapter 10; see also O'Donnell, Lydgate, & Fo, 1979).

CONCLUSIONS

Much past research on offending and antisocial behavior has been cross-sectional or correlational in design. The use of longitudinal and experimental studies represented a great step forward in methodology. The time is now ripe to combine these strong designs to capitalize on the advantages of both. Longitudinal–experimental studies should now be mounted that include at least 3 years of personal contacts with the subjects before and after an intervention, and that also include repeated, frequent data collection from a variety of sources. These kinds of studies would not be cheap, although one way of minimizing the cost might be to add an experimental intervention to an existing longitudinal study. They are not without methodological problems either, as I have pointed out in this chapter. However, the best ways of confronting and overcoming these problems are to continue the funding, data collection, and analysis of existing projects and to embark on new longitudinal–experimental studies. These studies hold out the best hope of advancing knowledge about the explanation, prevention, and treatment of offending and antisocial behavior.

REFERENCES

Ball, J. C., Rosen, L., Flueck, J. A., & Nurco, D. N. (1981). The criminality of heroin addicts: When addicted and when off opiates. In J. A. Inciardi (Ed.), *The drugs-crime connection* (pp. 39–65). Beverly Hills, CA: Sage.

Baltes, P. B., Reese, H. W., & Lipsitt, L. P. (1980). Life span developmental psychology. *Annual Review of Psychology, 31*, 65–110.

Bell, R. A. (1954). An experimental test of the accelerated longitudinal approach. *Child Development, 25*, 281–286.

Berrueta-Clement, J. R., Schweinhart, L. J., Barnett, W. S., Epstein, A. S., & Weikart, D. P. (1984). *Changed lives.* Ypsilanti, MI: High/Scope.

Blumstein, A., Cohen, J., & Farrington, D. P. (1988). Longitudinal and criminal career research: Further clarifications. *Criminology, 26*, 57–74.

Blumstein, A., Cohen, J., Roth, J. A., & Visher, C. A. (Eds.). (1986). *Criminal careers and "career criminals"* (Vol. 1). Washington, DC: National Academy Press.

Botvin, G. J., & Eng, A. (1982). The efficacy of a multicomponent approach to the prevention of cigarette smoking. *Preventive Medicine, 11*, 199–211.

Bursik, R. J. (1988). Social disorganization and theories of crime and delinquency: Problems and prospects. *Criminology, 26*, 519–551.

Campbell, D. T., & Stanley, J. C. (1966). *Experimental and quasi-experimental designs for research.* Chicago: Rand McNally.

Coie, J. D., & Krehbiel, G. (1984). Effects of academic tutoring on the social status of low-achieving, socially rejected children. *Child Development, 55*, 1465–1478.

Conner, R. F. (1977). Selecting a control group: An analysis of the randomization process in twelve social reform programs. *Evaluation Quarterly, 1*, 195–244.

Cook, T. D., & Campbell, D. T. (1979). *Quasi-experimentation.* Chicago: Rand-McNally.

Cornish, D. B., & Clarke, R. V. G. (1975). *Residential treatment and its effects on delinquency.* London: Her Majesty's Stationery Office.

Elliott, D. S., Huizinga, D., & Ageton, S. S. (1985). *Explaining delinquency and drug use.* Beverly Hills, CA: Sage.

Empey, L. T., & Erickson, M. L. (1972). *The Provo experiment.* Lexington, MA: D. C. Heath.

Empey, L. T., & Lubeck, S. G. (1971). *The Silverlake experiment.* Chicago: Aldine.

Erickson, M. F., Sroufe, L. A., & Egeland, B. (1985). The relationship between quality of attachment and behavior problems in preschool in a high-risk sample. In I. Bretherton & E. Waters (Eds.), Growing points of attachment theory and research. In *Monographs of the Society for Research in Child Development, 50* (Serial No. 209, pp. 147–166).

Evans, R. I., Rozelle, R. M., Maxwell, S. E., Raines, B. E., Dill, C. A., Guthrie, T. J., Henderson, A. H., & Hill, P. C. (1981). Social modeling films to deter smoking in adolescents: Results of a three-year field investigation. *Journal of Applied Psychology, 66*, 399–414.

Farrington, D. P. (1977). The effects of public labelling. *British Journal of Criminology, 17*, 112–125.

Farrington, D. P. (1983). Randomized experiments on crime and justice. In M. Tonry & N. Morris (Eds.), *Crime and justice* (Vol. 4, pp. 257–308). Chicago: University of Chicago Press.

Farrington, D. P. (1986). Age and crime. In M. Tonry & N. Morris (Eds.), *Crime and justice* (Vol. 7, pp. 189–250). Chicago: University of Chicago Press.

Farrington, D. P. (1988). Studying changes within individuals: The causes of offending. In M. Rutter (Ed.), *Studies of psychosocial risk* (pp. 158–183). Cambridge: Cambridge University Press.

Farrington, D. P. (1990a). Age, period, cohort and offending. In D. M. Gottfredson & R. V. Clarke (Eds.), *Policy and theory in criminal justice* (pp. 51–75). Aldershot, England: Avebury.

Farrington, D. P. (1990b). Implications of criminal career research for the prevention of offending. *Journal of Adolescence, 13,* 93–113.

Farrington, D. P. (1991a). Antisocial personality from childhood to adulthood. *Psychologist, 4,* 389–394.

Farrington, D. P. (1991b). Longitudinal research strategies: Advantages, problems, and prospects. *Journal of the American Academy of Child and Adolescent Psychiatry, 30,* 369–374.

Farrington, D. P., & Hawkins, J. D. (1991). Predicting participation, early onset, and later persistence in officially recorded offending. *Criminal Behavior and Mental Health, 1,* 1–33.

Farrington, D. P., Loeber, R., Elliott, D. S., Hawkins, J. D., Kandel, D. B., Klein, M. W., McCord, J., Rowe, D. C., & Tremblay, R. E. (1990). Advancing knowledge about the onset of delinquency and crime. In B. B. Lahey & A. E. Kazdin (Eds.), *Advances in clinical child psychology* (Vol. 13, pp. 283–342). New York: Plenum.

Farrington, D. P., Ohlin, L. E., & Wilson, J. Q. (1986). *Understanding and controlling crime.* New York: Springer-Verlag.

Farrington, D. P., Snyder, H. N., & Finnegan, T. A. (1988). Specialization in juvenile court careers. *Criminology, 26,* 461–487.

Finckenauer, J. O. (1982). *Scared straight.* Englewood Cliffs, NJ: Prentice-Hall.

Garrison, W. T., & Earls, F. (1987). *Temperament and child psychopathology.* Newbury Park, CA: Sage.

Gendreau, P., & Ross, R. R. (1987). Revivification of rehabilitation: Evidence from the 1980s. *Justice Quarterly, 4,* 349–407.

Glenn, N. D. (1977). *Cohort analysis.* Beverly Hills, CA: Sage.

Greenwood, P. W. (1986). Promising approaches for the rehabilitation or prevention of chronic juvenile offenders. In P. W. Greenwood (Ed.), *Intervention strategies for chronic juvenile offenders* (pp. 207–233). New York: Greenwood Press.

Hawkins, J. D., Von Cleve, E., & Catalano, R. F. (1991). Reducing early childhood aggression: Results of a primary prevention program. *Journal of the American Academy of Child and Adolescent Psychiatry, 30,* 208–217.

Kassebaum, G., Ward, D., & Wilner, D. (1971). *Prison treatment and parole survival.* New York: Wiley.

Ladd, G. W., & Asher, S. R. (1985). Social skill training and children's peer relations: Current issues in research and practice. In L. L. Abate &

M. A. Milan (Eds.), *Handbook of social skills training and research* (pp. 219–244). New York: Wiley.

Lichtman, G. M., & Smock, S. M. (1981). The effects of social service on probation recidivism: A field experiment. *Journal of Research in Crime and Delinquency, 18*, 81–100.

Lipsey, M. W. (1988). Juvenile delinquency intervention. In H. S. Bloom, D. S. Cordray, & R. J. Light (Eds.), *Lessons from selected program and policy areas* (pp. 63–84). San Francisco: Jossey-Bass.

Loeber, R., Stouthamer-Loeber, M., Van Kammen, W., & Farrington, D. P. (1991). Initiation, escalation and desistance in juvenile offending and their correlates. *Journal of Criminal Law and Criminology, 82*, 36–82.

Maxim, P. S. (1985). Cohort size and juvenile delinquency: A test of the Easterlin hypothesis. *Social Forces, 63*, 661–681.

McCord, J. (1978). A thirty year follow-up of treatment effects. *American Psychologist, 33*, 284–289.

McCord, J. (1979). Some child-rearing antecedents of criminal behavior in adult men. *Journal of Personality and Social Psychology, 37*, 1477–1486.

Multiple Risk Factor Intervention Trial Research Group. (1982). Multiple Risk Factor Intervention Trial: Risk factor changes and mortality results. *Journal of the American Medical Association, 248*, 1465–1477.

O'Donnell, C. R., Lydgate, T., & Fo, W. S. O. (1979). The buddy system: Review and follow-up. *Child Behavior Therapy, 1*, 161–169.

Patterson, G. R. (1982). *Coercive family process.* Eugene, OR: Castalia.

Reckless, W. C., & Dinitz, S. (1972). *The prevention of juvenile delinquency.* Columbus, OH: Ohio State University Press.

Schweinhart, L. J., & Weikart, D. P. (1980). *Young children grow up.* Ypsilanti, MI: High/Scope.

Severy, L. J., & Whitaker, J. M. (1982). Juvenile diversion: An experimental analysis of effectiveness. *Evaluation Review, 6*, 753–774.

Short, R. J., Simeonsson, R. J., & Huntington, G. S. (1990). Early intervention: Implications of Public Law 99-457 for professional child psychology. *Professional Psychology, 21*, 88–93.

Telch, M. J., Killen, J. D., McAlister, A. L., Perry, C. L., & Maccoby, N. (1982). Long-term follow-up of a pilot project on smoking prevention with adolescents. *Journal of Behavioral Medicine, 5*, 1–8.

Thornberry, T. P. (1989). Panel effects and the use of self-reported measures of delinquency in longitudinal studies. In M. Klein (Ed.), *Cross-national research in self-reported crime and delinquency* (pp. 347–369). Dordrecht, The Netherlands: Kluwer.

Tonry, M., Ohlin, L. E., & Farrington, D. P. (1991). *Human development and criminal behavior.* New York: Springer-Verlag.

Tremblay, R. E., McCord, J., Boileau, H., Charlebois, P., Gagnon, C., LeBlanc, M., & Larivée, S. (1991). Can disruptive boys be helped to become competent? *Psychiatry, 54*, 148–161.

Tremblay, R. E., McCord, J., Boileau, H., LeBlanc, M., Gagnon, C., Charlebois, P., & Larivée, S. (1990, November). *The Montreal prevention experi-*

ment: School adjustment and self-reported delinquency after three years of follow-up. Paper presented at the Annual Meeting of the American Society of Criminology, Baltimore.

Waldo, G. P., & Chiricos, T. A. (1977). Work release and recidivism: An empirical evaluation of a social policy. *Evaluation Quarterly, 1,* 87–108.

Waldo, G. P., & Griswold, D. (1979). Issues in the measurement of recidivism. In L. Sechrest, S. O. White, & E. D. Brown (Eds.), *The rehabilitation of criminal offenders: Problems and prospects* (pp. 225–250). Washington, DC: National Academy of Sciences.

Wolfgang, M. E., Figlio, R. M., & Sellin, T. (1972). *Delinquency in a birth cohort.* Chicago: University of Chicago Press.

Yamaguchi, K., & Kandel, D. B. (1984). Patterns of drug use from adolescence to young adulthood: 2. Sequences of progression. *American Journal of Public Health, 74,* 668–672.

Yarrow, M. R., Campbell, J. D., & Burton, R. V. (1970). Recollections of childhood: A study of the retrospective method. *Monographs of the Society for Research in Child Development, 35*(5, Serial No. 138).

Index

◆ ——— ◆

Activity Rating Scale, 96
Activity settings, 223–227
Adolescent Transitions Program
  background, 260
  implications, 275–279
  methods, 260–269
  results, 269–275
Adolescents. *See also* St. Louis Project
  aggressive behavior in, 283–284
  bonding theory, 324
  in Buddy System, 212–215
  differential association perspective, 317
  gangs, 220
  managing in discussion group, 295–296
  medication for, 110
  moral reasoning intervention with,
    292–300
  opportunity perspective, 314–315
  Peer Culture Development program
    for, 215–318, 320–321
  peer networks and intervention
    outcomes, 218–221
  pharmacotherapy for attention
    deficit hyperactivity disorder,
    110
  research needs, 371–372
  role of moral reasoning in
    rehabilitation, 305–306
  school bonding experiment, 312–
    313, 317, 319–320
  self-regulation in substance abuse
    intervention, 264–265

  self-reporting, 268
  social network formation, 223
  Student Training Through Urban
    Strategies program for, 313–
    315, 318, 321–324
  subcultural perspective, 317
  substance abuse prevention, 140
  teacher assessment of, 267–268
Adoption, 12
Adult Performance Level Survey, 79
Affective development
  maternal, and infant risk, 23–24
  moral reasoning and, 303
  mother–child interaction and, 25–26
Age of onset, 11, 130–131, 133, 139, 354
Aggression
  in adolescents, 283–284
  assessment, 124–125, 127–128, 175–
    178, 185
  Baltimore intervention in, 164
  as behavioral marker, 110
  etiological role of, 169
  Montréal Longitudinal-
    Experimental Study results,
    127–128
  pharmacotherapy for attention
    deficit hyperactivity disorder
    and, 110
  reinforcement model in families,
    91
  school variability, 175–177
  shy behavior and, 170

Alcohol. *See* Drug use; Substance abuse

Assessment. *See also* Aggression, assessment

antisocial behavior, teacher–parent convergence in, 267–268

attention deficit hyperactivity disorder, 92–93

automatic reaction patterns, 255–256

baseline modeling in, 178, 181–182

behavior gains from association with prosocial peers, 235, 237–240

beliefs/norms, regarding drug use, 150–151

child's goals, 38

classroom environments, 175–178

court records in, 200

disruptive behavior, 124–125

early onset delinquency, 151

family constructs, 149–150

family cooperation, 201–202

group dynamics, 247–250

IQ, 84

likability, 124–125

moral reasoning in adolescents, 291–292

mother–child relations, 30, 33–34

mother's motivation, 48

Novel Toy procedure, 37–38

outcome, considerations in, 4, 16, 117

parental behaviors, 256–258, 266–267, 276–277

by child, 132–133, 149–150

parenting skills, 132–135

peer interactions, 4 year olds, 36–38

preschool child behavior, 12

preschool intervention outcome, 74

of psychological well-being, 174

school achievement, 125

school constructs by student, 150

social adaptational status, 163, 166–167, 173–174

social adjustment, 125–126

social network, 221

social task response in classrooms, 173–174

social withdrawal, 124–125

structural equation modeling in, 269, 276–277

trained teaching practices, 148–149

videotaped family problem solving, 265

Assessment instruments

Activity Rating Scale, 96

Adult Performance Level Survey, 79

Baltimore How I Feel, 174

California Achievement Tests, 79, 155–156

Child Behavior Checklist, 268

Children's Depression Inventory, 174

Child's Behavior Traits, 54

Depression Self-Rating Scale, 174

Home Situations Questionnaire, 96

Hopelessness Scale for Children, 174

Issues Checklist, 265

Maternal Interactive Behavior, 53

Moral Judgement Interview, 291

Mother Negative Discipline construct, 266–267, 269–270

Parent Rating Scale-Revised, 96, 104

Peer Assessment Inventory, 174, 175

Preschool Behavior Questionnaire, 121

problems in, 84, 277–278

Prosocial Behavioral Questionnaire, 121

Pupil Evaluation Inventory, 124–125, 174

Response Class Matrix, 97, 105

Revised Children's Manifest Anxiety Scale, 174

role of, 256, 276–277

School Adjustment Index, 292, 293

Social Behavior Questionnaire, 121, 124

Strange Situation procedures, 33

Teacher Observation of Classroom Adaptation-Revised, 173

videotaped problem solving task, 265

Attachment theory, 26–28, 371
   assessment, 33–34
   peer relations and, 36–38
   relations to outcome, 27–28, 38
Attention deficit hyperactivity
      disorder
   age as variable in, 94
   assessment, 92–93
   follow-up research, 108–110
   methylphenidate in management of,
      90, 96–110
   Oppositional Defiant Disorder and, 94
   parent–child interactions, 93–94,
      96–100
   peer relations, 95, 103–106
   predictive of adult behavior, 89–90,
      108–110
   prevalence, 89
   social response to, 90
   subclinical concentration problems,
      179
   teacher–child interactions, 94–95,
      100–103
Attrition/accretion, in experiments,
      35, 152–153, 247–250, 262–263,
      334

B

Baltimore How I Feel self-report, 174
Baltimore preventive trials
   assessment procedures, 173–178
   baseline modeling in, 178–182
   controlling for effects, 186–189
   procedures, 182–186
   research design, 162, 170, 172–173
   results, 189–190
Behavioral therapy
   activity setting concept and, 223–
      225, 227
   adolescent self-regulation in
      substance abuse intervention,
      264–265
   assessing behavioral types, in peer
      groups, 237–239

Buddy System, 212–215, 218
coercion model, 253–256
environmental factors in theory,
      221–228
pharmacotherapy for attention
      deficit hyperactivity disorder
      and, 99–100, 107–108
theoretical development, 209–211,
      215–218
triadic model, 211
Boys, 175, 179. *See also* Gender
Buddy System, 212–215, 218, 227
Burnout, counselor, 347–348

C

California Achievement Tests, 79,
      155–156
Cambridge–Somerville Youth Study
   background, 196–198
   follow-up, 47, 200–204, 365–366
   goals, 4
   procedures, 198–200
   results, 200–203
Catch 'Em Being Good, parent
      training program, 146
Causal hypotheses. *See also* Risk
      factors
   adolescent subcultural values in,
      316–317
   attachment theory in, 26–28
   attention deficit hyperactivity
      disorder in, 89–90
   in childhood behavior research, 11–16
   childhood education in, 67, 75, 312,
      314–315
   community epidemiology in, 165–166
   epidemiologically based research
      on, 162–164
   family relationships in, 21, 23–24,
      45–46, 91–93
   Hawthorne effects and, 13, 346–348,
      349
   longitudinal research and, 7, 13,
      117, 353–358

Causal hypotheses (*continued*)
  moral development in, 284–285,
    288–290
  mother–child interactions in, 25–
    26
  parenting skills/behaviors in, 4, 11–
    12, 118–121, 253–256
  prevention experiments in testing,
    3–8, 11, 12–13, 358–361
  proving, 8–10
  role of field experimentation in
    testing, 324–327
  third variable effects on, 6–7, 11,
    16–17, 172
Child Behavior Checklist, 268
Child effects
  on adults, 26, 91–92, 97–99, 102–
    103, 106–108, 118–119
  on peers, 103–106
Child guidance movement,
    196–198
Children. *See also* Adolescents; Infants
  aggression in, 38
  attachment security and peer
    interaction, 36–38
  classroom assessments, 173–182
  in Montréal Longitudinal-
    Experimental Study, 121
  outcome indicators, 12, 67, 82–84
  in preschool programs, 67–68, 75,
    81–84
  research needs, 368–369
  standardized measurement of
    behavior, 12
Children's Depression Inventory, 174
Child's Behavior Traits, 54
Clinical Nursing Models, preventive
    intervention
  background, 29
  follow-up, peer relations, 36–38
  research subjects, 29–30
  results, 34–36, 38
  treatment procedures/goals, 30–34
Coercion model, 253–256. *See also*
    Adolescent Transitions Program
  data collection in, 265

experimental findings, 275–276
  family management training in,
    261
Cognitive development
  activity setting concept in, 223–224
  choosing behavior and, 284–285,
    288–289, 306–307
  curricula for advancing, 49–50
  early verbal interaction and, 45–48
  internal working model of self, 27
  moral development and, 285, 289,
    300–302, 307
  mother–child interaction and, 25–26
  role of setting in, 223
  siblings of research subjects, 53
  training program for children, 146
Cohort effects, 357
Communication skills. *See also*
    Mother–Child Home Program
  building, in adolescent discussion
    group, 296
  developmental role of, 45–47
  role in activity setting, 224, 226
Community psychology, 222–226
Competence, maternal, 31–32, 35
Concentration problems, 179
Context, 22
Correlational research design, 257–
    258, 359–360
Counselor training, status offender
    supervision, 336
Criminal behavior. *See also*
    Delinquency
  aggressive classroom behaviors as
    predictive of, 163
  control theory of, 204
  effect of probation on, 219
  familial factors in, 47, 196
  juvenile status offenders, 330–331
  levels of schooling and, 43
  outcomes in Cambridge–Somerville
    Study, 200–202
  paternal absence and, 204
  peer relations as predictor of, 28
  preschool education and, 67, 73–74,
    80, 366

prison visits as preventive intervention for, 219
program results on, 73–74, 79–80, 130–131, 153, 156, 164, 201–203, 214–215, 218, 221, 268, 298, 319–321, 330–349
recidivism, 197–198, 305, 333, 341
rehabilitation, 304–305
research needs, 368–372
sociomoral reasoning and, 301–302
substance abuse as predictor of, 139
Cross-lagged regression modeling, 178
Cross-sectional studies, 119, 353–354, 356, 357

D

Delinquency. *See also* Criminal behavior; Intensive Protective Supervision Project; Montréal Longitudinal-Experimental Study; Seattle Social Development Project
assessing early onset, 151
behavior modification in preventing, 209, 211
Buddy System in preventing, 212–215, 218, 227
child skills training in preventing, 146
early agressive behavior as predictive of, 163–164, 170
early onset, 139–140
early research in, 197–198
juvenile gang, 220
moral reasoning and, 288–290
multifactorial intervention, 141, 164
parent–child training and, 133
parenting and, 118, 120–121, 197
Peer Culture Development intervention for, 315–318, 320–321
peer relations as predictor of, 28, 29
Positive Action Through Holistic Education intervention for, 312–313, 317, 319–320
poverty as risk factor in, 4

preschool education and, 67, 68, 79–80, 366–367
probation supervision and recidivism, 331–333
prosocial peers in intervention for, 235
role of setting in planning interventions for, 225–227, 233–234
setting as risk factor for, 221–227
social network effects on, 218–221, 233–235
Student Training Through Urban Strategies intervention for, 313–315, 318, 321–324
teaching training in intervention for, 143–146
Depression Self-Rating Scale, 174
Design. *See* Research design
Developmental epidemiology
community epidemiology in, 165–166
development in, 166–168
outcome analysis in, 189–190
parallel design, 172–173
role of, 162–164
Differential association theory, 317, 324–325
Discipline, parental. *See also* Parents/parenting, training
child's assessment of, 132–133, 134
early substance abuse and, 260
measuring, 256–257, 266–267, 277–278
related to child antisocial behavior, 11, 258–259
in testing coercion model of antisocial behavior, 275–276
third variable effects in experiments on, 259
training, 12, 134, 263
Drug use, 140, 151–153, 164

E

Education. *See also* Teachers
child-centered, 76, 83

Education (*continued*)
  classroom assessments, 175–178
  cultural factors in, 217–218
  dysfunctional behaviors and, 43
  Mastery Learning program, 182–186
  open-framework approach, 76
  performance and early verbal
    interaction, 54
  Positive Action Through Holistic
    Education, 312–313, 317, 319–320
  preschool, role of, 44, 67, 72–73,
    82–83
  programmed-learning approach, 76
  in social development model, 141–142
  Student Training Through Urban
    Strategies, 313–315, 318, 321–324
Effect. *See* Results
Employment outcomes
  education and, 43, 67, 68
  preschool intervention and, 73
  social networks and, 217
Endpoint analyses, 240–241, 250
Environmental risk factors. *See also*
    Familial risk factors
  activity setting concept in, 223–227
  affecting verbal interaction, 46–47
  in behaviorism, 216–218, 221–228
  infant development and, 22–23
  micro/macrosettings, 222
  peer networking and, 223
  in research model, 259
  significance of, 226–227
  for substance abuse, 140–141
Epidemiologic research, role of, 4

F

Familial risk factors. *See also*
    Environmental risk factors;
    Mother–child relations; Parents/
    parenting; Risk factors
  adult competencies as, 23–24
  bonding as protection, 141–142
  Cambridge–Somerville data, 204
  communication skills and, 45–46

  early research on, 196–198
  field research, 259–260
  infant development and, 22–23
  insecure attachments, 26–28
  moral development and, 289
  negative reinforcement models, 91–92
  research models, 256–259
  for substance abuse, 140–141, 260
Father(s). *See also* Parents/parenting
  absence of, 204
  attention deficit hyperactivity
    disorder child and, 108
  behavior of, 132
  characteristics of, 68, 123
Females. *See* Gender as variable
Field experimentation, problems of,
    325–327
Follow-up research. *See also*
    Longitudinal research
  attention deficit hyperactivity
    disorder treatment, 108–110
  behavior modification interventions, 215
  Cambridge–Somerville Study, 200–
    203, 365–366
  changed circumstances affecting,
    364–365
  depression-poor achievement cycle,
    179–181
  developmental mapping in, 165
  family relationships and criminal
    behavior, 47
  of infants, 37–38
  in moral reasoning intervention,
    297–298, 300
  parent behavior training and child's
    school performance, 53–59
  parent–child training intervention
    (Montréal), 133
  peer-directed social competence,
    36–38
  preschool enrichment program, 44
  prospective, 6
  retrospective, 6
  role of, 13, 117–118
  in status offender supervision
    project, 341

G

Gangs, 220
Gender as variable
 adolescent arrest rate, 214
 adolescent self-reporting, 268
 assessing reciprocal relationships, 179
 attention deficit hyperactivity
  disorder, 93–94, 97
 classroom maladaptive behaviors,
  178–179
 effect of negative discipline
  practices, 267
 Mastery Learning intervention
  outcome, 186
 social development interaction, 153,
  155–156
 teacher-rated social behavior, 268,
  276
Girls, 175, 179. *See also* Gender
Good Behavior Game, 182–185
Group Integration Project. *See*
 St. Louis Experiment
Group work
 adolescent discussion group, 295–296
 adolescents in Peer Culture
  Development intervention,
  315–318, 320–321
 Good Behavior Game, 182
 Guided Group Interaction model,
  315, 323, 326–327
 traditional group work, 237, 244
Guided Group Interaction model, 315,
 323, 326–327

H

Hawthorne effects, 13, 346–348, 349
High/Scope Curriculum Study
 background, 75
 and Perry Preschool study, 70, 75
 research design, 76–78
 results, 78–84
Home Situations Questionnaire, 96
Hopelessness Scale for Children, 174

How to Help Your Child Succeed in
 School, 146–147
Hyperactivity. *See* Attention deficit
 hyperactivity disorder

I

Infants. *See also* Mother–child relations
 effects on parents, 26
 environmental risk factors, 22–23
 research on, 370–371
Intelligence
 Clinical Nursing Models program
  results, 35
 in Mother–Child Home Program
  results, 57–58
 predictive capacity of, 51, 84
 in preschool curriculum research
  program, 72, 77–78, 79, 82
Intensive Protective Supervision
 Project
 counselor selection, 336
 design, 333–334
 goals of, 332–333
 Hawthorne effects, 346–348
 procedures, 335–336
 research population, 337
 results, 337–346, 348–349
Interpersonal Cognitive Problem
 Solving training program, 146
Issues Checklist, 265

J

Juvenile Justice and Delinquency
 Prevention Act (1974), 330

L

Life-course development
 behavioral development in, 167
 in developmental epidemiology,
  162, 167–168

Longitudinal research. *See also* Follow-
   up research
   advantages of, 353–356
   Consortium of Longitudinal Studies, 67
   defining, 353–354
   experimental study concurrent
      with, 118, 361–368, 372
   future needs, 368–372
   overidentification of causes, 13
   preschool programs, 67
   problems in, 356–358
   role of, 5–6, 7, 117–118
   Seattle Social Development Project, 143
   structural equation modeling in,
      269, 276–277
   vs. cross-sectional studies, 119, 353–
      354, 356, 357

M

Males. *See also* Gender
   with attention deficit hyperactivity
      disorder, 93–94, 97
   gender, as risk factor, 11, 163
   predictors of offending by, 356
Mastery Learning program, 182–186
Matching treatment and clients, 36
Medication, effects, 96
Methylphenidate, 90, 96–100
Montréal Longitudinal-Experimental
   Study
   background, 120–121
   follow-up, 124–126
   goals of, 4
   procedures, 123–124
   research population, 121–123
   results, 126–135, 367
Moral Judgement Interview, 291
Moral reasoning
   adolescent discussion sessions, 294–
      296
   assessing in adolescents, 291–292
   assessing intervention outcome,
      297–300, 303–304
   behavior and, 288–290

   developmental aspects, 285–289
   in etiology of antisocial behavior,
      300–303
   experimental intervention in, 292–
      297
   research on, 290–291, 300
   role in rehabilitation, 304–307
Mother–Child Home Program
   background, 45–48
   goals of, 44–45
   problems in, 62–63
   procedures, 47–52
   replications, 54–57
   research population, 51–52
   results, 53–54, 57–61
Mother–child relations
   attachment theory of, 26–28, 371
   attention deficit hyperactivity
      disorder and, 93–94, 96–100
   cognitive development and, 25–26,
      45–46
   cue-sensitivity in, 25, 26
   discipline, 118–120, 132, 266–267,
      269–270
   distal factors affecting, 28–29
   moral development and, 289
   mutual adaptation process, 25
   peer interactions affected by, 36–37
   preventive interventions
      Clinical Nursing Models, 29–36
      Mother–Child Home Program,
         44–63
      Newborn Nursing Models, 29
   response to infant distress, 25
   setting conditions and, 22
   verbal interaction in, 45–47, 54
Multiple Risk Factor Intervention
   Trial, 363–364

N

Negative outcomes
   Buddy System, 215, 218
   Cambridge–Somerville Youth
      Study, 201–204, 365–366

interpretation, 203–204
Peer Culture Development
    program, 320–321
peer networks and, 218–221, 234
risks, 189
Newborn Nursing Models, 29
Novel Toy procedure, 37–38
Nursing services, 29, 30–31

O

Operant conditioning, 210
Oppositional Defiant Disorder, 94
Oregon Social Learning Center, 123
Oregon Youth Study, 257
Outcomes, preventive intervention.
    See also Follow-up research
    aggressive classroom behavior, 185–
        190
    attention deficit hyperactivity
        disorder, 106–110
    behavior modification, 214–215
    discipline training, 260, 269–270,
        276
    Hawthorne effects in, 13, 346–348,
        349
    in longitudinal–experimental
        research on behavior, 365–368
    maternal discipline, 270–275
    negative iatrogenic effects in, 189,
        201–203, 214–215, 365–366
    neighborhood-based delinquency
        programs, 218
    parent behavior training
        analysis of results in, 59–63
        positive results in, 53–57
        problematic results in, 57–58
    parent–child training (Montréal
        study), 133–135
    effect on aggressive behaviors,
        127–128
    effect on home adjustment, 131–
        132
    effect on onset of delinquent
        behavior, 130–131

effect on parenting behavior,
    132–133
effect on school achievement,
    126–127
effect on school adjustment, 128–
    130
Peer Culture Development, 320–321
Positive Action Through Holistic
    Education, 319–320
preschool curricula, 72–75, 79–82
prison visits, 219
prosocial peer group
    nonparticipant assessment of,
        243–245
    parent/referral agent assessment
        of, 247
    participant assessment of, 245–246
public policy implications, 82–84,
    367
return on investment and, 74–75,
    82–83
secure attachments, 34–36
social development, in drug abuse/
    delinquency protection, 155–
    157
sociomoral reasoning in, 297–300,
    302
status offender supervision
    during intervention, 337–341
    late effects in, 341–346
Student Training Through Urban
    Strategies, 321–324

P

Parent–Child Home Program, 56–57
Parent–child interaction. *See* Parents;
    Child effects
Parent Rating Scale–Revised, 96, 104
Parents/parenting. *See also* Child
    effects; Discipline, parental;
    Familial risk factors
    adolescents and, 253–279
    aggressive boys and, 122–135
    assessing role of, 132–135

Parents/parenting (*continued*)
   assessing via Mother Negative
      Discipline construct, 266–267,
      269–270
   as causal agent, 11–12, 25–26
   coercion model, 91, 253–256, 275–
      276
   early research on, 196–198
   in etiology of behavioral problems,
      22–24, 93–94, 118, 196
   experimental intervention, 29–38,
      123–135
   familial bonding, 141–142
   family management skills, 261, 263
   field research, 259–260
   infants at risk and, 21–38
   interaction with child, 254–255
   measurement in research of, 256–
      259, 276–278
   moral development and, 289
   pharmacotherapy for attention
      deficit hyperactivity disorder
      and, 99–100, 107–108
   practices, 260
   punishment, 274
   research design for assessing, 118–120
   research models, 256–259
   social interactional perspective, 26,
      254
   training, 71, 123, 132, 134, 146–147,
      260, 263
Peer Assessment Inventory, 174, 175
Peer Culture Development, 315–318,
   320–321
Peer group interactions
   and adolescent intervention
      outcomes, 218–221, 244–245, 250
   attachment security assessment and,
      36–38
   attention deficit hyperactivity
      disorder and, 95, 103–106
   classifying behavioral types, 237–
      239
   degrees of integration, 239–240
   early attachments affecting, 27–28
   gang research, 220
      negative outcomes and, 234
      as outcome indicator, 28
      parent–child relations and, 120
      peer counselors, 264–265
   Peer Culture Development
      intervention, 315–318, 320–321
      peer nominated assessments, 175–
      177
      preventive interventions, 221, 228,
      233–235
      prosocial, in treatment, 233–235,
      250
      reciprocal relationships, 179
      research needs, 369
      as research variable, 235–236
      setting and, 223, 227–228
Perry Preschool Project
   follow-up research, 71
   research design, 68–71
   results, 44, 68, 71–75, 81–84, 366–
      367
Pharmacotherapy
   for attention deficit hyperactivity
      disorder, 90, 96–110
   Ritalin, 90
Positive Action Through Holistic
   Education, 312–313, 317, 319–320
Preschool Behavior Questionnaire, 121
Preventive interventions. *See also*
   Research design
   Adolescent Transitions Program,
      260–279
   age considerations, 47–48
   attention deficit hyperactivity
      disorder, 90
   Baltimore preventive trials on
      aggressive behavior, 170, 172–
      190
   baseline modeling in, 178
   Buddy System, 212–215
   Cambridge–Somerville Youth
      Study, 198–204
   Clinical Nursing Models, 29–36
   compensation for participants, 14
   designing parent training
      experiments, 119–120

developmental epidemiology in, 162–165

dual trials in, 172–173

economic benefits, 68, 74–75, 82–83

epidemiologic research and, 4

evaluating, 16–17, 51

family-based, preschool, 44–45

Helping Relationship model, 31

High/Scope Curriculum Study, 75–84

High/Scope preschool research, 68–84

Intensive Protective Supervision Project, 332–348

interim effects, 15–16

lack of, for behavior problems, 8

in mental health, 163

Montréal Longitudinal-Experimental Study, 120–135

Mother–Child Home Program, 44–63

Newborn Nursing Models, 29

Parent–Child Home Program, 56–57

Peer Culture Development, 315–318, 320–321

in peer network formation, 221

Perry Preschool Study, 68–75, 81–84

Positive Action Through Holistic Education, 312–313, 317, 319–320

proving causality by, 8–10

recognizing causality, 13–14

research design suggestions, 369–372

role of, 3–4, 7–8, 17

role of experimentation in behavior research, 11–14

role of moral reasoning in, 305–306

Scared Straight program, 219

Seattle Social Development Project, 141–157

shy/aggressive behaviors, 182–186

social interaction as target of, 225–226

sociomoral reasoning development program, 290–307

St. Louis Experiment, 236–251

Student Training Through Urban Strategies, 313–315, 318, 321–324

subgroup analysis in, 168–169

substance abuse, 139–140, 260

Youth Development Project, 227–228

Probation. See Intensive Protective Supervision Project

Program Development Evaluation, 311, 326

Prosocial Behavior Questionnaire, 121

Prospective study, 6

Public assistance, preschool intervention and subsequent, 73

Punishment
child's assessment of, 149
physical, as assessment variable, 133

Punishment Density Score, 266

Pupil Evaluation Inventory, 124–125, 174

R

Randomization in experimentation, 178, 317–318, 358–359
in Cambridge-Somerville Youth Study, 198–199
in Montréal Longitudinal-Experimental Study, 121–123
in Perry Preschool study, 68–70
prevention experiment strategies, 15, 51–52
subject-randomized research, 52–53
unit-randomized research, 51–52

Recidivism research, 197–198, 305, 333, 341

Research design. See also Randomization in experimentation
accretion in, 152–153
Adolescent Training Program, 276
Adolescent Transitions Program, 260–269
assessing Buddy System, 213–215

Research design (*continued*)
assessing moral reasoning in
adolescents, 291–297
assessing role of parenting skills,
118–120
attrition and, 35, 247–250, 334
baseline modeling, 178–182
Cambridge–Somerville Youth
Study, 198–200
Clinical Nursing Models, 30–34
community epidemiology, 165–166
correlational, 257–258, 359–360
developmental epidemiology, 169–
170
dual trials, 172–173
future needs, 368–372
general principles, 14–16
Hawthorne effects, 13, 346–349
High/Scope Curriculum Study, 76–78
identifying causal effects, 7–10
Intensive Protective Supervision
Project, 333–334
longitudinal–experimental, 361–372
model development and
measurement techniques, 256–
259, 276–278
Montréal Longitudinal–
Experimental study, 121–123
Mother–Child Home Program, 48–
52
multistage assessment in, 168–169
Newborn Nursing Models, 29
peer influences as variable in, 235–
236
peer interactions, 4-year follow-up,
37–38
Perry Preschool study, 68–71
pharmacotherapy for attention
deficit hyperactivity disorder,
96–97, 100
Positive Action Through Holistic
Education, 312–313
prevention experiments, 5–8, 10–11,
50–51
Program Development Evaluation
method, 311

proximal/distal effects in, 187–188
redundant effects in, 188–189
researcher–practitioner
collaboration, 311
Seattle Social Development Project,
143–147
St. Louis Experiment, 237–241, 250
structural equation modeling in,
269, 276–277
Student Training Through Urban
Strategies, 313–315, 318
theory-testing methodology, 324–
327
Research populations
adolescent, referred and
nonreferred, 236
adolescents at risk for substance
abuse, 260–261
attention deficit hyperactivity
disorder, 96
attrition/accretion in, 35, 152–153,
247–250, 262–263, 334
in Cambridge–Somerville Youth
Study, 199
disadvantaged preschoolers, 68, 77,
121
four year olds, in follow-up, 36–38
in longitudinal–experimental
research, 364, 365
mothers/preschool children, 44–45
pregnant, high-risk women, 29–30
in preventive research, 170–171
school-age children, urban,
multiethnic, 143
status offenders, 334, 337
Response Class Matrix, 97, 105
Results
Adolescent Transitions Program,
269–276
Baltimore preventive trials, 189–
190
buddy system, 212–214
Cambridge–Somerville Youth
Study, 200–204
Clinical Nursing Models, 34–36
effects of methylphenidate, 96–106

High/Scope Curriculum, 78–84
holistic education, 319–321
Intensive Protective Supervision
    Project, 348–349
Montréal Longitudinal-
    Experimental study, 126–135
Mother–Child Home Program, 53–
    61
peer culture, 319–321
Perry Preschool Project, 71–75, 81–
    84, 366–367
Seattle Social Development Project,
    153–157, 367
sociomoral reasoning, 297–300
St. Louis Experiment, 241–247
student training, 319–321
successful, 16–17
Retrospective study, 6
Revised Children's Manifest Anxiety
    Scale, 174
Risk factors, 11–12, 22–23. *See also*
    Environmental risk factors;
    Familial risk factors
Cambridge–Somerville study, 4
Montréal study, 4
response to attention deficit
    hyperactivity disorder, 90
substance abuse, 139–141, 260

S

Scared Straight, 219
Schools/schooling. *See also* High/Scope
    Curriculum Study; Mother–Child
    Home Program; Teachers
aggressive behavior in, 163–164, 170
child-centered, 76, 83
classroom assessments, 175–178
classroom attitudes, 54
cooperative activities vs. individual
    performance emphasis in, 217–
    218
cultural factors in, 217–218
depression affecting performance
    in, 179

early cognitive development and
    performance in, 45, 54
Mastery Learning program, 182–186
open-framework approach, 76
parent behavior training and child's
    performance in, 53–61
parental discipline training and, 276
peer rejection as predictor of
    performance in, 28
performance in, as risk factor, 12,
    43
Positive Action Through Holistic
    Education, 312–313, 317, 319–
    320
preschool interventions and later
    performance in, 44, 67–68, 72–
    73, 79, 81–82, 366
programmed learning approach in,
    76
public policy and, 82–84
self-identity affected by tutoring,
    203
in social development model, 141–
    142
social networks of at-risk students,
    221
Student Training Through Urban
    Strategies, 240–241, 250
success, 72–73, 79, 126–129, 154,
    181–190, 290–300, 320–321
success/failure in, as third variable
    effect, 6–7
Seattle Social Development Project
data collection, 147–153
procedures, 143–147
results, 153–157, 367
theoretical background, 141–143
Self-esteem, 47, 326
Setting conditions. *See* Context
Shy behavior
aggressive behavior and, 170
assessing, 175–178
as outcome indicator, 172
Siblings, cognitive development, 53
Social Behavior Questionnaire, 121,
    124

Social control theory, 141, 324–325
Social development model, 141–142
Social learning theory, 141, 237, 263
Social skills/behavior
    adolescents, 221, 264
    children, 120, 124
    infant risk and, 23, 29, 31
    preschool education and, 73–74, 79–81
Socialization. *See* Parents/parenting
St. Louis Experiment
    attrition in, 247–250
    background, 236
    design, 237–241
    implications of, 250–251
    research population, 236
    results, 241–247
Status offenders. *See also* Intensive
        Protective Supervision Project
    defined, 330
    supervised deinstitutionalization
        program, 330–332
Stimulus–response theory, 210
Strain theory, 314–315, 324
Strange Situation procedures, 33
Stress, 24
Structural equation modeling, 269, 276–277
Student Training Through Urban
        Strategies, 313–315, 318, 321–324
Substance abuse. *See also* Seattle Social
        Development Project; Drug use
    adolescent self-regulation
        intervention, 264–265
    assessing student attitudes toward,
        150–151, 156
    attention deficit hyperactivity
        disorder treatment and, 109
    child skills training in preventive
        intervention, 146
    developmental paths leading to,
        164, 170
    early onset, risk factors for, 140,
        264
    early predictors of, 163–164
    family patterns in, 204

multifactorial interventions, 141,
        164
    parent training in preventive
        intervention, 146–147, 260, 263
    in parents, 11
    peer counselors in intervention for,
        264–265
    preschool curriculum types and
        subsequent, 80
    research needs, 369
    risk factors, 139–141, 260
    social development model
        intervention, 141–143
    teacher training in intervention for,
        143–146
Success. *See* Results

T

Teachers. *See also* Schools/schooling
    assessing student's social
        adaptational status, 173–174
    attention deficit hyperactivity
        disorder student and, 94–95,
        100–103, 108
    in child-centered approach, 76
    cooperative learning techniques,
        145
    gender differences in assessments
        by, 268, 276
    in High/Scope preschool
        curriculum, 70–71, 76–77
    interactive teaching methods, 144–145
    in open-framework approach, 76
    pay for, 84
    proactive classroom management,
        144
    programmed learning approach, 46
    student assessment of, 150
    Teacher Observation of Classroom
        Adaptation–Revised, 173
    training, in substance abuse
        intervention, 143–146
Token economies, 210, 211

Toys
  in assessment of child peer
    interactions, 37–38
  in cognitive development curricula,
    49
  Novel Toy procedure, 37–38
Treatment. *See* Preventive
    interventions
Treatment settings
  in behavioral therapy, 216
  in coercion model, 254
  importance of, vs. behavioral
    therapy, 227
  peer networks and, 220
  pharmacotherapy for attention
    deficit hyperactivity disorder,
    97–99

preschool interventions, 44
prosocial environments, 235
social network formation and, 225–
  228
structure of, 233
supervised probation, 333

V

Verbal Interaction Project, Inc., 45

Y

Youth Development Project, 221–228,
  227–228